Dr. Milling's work is a "must have" for practitioners looking to both better understand the underpinnings of hypnosis and to use hypnotic interventions with their clients. He has assembled a stellar team of leaders in the field who relay complex material in a way that allows readers to bring the science and efficacy of hypnosis to their patients. Bravo!

—**Guy H. Montgomery, PhD**, Past President, Society of Psychological Hypnosis (Division 30) of the American Psychological Association

This book includes some of the world's most authoritative authors providing clear, articulate support and instruction for the evidence-based use of clinical hypnosis. This should be on the bookshelf of students and experienced practitioners alike. Simply excellent!

—**Eric K. Willmarth, PhD**, Chair, Department of Applied Psychophysiology, College of Integrative Medicine and Health Sciences, Saybrook University, Pasadena, CA, United States; Past-President, American Society of Clinical Hypnosis, Society for Clinical and Experimental Hypnosis, and American Psychological Association Division 30: Society of Psychological Hypnosis

W0193383

EVIDENCE-BASED PRACTICE IN CLINICAL HYPNOSIS

EVIDENCE-BASED PRACTICE IN CLINICAL HYPNOSIS

LEONARD S. MILLING

EDITOR

 AMERICAN PSYCHOLOGICAL ASSOCIATION

Published by
American Psychological Association
750 First Street, NE
Washington, DC 20002
https://www.apa.org

Order Department
https://www.apa.org/pubs/books
order@apa.org

Typeset in Charter and Interstate by Circle Graphics, Inc., Reisterstown, MD

Printer: Gasch Printing, Odenton, MD
Cover Designer: Mercury Publishing Services, Rockville, MD

Library of Congress Cataloging-in-Publication Data

CIP Data has been applied for.
Library of Congress Control Number: 2023934121

https://doi.org/10.1037/0000347-000

Printed in the United States of America

10 9 8 7 6 5 4 3 2 1

Contents

Contributors

Erin L. Connors, PhD, Vanderbilt University Medical Center, Nashville, TN, United States

Shawn R. Criswell, PhD, Kaiser Permanente Northwest, Hillsboro, OR, United States

Gary R. Elkins, PhD, Baylor University, Waco, TX, United States

Joseph P. Green, PhD, Ohio State University, Lima, OH, United States

Lisa Lombard, PhD, Northwestern University Feinberg School of Medicine, Chicago, IL, United States

Steven Jay Lynn, PhD, Binghamton University–State University of New York, Binghamton, NY, United States

Lindsey C. McKernan, PhD, Vanderbilt University Medical Center, Nashville, TN, United States

Leonard S. Milling, PhD, University of Hartford, West Hartford, CT, United States

David B. Reid, PsyD, Saybrook University, Pasadena, CA, United States

Morgan Snyder, MA, Baylor University, Waco, TX, United States

Michael D. Yapko, PhD, private practice, Fallbrook, CA, United States

main section of the book were selected because they possess strong empirical support. For example, there are a large number of controlled studies demonstrating the efficacy of hypnosis for relieving clinical pain. Consequently, this book includes one chapter on acute and procedural pain, as well as another chapter on chronic pain. In contrast, hypnosis is frequently mentioned in clinical lore as a treatment for dissociative identity disorder and conversion disorder. However, there are few, if any, controlled studies of the use of hypnosis as a treatment for these problems. Therefore, the book does not include chapters on these topics.

The omission of chapters on particular topics like dissociative identity disorder and conversion disorder does not mean hypnosis is ineffective in treating these problems. As the APA Presidential Task Force on Evidence-Based Practice (2006) noted, "Specific interventions that have not been subjected to systematic empirical testing for specific problems cannot be assumed to be either effective or ineffective; they are simply untested to date. . . . Widely used psychological practices . . . should be rigorously evaluated" (p. 274). Indeed, the absence of chapters on popular uses of clinical hypnosis reveals potentially fruitful avenues for future research. Much remains to be done!

I thank the University of Hartford for providing a sabbatical that led to the inception of this book. I appreciate the guidance of Susan Reynolds of APA Books throughout the evolution of this project. I am indebted to Christine Bird, Interlibrary Services Coordinator at the University of Hartford, for her patience and help in obtaining many of the articles cited herein. Finally, my deep gratitude to the graduate and undergraduate students who have assisted me with my research throughout the years, which culminated in this book.

—Leonard S. Milling

REFERENCES

APA Presidential Task Force on Evidence-Based Practice. (2006). Evidence-based practice in psychology. *American Psychologist, 61*(4), 271–285. https://doi.org/10.1037/0003-066X.61.4.271

Chambless, D. L., & Hollon, S. D. (1998). Defining empirically supported therapies. *Journal of Consulting and Clinical Psychology, 66*(1), 7–18. https://doi.org/10.1037/0022-006X.66.1.7

Eysenck, H. J. (1952). The effects of psychotherapy: An evaluation. *Journal of Consulting Psychology, 16*(5), 319–324. https://doi.org/10.1037/h0063633

Milling, L. S., Valentine, K. E., LoStimolo, L. M., Nett, A. M., & McCarley, H. S. (2021). Hypnosis and the alleviation of clinical pain: A comprehensive meta-analysis. *International Journal of Clinical and Experimental Hypnosis, 69*(3), 297–322. https://doi.org/10.1080/00207144.2021.1920330

Milling, L. S., Valentine, K. E., McCarley, H. S., & LoStimolo, L. M. (2019). A meta-analysis of hypnotic interventions for depression symptoms. High hopes for hypnosis? *The American Journal of Clinical Hypnosis, 61*(3), 227–243. https://doi.org/10.1080/00029157.2018.1489777

Smith, M. L., & Glass, G. V. (1977). Meta-analysis of psychotherapy outcome studies. *American Psychologist, 32*(9), 752–760. https://doi.org/10.1037/0003-066X.32.9.752

Smith, M. L., Glass, G. V., & Miller, T. L. (1980). *The benefits of psychotherapy*. Johns Hopkins University Press.

Valentine, K. E., Milling, L. S., Clark, L. J., & Moriarty, C. L. (2019). The efficacy of hypnosis as a treatment for anxiety: A meta-analysis. *International Journal of Clinical and Experimental Hypnosis, 67*(3), 336–363. https://doi.org/10.1080/00207144.2019.1613863

EVIDENCE-BASED PRACTICE IN
CLINICAL
HYPNOSIS

1 AN INTRODUCTION TO THE PRACTICE OF CLINICAL HYPNOSIS

STEVEN JAY LYNN AND JOSEPH P. GREEN

We have devoted much of our careers to the study and clinical practice of hypnosis, not because hypnosis is an arcane or exotic method practiced by those with special powers of influence, or because we witnessed demonstrations of mind-boggling alterations of consciousness as dramatized in the media, or because we sought "quick fixes" in assisting our clients in embracing more fulfilling lives. Rather, the reason for our ongoing fascination with hypnosis is that it has opened doors for us in grappling with the mysteries of consciousness, the power of words in transforming our patients' lives, and how we could leverage a cost-effective, efficient method to harness their personal resources. More specifically, we have found hypnosis to be an efficacious means of modifying thoughts, feelings, and behaviors via suggestions; a vehicle to shift people's expectancies and models of themselves and the world; a method to evoke novel possibilities of thinking, feeling, doing, and circumventing ingrained and maladaptive habits; and a path to investigating the pliability of consciousness and a variety of psychological phenomena in the laboratory.

Hypnosis has come a long way since it inspired our curiosity many years ago. Today, hypnosis has carved out well-earned territory in the landscape of psychological science and clinical practice. Researchers probe intriguing

https://doi.org/10.1037/0000347-001
Evidence-Based Practice in Clinical Hypnosis, L. S. Milling (Editor)

hypnotic phenomena in laboratories across the world and share their findings with a wide audience via the most competitive and respected journals. These publications showcase contributions providing ample empirical rationales for practitioners to bring hypnosis into the purview of their interventions.

This volume underscores both how easy-to-implement hypnotic techniques can supplement science-based clinical interventions and how clinicians can use hypnosis with the assurance that it boasts a strong empirical foundation to guide their practice. We write this chapter in the hope that we will engage readers in new adventures in researching or threading hypnosis into their clinical endeavors, and that it will reinvigorate and inform researchers and practitioners already familiar with hypnosis.

ON THE NATURE OF HYPNOSIS

The following section of the chapter presents an overview of the definition of hypnosis and major theories of hypnotic responding.

Defining Hypnosis

Hypnosis falls within a broader domain of phenomena related to suggestion and suggestibility that encompasses waking imaginative suggestions, responses to cues and suggestions in forensic contexts, and placebo effects (Halligan & Oakley, 2014; Hilgard, 1973; Kihlstrom, 2008). Yet hypnosis occupies a unique niche within this broad conceptual space due to sociocultural views of hypnosis, the context in which it unfolds, and the procedures used to elicit hypnotic phenomena.

Comparisons between hypnosis and mindfulness and relaxation are not uncommon. Although it is accurate to say that relaxation and mindfulness can be achieved or guided via suggestion, hypnosis cannot be reduced to either. For example, people respond to hypnotic suggestions while wide awake and exercising on a stationary bicycle in which they experience a physiologically aroused rather than a relaxed state (see Bányai, 2018). Unlike hypnosis, mindfulness practice calls for observing the flow of consciousness with an accepting, nonjudgmental attitude. Not surprisingly, mindfulness practitioners display superior metacognition (Lush et al., 2016), whereas the opposite generally holds for highly suggestible individuals (Dienes et al., 2016). Still, mindfulness and hypnotic suggestions can be combined in clinical interventions (see Green & Lynn, 2019; Lynn et al., 2016; Raz & Lifshitz, 2016).

This idea that clinical hypnosis is tightly bound to the expectational and situational context in which it is practiced aligns most closely with the definition of hypnosis advanced decades ago by the Hypnosis Division (30) of the American Psychological Association (Kirsch, 1994b; based on Kihlstrom, 1985). This definition construes hypnosis as a process or procedure in which suggestions for imaginative experiences are provided for alterations in sensations, perceptions, thoughts, memories, or behaviors. In this light, what transpires during hypnosis depends very much on how the situation in which suggestions are embedded is presented to the participant (i.e., as hypnosis) and/or how people interpret the context (i.e., as "hypnotic").

Indeed, many hypnotic proceedings can be described in terms of multiple overlapping and often continuous elements that establish the context as clinical hypnosis. More specifically, prior to hypnosis, the hypnotist, in what we will refer to as prehypnotic communications, will set the stage for hypnosis by explicitly presenting the context as hypnosis and inculcate positive expectancies. A hypnotic induction follows, which is comprised of suggestions that further demarcate the context as hypnosis and precede specific suggestions for research or therapeutic purposes. In clinical situations, these suggestions are often developed in concert with the participant. Where the induction and suggestions begin and end is often a "strained, arbitrary, and artificial distinction" (Lynn et al., 2017, p. 371). It is the incredible diversity of creative suggestions utilized to alter subjective experiences in innumerable, targeted, and highly individualized ways that often lends appeal to hypnosis for clinicians and patients alike. Finally, hypnosis is terminated and a discussion of the experience ensues. In clinical hypnosis, these phases often merge seamlessly into a smooth conversational stream, and suggestions can be delivered formally (e.g., scripted) or interspersed more informally, with eyes open or closed.

The APA definition of hypnosis (Kirsch, 1994b), which emphasizes contextual and procedural aspects of hypnosis, (a) implies tremendous latitude in suggestions that come under the umbrella of hypnosis, (b) delineates a semblance of boundaries between what is "hypnotic" and what is "not hypnotic," (c) does not depend on the instantiation of a "trance" or special state of consciousness, and (d) facilitates scientific investigations insofar as empirical comparisons can be drawn across conditions that are "hypnotic" or "nonhypnotic." This definition of hypnosis is also conducive to studies using standardized scales that assess individual differences in hypnotic responding—variously referred to as hypnotic responsiveness, hypnotic susceptibility, hypnotizability, and hypnotic suggestibility—in contexts that are unambiguously defined as hypnotic. If the situation is neither defined nor perceived as such, then questions can arise concerning whether established test norms apply (and interpretation is possible) when valid and reliable scales of hypnotic responsiveness are used for clinical or research purposes.

A decade after the first definition was promulgated, the Executive Committee of the APA Division of Psychological Hypnosis (Green, Barabasz, et al., 2005) revised the definition to acknowledge that the "hypnotic induction is an extended initial suggestion for using one's imagination, and may contain further elaborations of the introduction" (p. 262). This aspect of the definition coincides with the fact that in clinical hypnosis there is often no sharp dividing line between the induction and the suggestions that follow.

The definition also took note of the widely used clinical technique of self-hypnosis, described as "the act of administering hypnotic procedures on one's own" (Green, Barabasz, et al., 2005, p. 262). Self-hypnosis, which we consider in greater detail later, can be a viable means of generalizing and maximizing treatment gains apart from the one-on-one hypnosis context and attune participants to their ongoing flow of spontaneous thoughts to steer them in a more positive, adaptive, and goal-directed manner. Self-hypnosis is also a means to illustrate how different psychological conditions can be the product of negative self-suggestions (e.g., I am a failure; I am helpless), which can be countered with self-suggestions.

The revised definition also noted that responsiveness to suggestion can be assessed with standardized scales, that scores can be aggregated into low, medium, and high categories, and that "the salience of evidence for having achieved hypnosis increases with the individual's score" (Green, Barabasz, et al., 2005, p. 263). Using such scales, researchers have determined that approximately 10% to 15% of participants exhibit low hypnotic suggestibility and respond to no or to only a few suggestions, 60% to 80% display moderate (medium) responsiveness, and 10% to 15% exhibit high hypnotic suggestibility and respond to the majority of the suggestions including those for hallucinations or amnesia that involve cognitive and perceptual alterations in consciousness (Terhune et al., 2017).

Most recently, yet another APA task force defined hypnosis as a "state of consciousness involving focused attention and reduced peripheral awareness characterized by an enhanced capacity for response to suggestion" (Elkins et al., 2015, p. 382). Across definitions of hypnosis, there is a strand of agreement that suggestions can alter the spontaneous and situationally activated flow of thoughts, feelings, action tendencies, and behaviors of individuals in situations that are typically defined as hypnosis by an external agent (e.g., clinician, researcher) or construed to be "hypnosis" by the participant.

Theories of Hypnosis

We next turn to major theories of hypnosis that capture important facets of hypnosis germane to clinical practice beyond the definition of hypnosis.

Psychodynamic Approaches

After Freud rejected hypnosis as a reliable treatment modality, hypnosis receded into the background as a therapeutic intervention until Erika Fromm (Fromm & Nash, 1997), Elgan Baker (1981), and Michael Nash (1997) revived interest in psychodynamic accounts. Psychodynamic theorists have called attention to a strong affective bond that can arise between the hypnotist and participant in a relationship in which fantasy, imagination, primary process mentation, and adaptive regression are important mediators of hypnotic responses and can be leveraged to facilitate emotion regulation and enhanced ego functioning for therapeutic purposes (Fromm & Nash, 1997). Psychodynamic approaches have not been systematically studied in controlled trials in which hypnosis is an adjunct to psychotherapy.

Neodissociation and Cold Control Theory

Dissociation theories of hypnosis address the nonvolitional quality of many hypnotic responses. In 1977, Hilgard argued that suggestion-related automaticity associated with hypnosis was produced by a dissociation of executive monitoring of actions from subsystems of control operational in everyday life (Hilgard, 1977). Hilgard's contentions were inspired by his discovery of the "hidden observer" phenomenon in which he argued the hypnotist uses suggestion to directly access a dissociated/observing aspect of the personality that can objectively report on pain, for example, while not experiencing suffering. Hilgard posited that during hypnosis an amnesic barrier segregates subsystems of control from executive functions. Accordingly, participants experience diminished behavioral control and respond automatically to suggested events. Hilgard's interpretation of the hidden observer stirred substantial controversy, as studies revealed that the nature of the hidden observer (e.g., reporting more vs. less pain) depended on the suggestions or cues inherent in the communications that elicited the seeming personality dissociation (see Green, Page, et al., 2005; Kirsch & Lynn, 1998). Regardless of the explanation for the hidden observer, the phenomenon highlights the ability of suggestion to facilitate a different and potentially more therapeutic perspective on one's experiences and actions (see Lynn et al., 1994).

Another version of dissociation theory—dissociative control theory (see Woody & Sadler, 2008) rejects the existence of the amnesic barrier that Hilgard proposed. Rather, hypnotic suggestions are argued to bypass higher-level executive voluntary control and access lower, more autonomous or involuntary levels of control. According to this view, this state of affairs creates the opportunity for the hypnotist to directly activate behaviors via suggestion that are consistent with therapeutic goals and to instantiate more adaptive coping responses.

Evidence indicates that much behavior in hypnotic and nonhypnotic contexts is executed on an automatic basis with little or no conscious control (see Kirsch & Lynn, 1998), that hypnosis is associated with a disruption of executive monitoring or metacognition, and that hypnosis may further automatize mental processes and behaviors (see Dienes & Perner, 2007; Lynn & Green, 2011; Kirsch & Lynn, 1999; Terhune et al., 2017). Because suggestions are conveyed in the context of hypnosis, participants are likely to attribute the involuntary "feel" of suggestions to the hypnotist or to the influence of hypnosis more globally (Dienes & Perner, 2007; Kirsch & Lynn, 1999; Martin & Pacherie, 2019).

While not explicitly a dissociation theory, but more rightly labeled a cognitive theory, *cold control theory* (Barnier et al., 2008; Dienes & Hutton, 2013; Dienes & Perner, 2007) argues that normal executive control during hypnosis is not compromised, but a lack of access to higher order thoughts (metacognitive states regarding one's mental representations) related to intentions degrades the everyday sense of agency. This view is consistent with testable claims that hypnotic responsiveness may be enhanced when monitoring and planning executive functions are decoupled from executive control (Jamieson & Sheehan, 2004; Lynn & Green, 2011). Research supports an important role for degraded metacognition in highly suggestible individuals, although the variables (e.g., eye closure, relaxation, focus on bodily sensations, expectancies, attributions of control to the hypnotist) linked with this finding have yet to be researched systematically (see Terhune et al., 2017).

There exists scant disagreement among theorists that highly suggestible individuals often experience hypnotic suggestions as "involuntary happenings." Yet involuntariness reports vary as a function of whether participants expect or are instructed that they will experience hypnotic responses as involuntary (Lynn et al., 1984), which is facilitated by the fact that hypnotic responses are often experienced as partly voluntary and partly involuntary, and many actions in both hypnotic and nonhypnotic situations are not deliberated prior to their execution (Kirsch & Lynn, 1999).

The Sociocognitve Model

The idea that expectancies modulate or mediate the subjective experience of hypnosis and corresponding behaviors is a cornerstone of the sociocognitive perspective. The *sociocognitive model* (SCM) is an open, evidence-based model that seeks to identify social and cognitive variables that stand in a functional relation with hypnotic responsiveness. This perspective locates hypnosis within a wide network of interacting variables that encompass beliefs, attitudes, expectancies, motivation, and ability to experience nonhypnotic imaginative suggestions. The SCM is also known as the cognitive behavioral model of hypnosis and is compatible with cognitive-behavioral psychotherapies that prioritize the influence of expectancies, cognitions, beliefs, and imaginings on behaviors and emotions. Kirsch, Montgomery et al.'s (1995) now classic meta-analysis revealed that the average client receiving cognitive-behavioral hypnotherapy exhibited greater improvement than at least 70% of clients receiving nonhypnotic cognitive-behavioral treatment.

The perspective has its roots in the early writings of Theodore Sarbin and T. X. Barber and their students William C. Coe, and Nicholas Spanos and John Chaves, respectively, and the later work of Irving Kirsch, Steven Jay Lynn, and Graham Wagstaff. These theorists vociferously challenged the existence of a special hypnotic state or trance and instead featured participants' often unconscious enactment of the social role of a hypnotized subject, "believed in imaginings," and the strategic, goal-directed nature of hypnotic responding (Coe & Sarbin, 1991; Lynn et al., 2008; Sarbin & Coe, 1972; Spanos, 1991; Wagstaff. 1991). The SCM has also highlighted the important role of imaginative suggestions, which can elicit profound changes in behavior and experience regardless of whether they are presented in a hypnotic or nonhypnotic context.

The SCM views hypnosis as a form of top-down regulation in which mental representations, including expectations, attitudes, and beliefs about hypnosis, cascade downstream to override or modulate perception, physiology, and behavior (see Terhune et al., 2017; see also Kirsch & Lynn 1998; Lynn et al., 1991; Spanos, 1986). Because hypnosis is widely viewed as a potent means of altering consciousness, in a therapeutic situation, positive expectancies can potentially enhance treatment outcomes. In fact, Kirsch has argued that hypnosis acts as a nondeceptive placebo, bolstering positive response expectancies that have a self-confirming nature (Kirsch, 1994a, response set theory; see also Kirsch & Lynn,1999).

According to *response set theory* (Kirsch & Lynn, 1998, 1999), much of what occurs during hypnosis is perceived as automatic, because actions, planned or unplanned, are viewed as initiated automatically at the time of activation by response sets (expectations and intentions). Hypnosis primes people to view the hypnotist or hypnosis as the source of their nonvolitional responses because of dominant cultural views that hypnotic responses are not self-initiated.

The SCM finds support in research showing that (a) expectancies, attitudes, beliefs, motivation, goal-directed fantasies and imaginings, and responsiveness to waking imaginative suggestions account for significant variability in hypnotic suggestibility (Barber, 1969; Barber et al., 1974; Lynn et al., 2010; Spanos, 1986, 1991) and that (b) hypnotic suggestibility can be substantially increased via social learning training programs (Gorassini & Spanos, 1986) that modify these mediating variables (e.g., enhance positive attitudes and expectancies, increase motivation and suggestion-directed imagining). Gfeller and Gorassini (2010) described how elements of such training programs can be exported to hypnotherapies to optimize treatment gains.

Phenomenological/Interactive Theories

Clinicians often use hypnosis to alter consciousness in meaningful and significant respects. Martin Orne (1959) was one of the first modern theorists to underscore the importance of subjective experiences and subtle as well as dramatic changes in cognitions and affects in hypnotic contexts in which individuals are especially sensitive to social and suggested cues and experimental demands (i.e., demand characteristics). More recently, researchers have documented profound changes in the experience of agency and perceptions of the self in responses to suggestions ranging from audio and visual hallucinations and to convincing out-of-body experiences, feelings of paralysis, and even delusions of a sex change (Connors et al., 2012; Noble & McConkey, 1995; Polito et al., 2014). These sorts of suggestions are experienced most compellingly on the part of highly suggestible individuals.

Phenomenological/interactive theories (like sociocognitive perspectives), view hypnotic responses as the by-product of multiple interacting variables (e.g., person, situation, rapport; McConkey, 1991; Nadon et al., 1987; Sheehan, 1991). However, in contrast with the SCM, they focus more on (a) differences between hypnotic and nonhypnotic waking behavior and the particular cognitive commitment people display to respond to suggestions in hypnotic situations (Sheehan, 1991) and (b) the meaning that participants ascribe to the hypnotist's communications that can activate highly diverse and idiosyncratic responses both within and across hypnotic sessions (McConkey, 1991; Sheehan & McConkey, 1982). Clinicians often encounter highly "individual" responses that are seemingly unrelated to the literal content of suggestions delivered, but nevertheless are emotionally salient, personally meaningful, and potentially worthy of exploration.

Ericksonian Hypnosis

Milton H. Erickson is widely regarded as the progenitor of modern clinical hypnosis. Erickson (Erickson et al., 1976; Haley, 1985) pioneered ingenious brief and strategic hypnotic approaches that used paradox, metaphors, analogies, indirect and permissive suggestions, and teaching stories to advantage. He appreciated the importance of creating positive expectancies for change and the automatic nature of thoughts and behaviors, antedating contemporary discussions of automaticity in hypnosis and everyday life. However, he is best known for his *utilization approach* that anticipated contemporary acceptance-based third wave approaches in championing radical acceptance of his patients and utilizing their innate resources and talents to foment change.

Rather than viewing hypnosis as a dissociative process, Erickson understood hypnosis as quite the opposite: an associative process that capitalized on shifting spontaneous and suggestion-related associations toward the realization of personal goals. As Erickson et al. (1976) wrote, "[M]ost people do not know that most mental processes are autonomous. . . . Hypnotic suggestions come into play when the therapist's directives have a significant effect on facilitating the expression of that flow in one direction or another" (p. 58).

Many of Erickson's creative stratagems and methods continue to be popular among clinicians and are promulgated in the recent writings of Stephen and Carol Lankton (2015), Michael Yapko (2018), and Jeffrey Zeig (2014). These authors have advocated effectively for tapping participants' acknowledged and unrecognized or underutilized personal resources, strengths, and motivations.

Ericksonian hypnotherapy (the addition of Ericksonian methods to psychotherapy) has not been investigated in controlled trials. However, many of his innovative techniques (e.g., paradoxical interventions, reframing) are grounded in principles of cognitive and behavioral change supported by research in social, clinical, and cognitive psychology (Lynn & Hallquist, 2004; Lynn & Sherman, 2000).

Psychophysiological Approaches
Elucidating the psychophysiological moderators and mediators of suggestions in hypnotic and nonhypnotic contexts promises to yield important insights across competing theoretical perspectives. Hypnotic responses, like all complex human behaviors and experiences that call for the deployment of attention and personal resources, will be reflected in cognitive, affective, and social domains and ultimately in the physiology of the participant. For the past three decades, researchers have been hot on the trail of the correlates and antecedents of hypnotic responsiveness. Evidence to date supports the idea that hypnosis and individual differences in responsiveness are associated with top-down regulation of lower brain structures and anterior cingulate, prefrontal, and parietal cortices (see Terhune et al., 2017).

Nevertheless, the ability to identify a unique psychophysiological state and the roles of different brain mechanisms reliably associated with hypnosis has so far proven elusive. This is probably the case because the subjective experience of hypnosis, including the experience of involuntariness and the reported "depth" of hypnosis, often vary substantially within a hypnotic session

(Cardeña, 2005; Cardeña et al., 2013) and in response to some suggestions but not others (Terhune et al., 2017). Even highly responsive people pass some suggestions but not others and different suggestions access different abilities, implying that multiple suggestion-related abilities underlie hypnotic responsiveness (Barnier et al., 2008; Woody et al., 2005). These different abilities likely reflect different neural correlates or antecedents of hypnotic responsivity. Thus, participants can be informed that even some highly responsive individuals discover that their experiences vary over the course of the session in interesting ways and that after the hypnosis they will have an opportunity to share what seemed to work best.

Psychophysiological research has borne fruit in an important respect: Studies have documented that hypnotic phenomena are "genuine" in that the effects of suggestions, such as a visual hallucination, for example (e.g., hallucinating an object), can be indexed by corresponding changes in physiology (e.g., visual cortex) among highly hypnotizable participants (Kosslyn et al., 2000; Szechtman et al., 1998). We have found it useful to share these sorts of findings with participants, which lend credibility to hypnosis as a means to effect change on multiple personal levels.

CONSIDERING INDIVIDUAL DIFFERENCES: DETERMINANTS OF HYPNOTIC RESPONSIVENESS

In the chapters that follow, readers will appreciate that hypnosis can be a potent instrument in affecting personal change. A burgeoning literature based on qualitative and meta-analytic findings documents the promise of hypnosis in treating medical and psychological conditions as diverse as irritable bowel syndrome, depression, and anxiety (see Terhune et al., 2017).

Yet individuals vary in their responses to hypnotic interventions. A keen awareness of potential individual differences in hypnotic responsiveness (e.g., alternative terms: hypnotic suggestibility, hypnotizability, hypnotic susceptibility) is prerequisite to optimizing the participants' experience of hypnosis. In fact, individual differences are the rule rather than the exception in hypnotic situations. Clinicians can benefit greatly from knowledge of the determinants of hypnotic responsiveness. Lynn et al. (2019) recently presented evidence pertaining to individual differences that we summarize here.

People who respond highly to hypnotic suggestions are likely to:

1. Expect they will respond to suggestions, be motivated to respond, and have the ability to respond to nonhypnotic as well as hypnotic imaginative suggestions. Expectancies consistently predict hypnotic responsiveness. Kirsch,

Silva et al. (1995) reported that response expectancy was the strongest predictor of hypnotic responsiveness among a pool of potential predictors including absorption, fantasy proneness, and personal motivation. Braffman and Kirsch (1999) found that the combination of expectancy, motivation, and nonhypnotic imaginative suggestibility accounted for slightly more than half the variance (i.e., 53%) in hypnotic responsiveness. Practitioners should keep in mind that while expectancies affect hypnotic suggestibility, responsiveness to suggestions in turn affect expectancies on a reciprocal and ongoing basis (Benham et al., 2006).

2. Become absorbed in suggestions, allocate attentional resources, and actively deploy imaginings to reify suggestion-related experiences that, in turn, bolster response expectancies (Kirsch & Lynn, 1999; Lynn, 1997).

3. Accurately interpret the intent of suggestions with minimal critique of their responses, interfering thoughts, and metacognitive awareness, and evidence a low threshold of response to hypnotic suggestions (Dienes & Perner, 2007; Lynn et al., 1991; Terhune et al., 2017).

4. Adopt "liberal" performance standards; that is, not so stringent or unattainable (e.g., believe a suggested hallucination must be perceived as lifelike in all respects; Lynn et al., 2003) as to dampen positive response expectancies and their belief that they "passed" a suggestion.

5. Experience rapport with the hypnotist (Gfeller et al., 1987; Lynn et al., 1991).

6. Score relatively high on measures of absorption, fantasy-proneness, dissociation, and positive attitudes about hypnosis. The correlations between such measures and hypnotic responsiveness are generally small-to-moderate and can be inflated artificially when measures are administered in the same test context. Although moderate levels of fantasy proneness, absorption, and imagery vividness contribute to the prediction of hypnotic responsiveness, very low levels of imaginative propensity are almost always associated with low responsivity (de Groh, 1989; Spanos, 1991), and strong negative attitudes about hypnosis suppress hypnotic responsiveness (Spanos et al., 1987).

THE PRACTICE OF CLINICAL HYPNOSIS

Clearly, a broad base of empirical knowledge is available to inform clinicians, beginning with the hypnotist sharing information prior to initiating hypnosis, to which we turn next.

Prehypnotic Information

Often prehypnotic information will flow directly into an induction, although it may be presented at any point in the contact with a participant and affect hypnotic responsiveness ranging from a small to a relatively large extent.

To set the stage for the proceedings, the practitioner typically will have (a) secured information about the participant's past experiences with hypnosis, if any; discussed the purpose and goals of the session; and solicited and/or reviewed potential suggestions with the participant; (b) attempted to instill positive attitudes, beliefs, and expectancies about hypnosis; (c) ascertained participant expectancies and knowledge about hypnosis and corrected myths and misconceptions; and (d) responded to questions. Mistaken beliefs include that people cannot resist or oppose suggestions, that they relinquish their willpower to the hypnotist, respond like an automaton, develop amnesia for what occurs and lose touch with their surroundings, not "come out of" hypnosis, and are gullible or of low intelligence (see Green et al., 2006; Lynn et al., 2010). Another myth of concern is that hypnosis increases the accuracy of memories. In fact, hypnosis is not a reliable method for improving memory and should not be used to retrieve relatively recent memories or excavate childhood memories, as hypnosis increases the risk of false memories and unwarranted confidence in memories independent of their veracity (Lynn et al., 2015).

The hypnotist would do well to actively encourage absorption and imaginal involvement in suggestions, enlist the cooperation of participants, and strive to cultivate a positive rapport. In engaging in these activities, clinicians will encourage a motivated cognitive commitment or preparedness to respond to suggestions that reflects response sets associated with highly suggestible individuals (e.g., Sheehan, 1991; Sheehan & McConkey, 1982; Tellegen, 1981).

Hypnosis Protocols: Are There Differences in Hypnotic Inductions?

Hypnotic inductions take many forms. Nevertheless, few if any differences in participant responsiveness exist across hypnotic inductions that vary in their length, whether suggestions are ordered from easy to difficult or vice versa; whether they are worded in permissive versus authoritative terms; or whether they call for relaxation or an alert–awake state of mind (Lynn et al., 2017; Terhune & Cardeña, 2016). Still, individuals we have treated have generally responded very favorably to the sorts of suggestions contained in the sample induction below.

The following example of a generic hypnotic induction via suggestions for eye fixation and closure combines multiple elements of calmness, feeling at ease, relaxation and attention to sensations and breathing, enhanced receptivity and ability to access personal resources, self-compassion and acceptance, and deepening of hypnotic experiences. These sorts of suggestions pave the way for treatment of a variety of conditions and for more tailored suggestions that follow the induction. The sample induction also includes reference to self-hypnosis, which is a useful method in itself and as a post-hypnotic method to enhance and maintain treatment gains. Readers will note that the suggestions in the sample induction are generally very permissive and neither authoritative (e.g., You *will* experience ___) nor particularly directive. Rather, they imply considerable latitude in responding in order to fulfill the task demands of the suggestions.

A Sample Hypnotic Induction Protocol

"Let's begin by you looking at the spot where the wall and ceiling meet. Just find that corner spot and stare at it for a little while. A spot of your choosing, actually any spot will do . . . as we begin hypnosis together, working together to help you discover all that you can learn in your hypnosis, what you can achieve . . . just continue looking at your spot.

Now, as you do so, it would be perfectly natural after a while for your eyelids to begin to become a bit heavy and tired from staring, and especially so as you pay attention to this happening, noticing it, directing your attention to the natural heaviness. Perhaps this sense of heaviness begins to be accompanied by a welcome release of tension you might have accumulated during the day as your body gets more comfortable and as you begin to unwind and relax and release as you notice the tiredness of your eyes . . . and the more you experience this heaviness . . . and as you discover just how heavy and tired you feel your eyes become . . . they can close easily and comfortably. In doing this, you can discover how bringing your attention to what I'm saying will help you to experience what is suggested.

But you don't need to focus on that right now. There's lots of time to go deeper into your experience . . . just the right level of hypnosis that is comfortable for you. Comfortable and at ease. Nothing to bother, nothing to disturb. As you listen to my voice and feel more calm, at ease, peaceful, perhaps even in synch with your breathing, perhaps you can also appreciate the value of taking a deep breath, a deep breath . . . how releasing it would be to let go of some of the tension accumulated in the natural course of daily life. Try it now, take a deep breath in. And let it go. Again, deep breath in . . . and out.

As you now pay some attention to your breathing—you may notice many sensations associated with your breathing. You may notice how your shoulders rise . . . and fall with each breath that you take. Or, how your chest expands . . . and then relaxes with each breath. Breathe in what you need. And, breathe out what you don't. Your body knows what to do . . . here and now . . . just being in the moment, breathing with ease, enjoying the comfort of just being in the moment with nothing to bother, nothing to disturb as you go deeper into hypnosis . . . exactly to the extent that's right for you. And you don't even have to think about it. Nothing more, nothing less, calm and at ease, perhaps noticing how some of the heaviness or maybe another feeling . . . perhaps warmth . . . is making its way through your body, easy, easy going . . . just let it happen if you wish. Or just maybe it's a cool sensation of comfort and calm . . . and, you know, some people even experience a certain lightness of being as they release and relax. As you go deeper, just as deep as you would like to go, you may discover that you feel more receptive, open, letting your experiences happen easy and effortlessly, while in the background of your awareness all the while knowing it's you who shape your experiences as you listen to the sound of my voice.

After all, hypnosis is really self-hypnosis; it is you who has the experience of calm and ease . . . you who thinks and imagines along with what I suggest . . . you who experiences suggestions . . . you who owns and can embrace your experiences . . . and it is you who after our time today can continue to experience suggestions . . . suited to you . . . to set your mind and intentions and plans to best achieve your goals.

IF EYES HAVE NOT CLOSED:

As you continue to go deeper and deeper into your hypnosis, into an open and receptive state of mind, just continue to hear my voice and think about what I share with you. You've done well to concentrate on the spot on the wall and listen to the sound of my voice going with you, but there is no need to stare at that spot any longer. Just let your eyes comfortably close. Please close your eyes now.

AFTER EYES HAVE CLOSED:

While you focused on your breathing and observed your body getting acquainted with what hypnosis is like for you, you closed your eyes, allowing for an internal focus and the presence of being to explore a bit what it would be like to be even more absorbed in your thoughts, feelings, and experiences . . . receptive . . . and focused on what I suggest as you draw upon a lifetime of learnings . . . joining in with the idea, images, and experiences that unfold, to encounter new possibilities of becoming . . . of being present . . . to develop compassion for yourself, empathy for yourself, loving-kindness toward yourself . . . opening yourself up to the excitement of self-discovery . . . open to new possibilities for creating the person you are capable of being . . . becoming . . . as you go just as deep as you wish . . . as you continue to hear my voice that will go with you . . . and you think about, imagine, and experience suggestions (for: insert purpose of suggestions) in your own unique way . . . with an openness to what is most helpful and what you need (insert goal or experience).

Now let's see; what if you were to go even deeper, enjoying the experience of thoughts, feelings, images, and intentions all coming together, merging in new or creative ways to achieve your goals? Yet bringing your lifetime of experiences with you . . . as you explore the depth of awareness and understanding needed to get in touch with your resources at a level you might not fully comprehend consciously . . . but these resources are gifts for yourself . . . to yourself . . . to be accessed during our hypnosis today and afterward with self-hypnotic techniques. I will share these with you. Wouldn't that be nice?"

Deepening the Experience of Hypnosis

Throughout the hypnotic induction and interspersed among suggestions, it is common for the hypnotist, as in the sample induction, to suggest that the client experience deeper, perhaps more intense, salient, or expansive feelings of relaxation, being at ease, or other suggested or desired states as stipulated by the participant in advance or developed "on the spot" at the judgment of the hypnotist. Such deepening suggestions can encourage refocusing or intensifying efforts to more fully experience any desired therapeutic state or suggested event (see Lynn et al., 2010). Deepening suggestions may also assist participants in experiencing suggestion-related phenomena that they might have previously struggled with or not fully achieved (Lynn & Kirsch, 2006).

Deepening suggestions may be accompanied by counts (e.g., ". . . with each count you will feel yourself going deeper and deeper into hypnosis . . . 1 . . . deeper, 2 deeper and deeper . . . 3 . . ."), such as counting breaths, simply "going deeper" with each count; waves breaking on the shore; steps toward a special place with properties of enhanced experience specified (e.g., relaxation, wisdom, insight, access to resources), and so forth. Yet another induction with deepening suggestions pivots around walking down a magnificent spiral staircase. The participant imagines the staircase first and reports how many steps they will descend until they reach the bottom. With each step down, the hypnotist suggests that they experience a deeper state of hypnosis and say aloud the step number (e.g., 1, 2, 3 . . .) in tandem with lifting an index finger to mark their progress (see Lynn & Kirsch, 2006, for another staircase induction).

Nevertheless, counting is not a requirement. Below is a short example of a suggestion to experience a deeper, more intensified level of hypnosis that does not rely on counting.

"As you become more familiar with your hypnosis, you may wish to go even deeper into hypnosis, deeper and deeper as you find a level that is just right for you. You may find yourself going deeper and deeper into hypnosis, your hypnosis . . . to a place within yourself, where you feel safe and secure. A place where you become increasingly aware of the possibilities within you, the potential for change, growth, confidence, empowerment, and the realization that you can live the life that you want to live. The life you choose to live . . . a life consistent with your values, your goals, and your intentions. Wouldn't it be nice to go just as deep into your hypnosis as you want to go. Deeply relaxed . . . calm and at ease. You can be deeply hypnotized but can still clearly hear what I am saying. Take a few minutes to do this, now. After a while, I will ask if you are ready to move forward and experience your hypnosis on an even deeper level?"

Another type of induction with deepening suggestions includes imagery focused on participants imagining their right or left hand rising off the resting surface, being lifted up gradually by brightly colored helium-filled balloons. As the hand rises, the person receives suggestions to experience deeper and deeper hypnosis and that when their hand moves upward and touches their face, they will experience a very deep level of hypnosis and feel even more relaxed when the hand returns to the resting surface.

The Diversity of Hypnotic Suggestions

What is more important in determining therapy outcome than the use of a particular induction or the deepening method is likely the salience of specific suggestions and their congruence with the goals and aims of the therapy enterprise, alongside the participants' beliefs, attitudes, expectancies, and ability to respond to suggestions in the context of hypnosis.

Hypnotic suggestions constrain the vast reservoir of spontaneous involuntary thoughts, fantasies, imaginings, and inchoate associations that mark much of our mental life and channels them in therapeutic directions to transform maladaptive beliefs, thoughts, and action tendencies into more adaptive schemas and goal-directed behaviors (see Lynn et al., 2019).

Hypnotic suggestions are different from instructions and lack their coercive quality (Terhune et al., 2017). Suggestions are typically verbal communications, but they can be nonverbal as well, explicit or implicit, imply a passive or automatic response or a deliberate conscious response, delivered in a permissive or an authoritative manner, or contain rich suggestion-related imagery or minimal imagery, affording substantial flexibility on the part of the hypnotist in crafting suggestions. In clinical contexts, suggestions often unwind in a reciprocal manner in which participant responses influence hypnotist interventions on a recursive unfolding basis.

Clinicians can titrate to some extent whether suggestions are experienced as mostly voluntary or not by modifying suggestion wording and participant expectancies (see Lynn et al., 1994). For example, involuntariness reports are related to suggestions worded in a traditional direct-authoritative manner. When suggestions are worded more permissively (e.g., You may begin to experience lightness in your hand vs. You will experience your hand getting lighter), responses are typically perceived as more voluntary (see Lynn et al., 1993). Clinicians can modify suggestions to accord with participant preferences to address concerns about relinquishing control during hypnosis. More permissive suggestions typically do not compromise behavioral responses to suggestions relative to authoritative suggestions (Lynn et al., 1993).

Practitioners can be reassured that many of the suggestions used for therapeutic purposes (e.g., relaxation, imagining events, imaginative rehearsal, ego strengthening) are not particularly challenging, demanding, or difficult to pass, other than by those considered "low hypnotizable" (Barber, 1985). Montgomery et al. (2011) reported that hypnotic ability accounts for only 6% of the variability in treatment outcomes in clinical care settings, although hypnotic responsiveness is still a statistically significant predictor of clinical utility.

These sorts of findings are consistent with our experience that it is often not necessary to conduct a formal assessment of hypnotic responsiveness for clinical purposes. Nevertheless, in rare and exceptional cases, such as when hypnosis is considered as a substitute for an anesthetic (i.e., due to prior allergic/anaphylactic response) for a dental extraction, it is prudent to determine that the candidate for hypnosis responds successfully to analgesia suggestions in advance of any procedure as well as to test for high levels of hypnotic responsiveness based on a standardized scale.

It is often obvious that some participants are especially low in hypnotic responsiveness when an actual induction is attempted, and in this case formal assessment of hypnotic responsiveness is not likely to yield incrementally useful information. However, some of these same individuals will both respond successfully to imaginative suggestions administered in a nonhypnotic context and express openness to this alternative. Fortunately, much can be accomplished with nonhypnotic imaginative suggestions, as hypnosis confers only a small advantage in responsiveness—on average approximately 1.5 suggestions out of a total of 12 suggestions (Kirsch & Lynn, 1995).

Self-Hypnosis and Posthypnotic Suggestions

Suggestions can be administered either by another person (i.e., hetero-hypnosis) or self-administered (i.e., self-hypnosis). The practitioner can legitimately convey the idea that all hypnosis can be considered "self-hypnosis." After all, it is the participant who chooses whether to respond to suggestions or squelch the response, actively participate during the session, and imagine the suggested state of affairs; similar to the reference to self-hypnosis in the sample induction in which it is emphasized that it is the client who is "doing the work." Self-hypnosis can be a powerful and portable tool to (a) instate new cognitive-affective-behavioral responses or (b) to challenge or replace existing negative self-suggestions that are at the core of diverse manifestations of psychopathology, including depression and anxiety (e.g., "I'm worthless," "I'll make a fool of myself at the party"), with more positive, goal-directed, self-administered suggestions in everyday life (see Lynn & Kirsch, 2006).

Sometimes self-hypnosis is administered in the absence of a prior hypnotic induction. That is, from the outset, the therapist contextualizes the situation as self-hypnosis. More commonly, self-hypnosis can be utilized on a post-hypnotic basis after an initial session in which the hypnotist induces hypnotic responses. When this occurs, the suggestion to engage in self-hypnosis after the session is a good example of a posthypnotic suggestion: A suggestion to engage in a mental or behavioral activity following hypnosis (Barnier & McConkey, 1999). Posthypnotic suggestions often prime certain responses in certain circumstances. For example, Hammond (1992) recommends the following format for posthypnotic suggestions: "When I feel _____, I will _____." Many different cues can be attached to posthypnotic suggestions that include visual cues (e.g., "When I see a person smoking, I will remind myself that smoking is bad for my health"), sounds ("Whenever I hear _____ on the radio, I will list five reasons to not smoke"), thoughts ("When I think I need to smoke, I will have an image of myself as a nonsmoker"), and physical sensations and emotions ("When I feel an urge to smoke, I will tell myself that the urge will pass"). Each of these suggestions can be anchored with a sense of strength and resolve to resist any urge to smoke, as we describe in Chapter 7.

Characterizing hypnotic experiences as self-generated can encourage participants to create and embellish their own suggestions tailored to their specific needs and goals. The brief script below expands on the metaphor of Lynn and Kirsch (2006), which links self-hypnosis skills with the common experience of riding a bicycle.

"Remember when you first learned to ride a bike? If you were like me, you might have been a little scared, uncertain of what to do, and lacking

confidence that you could master the task. You might have been concerned that you would fail. Maybe you feared that you'd not be able to experience the thrill of coasting along on your bike, with the cool breeze blowing through your hair, joining in the fun with your friends or family members or just riding around yourself.

But you did learn. You could do it, and you did do it. And, after a little practice, you learned that not only could you ride, but you could do so without much effort, even without much thinking. You just jumped on your bike and took off. You let your mind and body work together to do all the things needed to maintain your balance, steer the bike, going from place to place, at your own pace, in control, and enjoying the ride. Soon, you were able to move in the direction that you wanted to move.

Isn't it amazing that you were in such control—doing all the things you needed to do—yet the act of riding a bike was easy, effortless, and seemingly automatic. You didn't have to think about controlling the bike. It became so effortless, right? Your mind and body working together to achieve a goal. Without effort, without stress, easy and effortless.

It's the same with hypnosis. You are in control and you go in the direction you choose. You imagine along with the suggestion, to respond or to make suggestions seem real. It's your choice, your decision, your work. And, just like riding a bike, it gets easier with time. Easier and easier with time and practice.

Given this understanding that you are the one making things happen, you are the one creating your experiences, you can see how all hypnosis is, in fact, self-hypnosis. After a little practice listening to me guiding you with my suggestions, you will gain confidence that you can give yourself suggestions, and create your own suggestions. The beauty of this realization is that you can personalize suggestions that are just right for you, as you know best what you need, what you want, and what works best for you."

CONCLUSION

Hypnosis affords clinicians with a brief, efficient, and cost-effective methodology to alleviate or address a wide range of psychological conditions and disorders. Clinicians of diverse stripe should consider adding hypnosis to their repertoire of evidence-based interventions as a potential catalyst of treatment effects. Self-hypnosis and posthypnotic suggestions can be utilized to maximize the transfer and generalization of treatment gains outside the hypnotic context. The chapters that follow provide substantial documentation of the salutary effects of hypnosis, along with guidance to facilitate the use of hypnosis in a wide range of clinical contexts. After reading this volume, it is our hope that readers will share our fascination with hypnosis and integrate it into their clinical work to explore how it can impact the lives of their patients and assist them in achieving their goals.

REFERENCES

Baker, E. L. (1981). An hypnotherapeutic approach to enhance object relatedness in psychotic patients. *International Journal of Clinical and Experimental Hypnosis, 29*(2), 136–147. https://doi.org/10.1080/00207148108409154

Bányai, É. I. (2018). Active-alert hypnosis: History, research, and applications. *The American Journal of Clinical Hypnosis, 61*(2), 88–107. https://doi.org/10.1080/00029157.2018.1496318

Barber, T. X. (1969). An empirically-based formulation of hypnotism. *The American Journal of Clinical Hypnosis, 12*(2), 100–130. https://doi.org/10.1080/00029157.1969.10734313

Barber, T. X. (1985). Hypnosuggestive procedures as catalysts for psychotherapies. In S. J. Lynn, & J. P. Garske (Eds.), *Contemporary psychotherapies: Models and methods* (pp. 333–376). Charles E. Merrill.

Barber, T. X., Spanos, N. P., & Chaves, J. F. (1974). *Hypnosis, imagination, and human potentialities.* Pergamon Press.

Barnier, A. J., Dienes, Z., & Mitchell, C. J. (2008). How hypnosis happens: New cognitive theories of hypnotic responding. In M. Nash & A. J. Barnier (Eds.), *The Oxford handbook of hypnosis: Theory, research, and practice* (pp. 141–178). Oxford University Press. https://doi.org/10.1093/oxfordhb/9780198570097.001.0001

Barnier, A. J., & McConkey, K. M. (1999). Hypnotic and posthypnotic suggestion: Finding meaning in the message of the hypnotist. *International Journal of Clinical and Experimental Hypnosis, 47*(3), 192–208. https://doi.org/10.1080/00207149908410032

Benham, G., Woody, E. Z., Wilson, K. S., & Nash, M. R. (2006). Expect the unexpected: Ability, attitude, and responsiveness to hypnosis. *Journal of Personality and Social Psychology, 91*(2), 342–350. https://doi.org/10.1037/0022-3514.91.2.342

Braffman, W., & Kirsch, I. (1999). Imaginative suggestibility and hypnotizability: An empirical analysis. *Journal of Personality and Social Psychology, 77*(3), 578–587. https://doi.org/10.1037/0022-3514.77.3.578

Cardeña, E. (2005). The phenomenology of deep hypnosis: Quiescent and physically active. *International Journal of Clinical and Experimental Hypnosis, 53*(1), 37–59. https://doi.org/10.1080/00207140490914234

Cardeña, E., Jönsson, P., Terhune, D. B., & Marcusson-Clavertz, D. (2013). The neurophenomenology of neutral hypnosis. *Cortex, 49*(2), 375–385. https://doi.org/10.1016/j.cortex.2012.04.001

Coe, W. C., & Sarbin, T. R. (1991). Role theory: Hypnosis from a dramaturgical and narrational perspective. In S. J. Lynn & J. W. Rhue (Eds.), *Theories of hypnosis: Current models and perspectives* (pp. 303–323). Guilford Press.

Connors, M. H., Barnier, A. J., Coltheart, M., Cox, R. E., & Langdon, R. (2012). Mirrored-self misidentification in the hypnosis laboratory: Recreating the delusion from its component factors. *Cognitive Neuropsychiatry, 17*(2), 151–176. https://doi.org/10.1080/13546805.2011.582287

de Groh, M. (1989). Correlates of hypnotic susceptibility. In N. P. Spanos & J. F. Chaves (Eds.), *Hypnosis: The cognitive behavioral perspective* (pp. 32–63). Prometheus Books.

Dienes, Z., & Hutton, S. (2013). Understanding hypnosis metacognitively: rTMS applied to left DLPFC increases hypnotic suggestibility. *Cortex, 49*(2), 386–392. https://doi.org/10.1016/j.cortex.2012.07.009

Dienes, Z., Lush, P., Semmens-Wheeler, R., & Naish, P. (2016). Hypnosis as self-deception: Meditation as self-insight. In A. Raz & M. Lifshitz (Eds.), *Hypnosis and meditation: Toward an integrative science of conscious planes* (pp. 107–128). Oxford University Press.

Dienes, Z., & Perner, J. (2007). Executive control without conscious awareness: The cold control theory of hypnosis. In G. A. Jamieson (Ed.), *Hypnosis and conscious states: The cognitive neuroscience perspective* (pp. 293–314). Oxford University Press.

Elkins, G. R., Barabasz, A. F., Council, J. R., & Spiegel, D. (2015). Advancing research and practice: The revised APA Division 30 definition of hypnosis. *International Journal of Clinical and Experimental Hypnosis, 63*(1), 1–9. https://doi.org/10.1080/00207144.2014.961870

Erickson, M. H., Rossi, E. L., & Rossi, S. I. (1976). *Hypnotic realities: The induction of clinical hypnosis and forms of indirect suggestion.* Irvington Publishers.

Fromm, E., & Nash, M. R. (1997). *Psychoanalysis and hypnosis.* International Universities Press.

Gfeller, J. D., & Gorassini, D. R. (2010). Enhancing hypnotizability and treatment response. In S. J. Lynn, J. W. Rhue, & I. Kirsch (Eds.), *Handbook of clinical hypnosis* (2nd ed., pp. 339–355). American Psychological Association. https://doi.org/10.2307/j.ctv1chs5qj.17

Gfeller, J. D., Lynn, S. J., & Pribble, W. E. (1987). Enhancing hypnotic susceptibility: Interpersonal and rapport factors. *Journal of Personality and Social Psychology, 52*(3), 586–595. https://doi.org/10.1037/0022-3514.52.3.586

Gorassini, D. R., & Spanos, N. P. (1986). A social–cognitive skills approach to the successful modification of hypnotic susceptibility. *Journal of Personality and Social Psychology, 50*(5), 1004–1012. https://doi.org/10.1037/0022-3514.50.5.1004

Green, J. P., Barabasz, A. F., Barrett, D., & Montgomery, G. H. (2005). Forging ahead: The 2003 APA Division 30 definition of hypnosis. *International Journal of Clinical and Experimental Hypnosis, 53*(3), 259–264. https://doi.org/10.1080/00207140590961321

Green, J. P., & Lynn, S. J. (2019). *Cognitive behavioral therapy, mindfulness, and hypnosis for smoking cessation: A scientifically informed intervention.* Wiley-Blackwell.

Green, J. P., Page, R. A., Handley, G. W., & Rasekhy, R. (2005). The 'hidden observer' and ideomotor responding: A real-simulator comparison. *Contemporary Hypnosis, 22*(3), 123–137. https://doi.org/10.1002/ch.8

Green, J. P., Page, R. A., Rasekhy, R., Johnson, L. K., & Bernhardt, S. E. (2006). Cultural views and attitudes about hypnosis: A survey of college students across four countries. *International Journal of Clinical and Experimental Hypnosis, 54*(3), 263–280. https://doi.org/10.1080/00207140600689439

Haley, J. (1985). *Conversations with Milton H. Erickson, MD: Vol. 1. Changing individuals.* W. W. Norton & Co.

Halligan, P. W., & Oakley, D. A. (2014). Hypnosis and beyond: Exploring the broader domain of suggestion. *Psychology of Consciousness: Theory, Research, and Practice, 1*(2), 105–122. https://doi.org/10.1037/cns0000019

Hammond, D. C. (1992). *Manual for self-hypnosis.* American Society of Clinical Hypnosis.

Hilgard, E. R. (1973). The domain of hypnosis. With some comments on alternative paradigms. *American Psychologist, 28*(11), 972–982. https://doi.org/10.1037/h0035452

Hilgard, E. R. (1977). *Divided consciousness: Multiple controls in human thought and action.* Wiley.

Jamieson, G. A., & Sheehan, P. W. (2004). An empirical test of Woody and Bowers's dissociated-control theory of hypnosis. *International Journal of Clinical and Experimental Hypnosis, 52*(3), 232–249. https://doi.org/10.1080/0020714049052349

Kihlstrom, J. F. (1985). Hypnosis. *Annual Review of Psychology, 36*(1), 385–418. https://doi.org/10.1146/annurev.ps.36.020185.002125

Kihlstrom, J. F. (2008). The domain of hypnosis, revisited. In M. R. Nash & A. J. Barnier (Eds.), *The Oxford handbook of hypnosis: Theory, research, and practice* (pp. 21–52). Oxford University Press.

Kirsch, I. (1994a). Clinical hypnosis as a nondeceptive placebo: Empirically derived techniques. *The American Journal of Clinical Hypnosis, 37*(2), 95–106. https://doi.org/10.1080/00029157.1994.10403122

Kirsch, I. (1994b). Defining hypnosis: A core of agreement in the apple of discord. *Contemporary Hypnosis, 11*(3), 160–162.

Kirsch, I., & Lynn, S. J. (1995). Altered state of hypnosis: Changes in the theoretical landscape. *American Psychologist, 50*(10), 846–858. https://doi.org/10.1037/0003-066X.50.10.846

Kirsch, I., & Lynn, S. J. (1998). Social–cognitive alternatives to dissociation theories of hypnotic involuntariness. *Review of General Psychology, 2*(1), 66–80. https://doi.org/10.1037/1089-2680.2.1.66

Kirsch, I., & Lynn, S. J. (1999). Automaticity in clinical psychology. *American Psychologist, 54*(7), 504–515. https://doi.org/10.1037/0003-066X.54.7.504

Kirsch, I., Montgomery, G., & Sapirstein, G. (1995). Hypnosis as an adjunct to cognitive–behavioral psychotherapy: A meta-analysis. *Journal of Consulting and Clinical Psychology, 63*(2), 214–220. https://doi.org/10.1037/0022-006X.63.2.214

Kirsch, I., Silva, C. E., Comey, G., & Reed, S. (1995). A spectral analysis of cognitive and personality variables in hypnosis: Empirical disconfirmation of the two-factor model of hypnotic responding. *Journal of Personality and Social Psychology, 69*(1), 167–175. https://doi.org/10.1037/0022-3514.69.1.167

Kosslyn, S. M., Thompson, W. L., Costantini-Ferrando, M. F., Alpert, N. M., & Spiegel, D. (2000). Hypnotic visual illusion alters color processing in the brain. *The American Journal of Psychiatry, 157*(8), 1279–1284. https://doi.org/10.1176/appiajp.157.8.1279

Lankton, S. R., & Lankton, C. H. (2015). *The answer within: A clinical framework of Ericksonian hypnotherapy.* Routledge. https://doi.org/10.4324/9781315803937

Lush, P., Naish, P., & Dienes, Z. (2016). Metacognition of intentions in mindfulness and hypnosis. *Neuroscience of Consciousness, 2016*(1), niw007. https://doi.org/10.1093/nc/niw007

Lynn, S. J. (1997). Automaticity and hypnosis: A sociocognitive account. *International Journal of Clinical and Experimental Hypnosis, 45*(3), 239–250. https://doi.org/10.1080/00207149708416126

Lynn, S. J., & Green, J. P. (2011). The sociocognitive and dissociation theories of hypnosis: Toward a rapprochement. *International Journal of Clinical and Experimental Hypnosis, 59*(3), 277–293. https://doi.org/10.1080/00207144.2011.570652

Lynn, S. J., Green, J. P., Elinoff, V., Baltman, J., & Maxwell, R. (2016). When worlds combine: Synthesizing hypnosis, mindfulness, and acceptance-based approaches to psychotherapy and smoking cessation. In A. Raz & M. Lifshitz (Eds.), *Hypnosis and meditation: Towards an integrative science of conscious planes* (pp. 427–442). Oxford University Press.

Lynn, S. J., Green, J. P., Jaquith, L., & Gasior, D. (2003). Hypnosis and performance standards. *International Journal of Clinical and Experimental Hypnosis, 51*(1), 51–65. https://doi.org/10.1076/iceh.51.1.51.14062

Lynn, S. J., Green, J. P., Polizzi, C. P., Ellenberg, S., Gautam, A., & Aksen, D. (2019). Hypnosis, hypnotic phenomena, and hypnotic responsiveness: Clinical and research foundations—A 40-year perspective. *International Journal of Clinical and Experimental Hypnosis, 67*(4), 475–511. https://doi.org/10.1080/00207144.2019.1649541

Lynn, S. J., & Hallquist, M. N. (2004). Toward a scientifically based understanding of Milton H. Erickson's strategies and tactics: Hypnosis, response sets and common factors in psychotherapy. *Contemporary Hypnosis, 21*(2), 63–78. https://doi.org/10.1002/ch.292

Lynn, S. J., & Kirsch, I. (2006). *Essentials of clinical hypnosis: An evidence-based approach.* American Psychological Association.

Lynn, S. J., Kirsch, I., & Hallquist, M. N. (2008). Social cognitive theories of hypnosis. In M. R. Nash & A. J. Barnier (Eds.), *The Oxford handbook of hypnosis: Theory, research, and practice* (pp. 111–139). Oxford University Press.

Lynn, S. J., Lemons, P., Green, J. P., Mazzoni, G., Lilienfeld, S. O., & Kirsch, I. (2015). Forensic hypnosis. In R. Cautin & S. O. Lilienfeld (Eds.), *Encyclopedia of clinical psychology* (pp. 1262–1264). Wiley. https://doi.org/10.1002/9781118625392.wbecp363

Lynn, S. J., Maré, C., Kvaal, S., Segal, D., & Sivec, H. (1994). The hidden observer, hypnotic dreams, and age regression: Clinical implications. *The American Journal of Clinical Hypnosis, 37*(2), 130–142. https://doi.org/10.1080/00029157.1994.10403125

Lynn, S. J., Maxwell, R., & Green, J. P. (2017). The hypnotic induction in the broad scheme of hypnosis: A sociocognitive perspective. *The American Journal of Clinical Hypnosis, 59*(4), 363–384. https://doi.org/10.1080/00029157.2016.1233093

Lynn, S. J., Nash, M. R., Rhue, J. W., Frauman, D. C., & Sweeney, C. A. (1984). Nonvolition, expectancies, and hypnotic rapport. *Journal of Abnormal Psychology, 93*(3), 295–303. https://doi.org/10.1037/0021-843X.93.3.295

Lynn, S. J., Neufeld, V., & Maré, C. (1993). Direct versus indirect suggestions: A conceptual and methodological review. *International Journal of Clinical and Experimental Hypnosis, 41*(2), 124–152. https://doi.org/10.1080/00207149308414543

Lynn, S. J., Rhue, J. W., & Kirsch, I. (Eds.). (2010). *Handbook of clinical hypnosis* (2nd ed.). American Psychological Association. https://doi.org/10.2307/j.ctv1chs5qj

Lynn, S. J., & Sherman, S. J. (2000). The clinical importance of sociocognitive models of hypnosis: Response set theory and Milton Erickson's strategic interventions. *American Journal of Clinical Hypnosis, 42*(3–4), 294–315. https://doi.org/10.1080/00029157.2000.10734363

Lynn, S. J., Weekes, J., Brentar, J., Neufeld, V., Zivney, O., & Weiss, F. (1991). Interpersonal climate and hypnotizability level: Effects on hypnotic performance, rapport, and archaic involvement. *Journal of Personality and Social Psychology, 60*(5), 739–743. https://doi.org/10.1037/0022-3514.60.5.739

Martin, J. R., & Pacherie, E. (2019). Alterations of agency in hypnosis: A new predictive coding model. *Psychological Review, 126*(1), 133–152. https://doi.org/10.1037/rev0000134

McConkey, K. M. (1991). The construction and resolution of experience and behavior in hypnosis. In S. J. Lynn & J. W. Rhue (Eds.), *Theories of hypnosis: Current models and perspectives* (pp. 542–563). Guilford Press.

Montgomery, G. H., Schnur, J. B., & David, D. (2011). The impact of hypnotic suggestibility in clinical care settings. *International Journal of Clinical and Experimental Hypnosis, 59*(3), 294–309. https://doi.org/10.1080/00207144.2011.570656

Nadon, R., Laurence, J-R., & Perry, C. (1987). Multiple predictors of hypnotic susceptibility. *Journal of Personality and Social Psychology, 53*(5), 948–960. https://doi.org/10.1037/0022-3514.53.5.948

Nash, M. R. (1997). Why scientific hypnosis needs psychoanalysis (or something like it). *International Journal of Clinical and Experimental Hypnosis, 45*(3), 291–300. https://doi.org/10.1080/00207149708416130

Noble, J., & McConkey, K. M. (1995). Hypnotic sex change: Creating and challenging a delusion in the laboratory. *Journal of Abnormal Psychology, 104*(1), 69–74. https://doi.org/10.1037/0021-843X.104.1.69

Orne, M. T. (1959). The nature of hypnosis: Artifact and essence. *The Journal of Abnormal and Social Psychology, 58*(3), 277–299. https://doi.org/10.1037/h0046128

Polito, V., Barnier, A. J., Woody, E. Z., & Connors, M. H. (2014). Measuring agency change across the domain of hypnosis. *Psychology of Consciousness: Theory, Research, and Practice, 1*(1), 3–19. https://doi.org/10.1037/cns0000010

Raz, A., & Lifshitz, M. (Eds.). (2016). *Hypnosis and meditation: Toward an integrative science of conscious planes.* Oxford University Press.

Sarbin, T. R., & Coe, W. C. (1972). *Hypnosis: A social psychological analysis of influence communication.* Holt, Rinehart and Winston.

Sheehan, P. W. (1991). Hypnosis, context, and commitment. In S. J. Lynn & J. W. Rhue (Eds.), *Theories of hypnosis: Current models and perspectives* (pp. 520–541). Guilford Press.

Sheehan, P. W., & McConkey, K. M. (1982). *Hypnosis and experience: The exploration of phenomena and process.* Lawrence Erlbaum Associates.

Spanos, N. P. (1986). Hypnotic behavior: A social–psychological interpretation of amnesia, analgesia, and "trance logic." *Behavioral and Brain Sciences, 9*(3), 449–467. https://doi.org/10.1017/S0140525X00046537

Spanos, N. P. (1991). A sociocognitive approach to hypnosis. In S. J. Lynn & J. W. Rhue (Eds.), *Theories of hypnosis: Current models and perspectives* (pp. 324–361). Guilford Press.

Spanos, N. P., Brett, P. J., Menary, E. P., & Cross, W. P. (1987). A measure of attitudes toward hypnosis: Relationships with absorption and hypnotic susceptibility.

American Journal of Clinical Hypnosis, 30(2), 139–150. https://doi.org/10.1080/00029157.1987.10404174

Szechtman, H., Woody, E., Bowers, K. S., & Nahmias, C. (1998). Where the imaginal appears real: A positron emission tomography study of auditory hallucinations. *Proceedings of the National Academy of Sciences of the United States of America, 95*(4), 1956–1960. https://doi.org/10.1073/pnas.95.4.1956

Tellegen, A. (1981). Practicing the two disciplines for relaxation and enlightenment: Comment on "Role of the feedback signal in electromyograph biofeedback: The relevance of attention" by Qualls and Sheehan. *Journal of Experimental Psychology: General, 110*(2), 217–226. https://doi.org/10.1037/0096-3445.110.2.217

Terhune, D. B., & Cardeña, E. (2016). Nuances and uncertainties regarding hypnotic inductions: Toward a theoretically informed praxis. *American Journal of Clinical Hypnosis, 59*(2), 155–174. https://doi.org/10.1080/00029157.2016.1201454

Terhune, D. B., Cleeremans, A., Raz, A., Lynn, S. J. (2017). Hypnosis and top-down regulation of consciousness. *Neuroscience & Biobehavioral Reviews, 81*(Pt. A), 59–74. https://dx.doi.org/10.1016/j.neubiorev.2017.02.002

Wagstaff, G. F. (1991). Compliance, belief, and semantics in hypnosis: A nonstate, sociocognitive perspective. In S. J. Lynn & J. W. Rhue (Eds.), *Theories of hypnosis: Current models and perspectives* (pp. 362–396). Guilford Press.

Woody, E. Z., Barnier, A. J., & McConkey, K. M. (2005). Multiple hypnotizabilities: Differentiating the building blocks of hypnotic response. *Psychological Assessment, 17*(2), 200–211. https://doi.org/10.1037/1040-3590.17.2.200

Woody, E. Z., & Sadler, P. (2008). Dissociation theories of hypnosis. In M. R. Nash & A. J. Barnier (Eds.), *The Oxford handbook of hypnosis: Theory, research, and practice* (pp. 81–110). Oxford University Press.

Yapko, M. D. (2018). *Trancework: An introduction to the practice of clinical hypnosis* (5th ed.). Routledge. https://doi.org/10.4324/9781351246309

Zeig, J. K. (2014). *The induction of hypnosis: An Ericksonian elicitation approach.* The Milton H. Erickson Foundation Press.

2 HYPNOSIS AND ANXIETY

DAVID B. REID

INTRODUCTION

Anxiety is a universal human emotion that alerts us to potential threats and motivates us to prepare for anticipated life challenges. Anxiety can be an appropriate reaction to a stressful circumstance, yet for many, excessive anxiety becomes counterproductive, and at times debilitating. Considered a diffuse mood state, anxiety involves unpleasant emotional experiences marked by a significant degree of apprehension about the potential appearance of future aversive or harmful events (Barlow & Cerny, 1988).

Anxiety disorders are the most common of the classified mental disorders and frequently co-occur with other mental or medical disorders, including alcohol or substance abuse (American Psychiatric Association, 2013). Anxiety disorders occur more frequently in females than in males at approximately a 2:1 ratio. Each of the five anxiety disorders discussed below—specific phobia, social anxiety disorder, panic disorder, agoraphobia, and generalized anxiety disorder—is diagnosed only when symptoms cannot be attributable to the physiological effects of a substance/medication or to another medical condition or not better explained by another mental disorder.

https://doi.org/10.1037/0000347-002
Evidence-Based Practice in Clinical Hypnosis, L. S. Milling (Editor)

Individuals with specific phobia are fearful and avoidant of specific objects or situations. Symptoms of anxiety are almost always immediately induced by the phobic situation, to a degree that is persistent and out of proportion to any actual risk. Social anxiety disorder (social phobia) involves fear and avoidance of social interactions and situations usually due to concerns associated with the possibility of being scrutinized. Individuals with social anxiety disorder are excessively concerned about being negatively evaluated by others, embarrassed, humiliated, rejected, or offending others. Panic disorder involves recurrent, unexpected panic attacks with persistent worry about having future panic attacks. Panic attacks are abrupt surges of intense fear associated with intense physical discomfort that rapidly peaks within a matter of minutes. Panic attacks may occur with identified precipitators or without any apparent source that brings about panic. Individuals with agoraphobia fear using public transportation, being in open spaces, being in enclosed places, waiting in line, being in a crowd, or away from home alone in other situations. These situations are typically feared as the individual experiences heightened worry that they will not be able to escape a situation, especially if panic-like symptoms manifest or other embarrassing symptoms arise. Finally, generalized anxiety involves persistent and excessive worry about various situations that people believe are uncontrollable, such as school and work performance. Individuals diagnosed with generalized anxiety disorder are usually restless, on edge, tense, and irritable.

In the United States, there is a reported 29% lifetime prevalence for anxiety disorders with an estimated 40 million American adults suffering from an anxiety-related disorder within a given year (Kessler et al., 2005). Accordingly, anxiety disorders in the United States generate a staggering annual economic burden of $42.3 billion to $46.6 billion, with nearly 75% of these costs attributable to morbidity, mortality, and reduced productivity (DuPont et al., 1996; Greenberg et al., 1999).

REVIEW OF OUTCOME RESEARCH

Several narrative reviews have suggested that hypnosis may be effective for treating anxiety and anxiety-related disorders (Flory et al., 2007; Hammond, 2010). Numerous case studies have demonstrated the benefits of hypnosis for treating dental anxiety (Eitner et al., 2006), needle phobia (Abramowitz & Lichtenberg, 2009), fear of flying (Hirsch, 2012), fear of swallowing or choking (Epstein & Deyoub, 1981; Reid, 2016), blood phobia (Noble, 2002), claustrophobia (Simon, 1999; Steggles, 1999), and panic disorder (Reid, 2017).

Importantly and of relevance to this book, a number of controlled studies (including randomized controlled studies) have been conducted that provide ample support for hypnosis as an evidence-based intervention for treating anxiety associated with dental procedures (Eitner et al., 2011; Glaesmer et al., 2015; Huet et al., 2011), surgery and medical interventions (Akgul et al., 2016; de Klerk et al., 2004; Lang et al., 2008; Saadat et al., 2006; Schupp et al., 2005), test-taking and performance situations (Boutin & Tosi, 1983; Stanton, 1994; Wojcikiewicz & Orlick, 1987), as well as general anxiety (Allen, 1998; Stanton, 1984; Whitehouse et al., 1996).

In the first meta-analysis quantifying the efficacy of hypnosis for treating anxiety, Valentine et al. (2019) demonstrated that individuals treated with hypnosis improved more than about 79% of control subjects. The authors reported an overall mean weighted effect size of 0.79 (95% CI [0.61 to 0.97]) when hypnosis was compared with contact (i.e., standard care and attention controls) and no-contact (i.e., no-treatment and waitlist controls) control conditions, as well as a mean weighted effect size of 1.12 (95% CI [0.83 to 1.41]) when hypnosis was compared with only no-contact control conditions. These findings, when compared with meta-analyses of other common therapeutic interventions, reveal that hypnosis is as effective as cognitive-behavioral therapy (CBT), progressive muscle relaxation (PMR), and psychodynamic therapy for treating anxiety disorders.

Furthermore, Valentine et al. (2019) determined that hypnosis was more effective in reducing anxiety symptoms when it was combined with other psychotherapeutic interventions including cognitive-behavioral therapy (Schoenberger et al., 1997) and biofeedback (Allen, 1998). The meta-analysis reported a mean weighted effect size of 1.25 (95% CI [0.82 to 1.68]) when hypnosis was combined with other treatments versus a mean weighted effect size of 0.70 (95% CI [0.52 to 0.88]) when hypnosis was used as the only intervention. These results are consistent with those reported by Milling et al. (2018), who determined that hypnosis was significantly more effective in treating obesity when combined with CBT than when applied as a stand-alone intervention.

Mindfulness, an alternative intervention for treating anxiety, has steadily gained interest and attention in recent years amongst the general mental health and hypnosis communities (Grover et al., 2018; Otani, 2016, 2020; Shenefelt, 2018). Some have proposed and encouraged the inclusion of mindfulness within hypnosis treatment protocols (Olendzki & Elkins, 2017; Yapko, 2011). Hofmann et al. (2010) observed an effect size of 0.41 (CI [0.23 to 0.59]) when mindfulness was compared with contact and no-contact control groups in treating individuals with a variety of medical and psychological conditions. Blanck et al. (2018) reported an effect size of 0.39 (CI [0.22

to 0.56]) when mindfulness was compared with no-contact control conditions in reducing anxiety experienced by student volunteers. In contrast, Valentine et al. (2019) obtained an effect size of 0.79 (CI [0.61 to 0.97]) when hypnosis was compared with contact and no-contact control conditions. This suggests that hypnosis may be more effective than mindfulness in treating anxiety.

Self-hypnosis, including the use of audio-recorded assisted and self-directed guidance, has been espoused as an essential and beneficial ancillary intervention to heterohypnosis for enhancing treatment efficacy (American Society of Clinical Hypnosis, 2019; Elkins, 2017) despite equivocal findings in the clinical literature. Furthermore, Valentine et al. (2019) reported that the effect of hypnosis interventions which incorporated self-hypnosis training was no different from those that did not. A recent meta-analysis may help to explain the inconsistency of findings regarding the benefits of self-hypnosis. Eason and Parris (2019) recently reported a systematic review and meta-analysis of the efficacy of 22 trials of self-hypnosis for a range of concerns including anxiety. These authors concluded that self-hypnosis was more likely to be effective when taught as an independent self-directed skill and when it involved at least three practice sessions.

CASE EXAMPLE

Treating anxiety, regardless of the specific disorder, should begin by educating a patient about their anxious symptoms and how they involve an adaptive response to what usually amounts to a *perceived* danger. When perceiving a threat to one's well-being (real or imagined), the body responds in predictable ways (e.g., rapid heartbeat, tightness in the chest, perspiration) once adrenaline and cortisol pump into the blood stream. When anxiety persists and disrupts daily functioning, an anxiety disorder is usually evident, and professional intervention is warranted.

Explaining how unwanted and bothersome anxiety symptoms are natural responses to certain life circumstances can mitigate any secondary fears a patient maintains about losing control. Furthermore, helping patients appreciate *how* anxiety symptoms are the byproduct of natural unconscious processes can foster an understanding that their body is actually not losing control, but behaving precisely as it should. Informing someone that their fight-or-flight system is functioning fine, but unfortunately "acting out" at inappropriate and inconvenient times, can encourage an appreciation that control to some extent is possible, and that learning more adaptive ways of managing stress and anxiety can be personally empowering. Such empowerment promotes a sense of autonomy and confidence in managing one's physiology and ultimately reducing symptoms of anxiety.

When treating people with anxiety disorders, I frequently share a personal story and relate their symptoms to a smoke alarm. The story goes something like this: One Thanksgiving morning while preheating my oven in preparation for the big feast, I noticed smoke seeping from the oven door. I jerked the door open as black smoke filled the kitchen, prompting other family members to throw open nearby windows. The fire alarm screeched and unnecessarily did its job. There was no fire, and my house was never in threat of burning to the ground. The alarm, however, had no way of knowing if the smoke billowing from the oven was benign or a life threatening matter.

Physiological responses to stress and anxiety are quite similar to my smoke detector. The mind cannot distinguish between real and imagined threats, and at times, it emits "false alarms." Through hypnosis, the patient's unconscious mind can help manage any unwanted symptoms, and promote healthier and more adaptive responses to any triggering stimuli.

Hypnosis has been identified and considered by some as an adjunctive tool among other therapeutic tools (e.g., cognitive-behavior therapy, psycho-dynamic therapy) within a metaphorical therapeutic toolbox (Saadat & Kain, 2007; Yapko, 2014; Zarren & Eimer, 2002). Rather than a single tool, I conceptualize hypnosis as a set of *versatile tools* within a therapeutic toolbox. As such, there are many tools or hypnotic interventions at our disposal for helping patients manage anxiety. As you will see below in my selected case study for this chapter, I employed a number of interventions including, but not limited to: fractionation (shifting depth of trance experiences), permissiveness (offering multiple options for trance experiences), ego strengthening (reinforcing confidence, esteem, personal value), deepening (enhancing trance, usually associated with increased absorption and relaxation), linking (pairing experiences during trance), interspersal (embedding suggestive messages into the trancework), ratification (verifying and validating that therapeutic trance indeed occurred and is helpful), posthypnotic suggestions, and anchors.

The Case

"Evaluate and treat anxiety/insomnia." These were the words scribbled on a faxed prescription pad I received 1 week prior to Jenny's initial appointment.

Jenny (pseudonym) was a 23-year-old, single, never married woman. She graduated with honors from a local university and was working on her MBA at the time of the initial consultation. Jenny said she "struggled with anxiety just about all my life" was a "chronic worrier" and added, "I just can't shut off mind especially when it's time to go to bed. It's out of my control." Despite initiating and practicing good sleep hygiene habits (e.g., no electronic devices after 10 p.m., 20-minute sleep efforts, no television in her bedroom, no late evening alcohol consumption), over the course of the prior year, Jenny awakened, on average, two to three times per night. She was usually able to fall back to sleep within 10 minutes, but she rarely slept more than 3 consecutive hours per night.

Jenny denied a history of panic attacks though acknowledged that she frequently felt "on edge," experienced intermittent rapid heart rate, shortness of breath, and episodic nausea. Jenny also reported that she avoided social engagements whenever possible, as she was worried about being judged by others and concerned she would say or do "something stupid, especially in class."

She denied a history of emotional, physical, or sexual trauma, and she also denied any concerns associated with phobias. There were no indications of an underlying mood disorder, and she denied a history of substance use other than consuming "a couple glasses of wine now and again."

At the time of the initial consultation, Jenny resided with her parents. She reported that she had good relations with her parents and denied that they were a source of her anxiety. She had an older sister who was married with one child, living in Pennsylvania. Her medical history was noncontributory, and she was not taking any prescribed medication. She was previously prescribed Prozac—titrated to 20 mg without therapeutic benefit over 3 months—that had been discontinued. Jenny had never participated in therapy before and said she knew "very little and probably nothing accurate" about hypnosis.

Jenny enjoyed reading, skiing, paddle boarding, and kayaking, all activities that require physical coordination and balance.

HYPNOSIS PROTOCOL

The hypnosis protocol provided below offers a summation of my hypnosis work with Jenny.

Introducing Hypnosis: A Trance-Forming Opportunity

Sometimes, it has been my experience that just by introducing hypnosis and describing what it is and isn't permits a wonderful opportunity for a beneficial trance experience. That is precisely what happened with Jenny during her second session as reported in portions of the transcript below. Comments are shown in parentheses.

After explaining how trance (an altered and altering state of consciousness) is a natural human experience (e.g., daydreaming, absorption in an engaging movie or novel, losing track of time) and that hypnosis essentially involves a set of skills and interventions utilizing trance to help people help themselves, Jenny expressed a sense of intrigue and curiosity. I asked her if she would like to experience a demonstration of hypnosis that I could record for her. Taking in a deep breath followed by an exhaled sigh, she said, "Sure. That sounds great."

"Very good." I said. *"So I invite you now to allow your eyes to wander around the room a bit and eventually settle on a spot wherever it may be. It could be on the wall behind me. Off to the side. Right or left. Anywhere it feels just right. Part of your unconscious mind might even find a spot for you."* As her eyes settled on a spot of the wall behind me, I said, *"That's great* (ratification). *So right now as those eyes* (dissociation by saying "those eyes") *focus on that spot, you may notice that your vision becomes a bit blurry; perhaps the spot moves around a bit, I don't know. And as those eyes settle, perhaps you can see yourself being somewhere else. Maybe it's a place you would like to visit. A place you are intimately familiar with . . . a place you would like to create . . . a place your unconscious mind creates for you. It doesn't matter* (permissiveness). *Notice how with each breath you inhale and then release, how much clearer you can see* (deepening) *and as things become clearer, notice how much more relaxed you can be* (linking). *Maybe colors or textures, or even things that are close to you become even more vivid. Notice what's there in the distance that you can't quite make out. Some people can even hear things. Sounds in the distance . . . sounds that are near you. Maybe with one of your next breaths you take in, certain aromas and fragrances* (multisensory suggestions) *come to you. Just being there now."*

As her breathing slowed, I said, *"That's right, just like that* (ratification). *Isn't it interesting how your eyes can focus on a spot yet you can see something else. How you can be somewhere else. Even as part of you is here, sitting in that chair, listening to my voice, part of you can be somewhere else, taking care of you* (ego strengthening). *And I think it is also interesting how some people can see even better with their eyes closed* (dissociation). *I wonder if you can see better with your eyes closed. So anytime it feels right, those eyes* (dissociation) *can close, so you can see whatever it is that you can see."*

Jenny closed her eyes, took in a slow breath, and as she gently exhaled, I invited her to *"be wherever you would like to be. Notice any difference with your experience with those eyes open . . . and now closed."* I offered suggestions for deepening, linking, and multiple sensory experiences and then said, *"If you want* (permissiveness), *you can allow those eyes to open again and see what you can see. Maybe see if you see better that place in your mind with those eyes open versus those eyes closed. And then gently close them again and see what you see"* (fractionation).

Jenny slowly opened her eyes and then closed them as her breathing slowed even more. *"That's great,"* I said. Knowing we had less than 5 minutes remaining for the session, I wanted to avoid an abrupt and direct countdown from five to one, and so initiated a permissive realert: *"How nice for you to take this time to take care of yourself* (ego strengthening). *Taking time from your day to create this experience for you. Noticing how you feel now compared to how you felt when we first started. And in a moment I will encourage you to become more alert and aware of all that is going on around you. But first, I invite you to take some time to internalize your experience. To put it somewhere for future access to use when you need it. And realize the changes that you have created in this brief period of time* (ego strengthening). *So when you appreciate that all that you created in this time . . . all that you did to not only help you now . . . but later . . . and knowing that it stays with you . . . when you are confident that this has been a helpful experience for you . . . then start to become more alert and aware . . . as alert perhaps as you were when you first came into my office but perhaps more comfortable as you leave."*

Jenny slowly opened her eyes, blinked several times while momentarily staring at the floor. She took in a deep breath, looked at me, smiled and said, "Wow, that was really nice."

I asked Jenny what experience seemed clearer or easier—eyes open, eyes closed, or perhaps it didn't matter. She said it was easier for her with her eyes closed, but it was also fine with her eyes open. She said, "Even with my eyes open, I could still see myself at the beach. The waves, the sand, clouds, all of it. I was in a kayak, just floating down the Sound." Since most natural trance experiences involve eyes being open (e.g., driving, reading, watching a movie, engaged in conversation) her response was not at all surprising.

Using Anchors

Jenny returned to my office 1 week later. It was during this third session that we focused on enhancing her ability to manage and "control" (her term as noted above) her generalized and social anxiety. This session was also recorded for Jenny to listen to at her convenience and involved the introduction and utilization of an anchor, which I frequently include during hypnosis.

Incorporating anchors during hypnosis serves as a wonderful opportunity for calming the wild beast of anxiety. Repeated and frequent pairing of calm, comforting, soothing relaxation with a conditioned stimulus like a smooth rock or gemstone, a comfortable positioning of the fingers, or rubbing one's fingertips across the thumb promotes opportunities for an individual to generate calm and comfort at any time in the future when stressful experiences arise. Over time, utilization of an anchor promotes a sense of comfort and calm, minimizing the activation of the sympathetic nervous system.

I prefer to introduce the concept of anchors to patients prior to initiating any formal hypnosis induction. After reviewing basic tenants of classical conditioning, I encourage my patients to consider a possible anchor to include during the hypnosis session. In fact, sometimes it is helpful to encourage people to find their own anchor and bring it to their next session. Once an anchor has been selected, I encourage them to apply the anchor as the hypnotic induction ensues allowing the pairing to be immediate and persist throughout the session. As you will see below, during my work with Jenny, I offered her some silent time to practice pairing her anchor with relaxation. A posthypnotic suggestion for using the anchor and experiencing success with practice over time was also provided. Finally, as with Jenny, I encourage my patients to refrain from using their anchor in the midst of the onset of a significant anxiety like a panic attack. Doing so will likely be met with failure (due to limited pairing and practice) and result in a premature abandonment of an anchor.

Jenny brought a gemstone to her next session. I encouraged her to close her eyes while holding the gemstone in her right hand. I then invited her to inspect the stone with her thumb and fingers, to *"notice the smoothness and perhaps the coolness of that stone."* A simple induction then followed: *"Very good. Just like that . . . as you notice everything you can notice about that stone, there in that hand* (dissociation with "that hand"). *Knowing just how it is that you can go into trance* (interspersal of a suggestion to go into trance) *in a way that is comfortable for you. Maybe notice things about the stone you didn't notice before and how much more comfortable and calm things can be with each breath you gently release . . . and the smoothness of the stone providing a sense of comfort . . . now. And I wonder how much more comfortable you will be in another five, or ten, or fifteen breaths. And even deeper, if you want* (permissiveness). *And as I talk to you and you can hear the words I am saying, and as your conscious mind hears these words and understands these words, another part of your mind, the unconscious part, is already helping you . . . already helping generate a comfortable and calm experience because it knows how to do that. It has been doing that for many years . . . calming and comforting. Your unconscious mind is very familiar with creating comfort and calm. Notice with each breath you bring in through your nose how that cool air calms things within, cools things within* (stated on the in-breath) *and how that . . . warm air you exhale* (stated on the out-breath) *allows you to release any tension within . . . just like that"* (stated on the out-breath).

Following some additional suggestions for enhancing comfort and relaxation, I introduced some silent time: *"You are doing great, Jenny. And right now, I would like to offer you some quiet time. Time to just take care of you . . . your unconscious mind can continue to assist as it knows how to assist and comfort you. So I will be quiet for about two minutes and I will keep an eye on the clock so you don't have to worry about the time because the time isn't important for you right now. Right now is time for you to take care of you. To notice how that stone there in that hand* (dissociation) *may feel different, as you feel different, calm and comfortable. I will be quiet starting now."*

After 2 minutes passed, I began to speak again: *"That's right. Very good. How nice for you to take time to take care of you* (ego-strengthening). *How holding that stone and connecting with comfort just comes together for you. And how helpful it has been for you . . . not just now but even later. How you have taken this time, invested this time* (utilization—Jenny was an MBA student) *in you . . . and how over time, things can change, you can change, and evolve* (utilization—Jenny was a biology major). *And how nice it will be . . . how your unconscious mind will provide you with a sudden experience of comfort and relaxation, maybe later today, or tomorrow, or some other time* (posthypnotic suggestion). *And how with practice and each and every time you take the time to do this . . . to shift to comfort, to hold that stone, and continue to shift and transform* (utilization) *to even more comfort . . . how nice that will be for you. There is a part of you that realizes just how you were able to make that shift, that transformation, today in such a brief period of time. What a wonderful skill you have there"* (ego strengthening).

With my guidance, Jenny eventually realerted. I encouraged her to listen to the recording that was made, once daily if possible. I also encouraged her to hold her gemstone to promote comfort when she was not in hypnosis by reinforcing the connection of her anchor with comfort and relaxation. Eventually, Jenny reported that she used her anchor to "settle my nerves while I was studying and when I was taking an exam."

One day, Jenny went to school and after arriving to class realized she left her gemstone behind. She had an accounting exam later that morning, but not enough time between classes to drive home and back to school. At first, she said she "felt a little panic creep in," but then recalled my prior suggestion of using her fingers and rubbing them against her thumb as an alternative anchor. This little port in the storm worked fine, as she reported an ability to ground herself and take the exam without further physiological disruption. One week later she was reinforced with a B+.

Promoting Sound Sleep

For the past year, if not longer, Jenny suffered from frequent bouts of terminal insomnia. While she was able to fall asleep adequately (at times with the assistance of melatonin or a rare shot of NyQuil), she would frequently awaken in the middle of the night. There were no apparent triggers for her premature awakening, and she also denied a history of intrusive dreams or nightmares. According to Jenny, she had a very clear appreciation of the source of her sleep disruption: "My mind won't shut off. It's like it just won't shut up."

Knowing that individualized interventions enhance productive outcomes when using hypnosis, I worked with her words. And so began her fifth session. (Please note that Jenny's fourth session is not discussed here as it was generally a repeat of session three and involved reinforcement of her use of an anchor.)

"I believe you are on to something there, Jenny," I said. *"Your mind . . . that is your conscious mind won't shut up. It's like it's not done for the day. There's unfinished business. The problem is you don't need to tend to unfinished business at 2 a.m. and again at 4 a.m. or 5 a.m. Right?"* She nodded in agreement.

I told her that I thought it was time for her conscious and unconscious minds to have a Come-to-Jesus meeting. I said, *"They need to work out some details about job duties, so to speak. Awake time, should be more conscious time . . . sleep time . . . that belongs to the unconscious mind. I think hypnosis would provide a perfect venue for that meeting. It could permit an opportunity for a terms-of-agreement understanding. A contract if you will"* (utilization). Jenny said, "Sounds like a plan."

I invited Jenny to be as comfortable as she could be and to just go into trance in a way that was beneficial for her (permissiveness). I told her to take her time and allow her head to gently nod when she was ready for me to assist.

After a slow head nod expressed her readiness, I offered opportunities for deepening: *"Isn't it nice to see just how well you are able to take care of yourself like that? To just close those eyes, taking some comforting breaths in. To realize how that cool air in is so comforting and calming*

*and cooling and the warm air out releases any tension, any stress . . .
if any? So each breath in . . . and out* (timed with her in-breath and out-
breath, respectively) *allows you to go . . . even deeper. As deep as you
would like. Allowing the unconscious mind to be more present. More
present to assist in a way that it knows how to. Having such a vast
resource of skills and abilities to be helpful now. And the conscious mind
to be a bit quieter or somehow in the distance. Like when you are drifting
out into the water, and the conscious mind just stays behind on a dock.
Still there. Not gone. But just quieter. Not as active. Not as involved . . .
for now."*

After a few minutes passed and additional deepening experiences were
linked with relaxation suggestions, I asked Jenny to allow her unconscious
mind to nod her head when she was in a "comfortable place." A few seconds
passed and she gently nodded her head. I replied, *"Very good. So you know
you have a conscious mind . . . and you know you have an unconscious
mind. And your conscious mind can be very active during the day while
you are awake. It thinks, evaluates, processes information, sometimes
worries, judges and criticizes, sometimes it just gets in the way. And
your unconscious mind is there . . . during your waking day, usually
working in the background taking care of things like your heart beating
and your breathing, and knowing how to move your body just right and
keep things nice and regulated internally without your conscious mind
knowing anything about that. In fact, your conscious mind isn't usually
aware of things your unconscious mind takes care of . . . unless there is
a problem. For instance, your conscious mind does not need to be aware
of every time you blink your eyes. There's no need for it to keep track of
such things. But if you had something in your eye that was bothersome . . .
well then your conscious mind might be very active and involved. Same
thing with swallowing. There is no need for your conscious mind to concern itself with swallowing, even though you swallow many times during
the day without conscious awareness. Until you have a sore throat.*

*So your conscious mind has certain job responsibilities and your
unconscious mind has its job duties too. Like during sleep. Your conscious
mind has no business being involved in sleep. That's up to your unconscious mind to take care of. Your unconscious mind will move your body
during the night allowing you to continue to rest and be comfortable . . . to
create some pleasant dreams . . . some you may remember, some you may
not . . . keeping you comfortable, allowing your body to rest and recover.
But it seems your conscious mind just has this sense that it has business
to take care of when it can . . . wait . . . yeah, just wait until morning.*

So right now as your conscious mind is listening in, it's important for it to understand that it will be able to take care of that business . . . but not when the unconscious mind is on duty for sleep. The conscious mind needs a break too and sleep is a wonderful time for it to take a break. So right now, I would like you to be able to invite your conscious mind and your unconscious mind to just come together for a moment . . . to come to an understanding that when it's time for your body to sleep, it's time for your unconscious mind to take a break. It's a nice balance (utilization) *. . . a healthy balance . . . just like your body knows how to balance in a kayak or on a set of skis, a nice healthy balance. So just take some time now. I will be quiet for two to three minutes and you can allow the conscious and unconscious mind to have that meeting. So they can come to terms and have an understanding that the conscious mind rests and is quiet and waits until it is time to awake in the morning. That the unconscious mind does what it knows what to do as it has always known how and what to do. After all, for nearly 20 years or more, your unconscious mind has provided you with restful and sound sleep through the night. And how nice it will be* (posthypnotic suggestion) *for your body to get the kind of sleep and rest it needs after your conscious and unconscious minds come to terms with each other. So I will be quiet starting now."*

Following a 3-minute period of silence, I began to speak again, and soon after, initiated a permissive realert intervention. A recording of the session was provided to Jenny and she was encouraged to listen to it daily, if possible, until our next session. She could listen to it at night, though she was informed that the intervention was not to facilitate sleep onset (this was not a problem for Jenny), it was to enhance sleep maintenance through the night.

Jenny returned to my office 10 days later and reported that the evening of her last session, she was "amazed" that she slept through the night, though she did awaken at 5 a.m. She listened to the recording every evening, and out of the other nine nights since we had last met, she slept through four of them (still awaking about 5 a.m.) and woke up "just once about 3 a.m. each time" and eventually awoke for the day between 7 and 7:30 a.m. She also reported that "sleeping better has helped my anxiety."

I met with Jenny for three additional sessions over the course of 2 months. She continued to listen to the recordings from her hypnosis sessions and also reported during her final session that she had been using her fingers and thumb as her anchor for enhancing comfort and calm. She would occasionally use her gemstone, but found it far more discrete and pragmatic to use that which was always readily accessible.

CONCLUSION

Many readers of this chapter have anecdotally witnessed and appreciated the benefits of hypnosis for treating individuals suffering from anxiety and anxiety-related disorders. As reviewed in this chapter, there is ample empirical data derived from randomized controlled studies published in peer-reviewed journals indicating clinical hypnosis is an evidence-based treatment intervention for anxiety and anxiety-related disorders. Indeed, the efficacy of hypnosis for treating anxiety associated with numerous medical, dental, and mental health concerns, as well as enhancing athletic and scholastic performance by minimizing anxiety has been well-supported.

When compared with other therapeutic interventions, hypnosis appears to be as effective for treating anxiety as CBT, PMR, and psychodynamic psychotherapy and perhaps more effective than mindfulness meditation. Hypnosis is also more effective when included as an adjunct with other treatment interventions such as CBT and biofeedback versus when employed as a stand-alone treatment.

Self-hypnosis, regardless of how it is delivered (i.e., audio-recording, self-directed), has received some attention in the literature over the years, though few controlled studies have adequately assessed its efficacy. Of the limited number of studies included in their meta-analysis, Valentine et al. (2019) reported that while self-hypnosis is beneficial for reducing anxiety it does not differ from the benefits offered by heterohypnosis alone. Self-hypnosis is more likely to be effective when it is taught as an independent self-directed skill and involves at least three practice sessions (Eason & Parris, 2019). Additional research is certainly warranted, though in the meantime, there do not appear to be any significant contraindications for including self-hypnosis in a treatment plan for reducing anxiety.

I believe it warrants mention that for most practicing clinicians, hypnosis is individualized and specifically tailored during treatment, as it was for Jenny. Clinical hypnosis, therefore, does not involve the reading of "standardized scripts" or prerecorded inductions that are generally employed (and warranted) in controlled studies. However, the findings of controlled studies can help to inform how a clinician might tailor hypnosis for a particular patient.

Whether employed in isolation or as an adjunct therapeutic intervention, hypnosis has been shown to effectively alleviate anxiety by facilitating adaptive coping skills, fostering more realistic thinking, improving stress management, enhancing control of one's physiology, and improving effective problem-solving skills. Clinical hypnosis can be conceptualized as an array of tools (e.g., interspersal, fractionation, anchors, posthypnotic suggestions, ego strengthening) within a therapeutic toolbox that are at the ready for clinicians to select from that empower their patients to help themselves by alleviating suffering from anxiety.

REFERENCES

Abramowitz, E. G., & Lichtenberg, P. (2009). Hypnotherapeutic olfactory conditioning (HOC): Case studies of needle phobia, panic disorder, and combat-induced PTSD. *International Journal of Clinical and Experimental Hypnosis, 57*(2), 184–197. https://doi.org/10.1080/00207140802665450

Akgul, A., Guner, B., Çırak, M., Çelik, D., Hergünsel, O., & Bedirhan, S. (2016). The beneficial effect of hypnosis in elective cardiac surgery: A preliminary study. *The Thoracic and Cardiovascular Surgeon, 64*(7), 581–588. https://doi.org/10.1055/s-0036-1580623

Allen, B. T. (1998). *A design of a combined cognitive-behavioral, biofeedback, and hypnosis training protocol for the reduction of generalized anxiety disorder* [Unpublished doctoral dissertation]. Adler School of Professional Psychology (Adler University).

American Psychiatric Association. (2013). *Diagnostic and statistical manual of mental disorders* (5th ed.). https://doi.org/10.1176/appi.books.9780890425596

American Society of Clinical Hypnosis. (2019). *Standards of training. Level 1: Fundamentals of clinical hypnosis* [Workshop]. American Society of Clinical Hypnosis Education and Research Foundation.

Barlow, D. H., & Cerny, J. A. (1988). *Psychological treatment of panic.* Guilford Press.

Blanck, P., Perleth, S., Heidenreich, T., Kröger, P., Ditzen, B., Bents, H., & Mander, J. (2018). Effects of mindfulness exercises as stand-alone intervention on symptoms of anxiety and depression: Systematic review and meta-analysis. *Behaviour Research and Therapy, 102*, 25–35. https://doi.org/10.1016/j.brat.2017.12.002

Boutin, G. E., & Tosi, D. J. (1983). Modification of irrational ideas and test anxiety through rational stage directed hypnotherapy [RSDH]. *Journal of Clinical Psychology, 39*(3), 382–391. https://doi.org/10.1002/1097-4679(198305)39:3<382::AID-JCLP2270390312>3.0.CO;2-L

de Klerk, J. E., du Plessis, W. F., Steyn, H. S., & Botha, M. (2004). Hypnotherapeutic ego strengthening with male South African coronary artery bypass patients. *American Journal of Clinical Hypnosis, 47*(2), 79–92. https://doi.org/10.1080/00029157.2004.10403627

DuPont, R. L., Rice, D. P., Miller, L. S., Shiraki, S. S., Rowland, C. R., & Harwood, H. J. (1996). Economic costs of anxiety disorders. *Anxiety, 2*(4), 167–172. https://doi.org/10.1002/(SICI)1522-7154(1996)2:4<167::AID-ANXI2>3.0.CO;2-L

Eason, A. D., & Parris, B. A. (2019). Clinical applications of self-hypnosis: A systematic review and meta-analysis of randomized controlled trials. *Psychology of Consciousness: Theory, Research, and Practice, 6*(3), 262–278. https://doi.org/10.1037/cns0000173

Eitner, S., Schultze-Mosgau, S., Heckmann, J., Wichmann, M., & Holst, S. (2006). Changes in neurophysiologic parameters in a patient with dental anxiety by hypnosis during surgical treatment. *Journal of Oral Rehabilitation, 33*(7), 496–500. https://doi.org/10.1111/j.1365-2842.2005.01578.x

Eitner, S., Sokol, B., Wichmann, M., Bauer, J., & Engels, D. (2011). Clinical use of a novel audio pillow with recorded hypnotherapy instructions and music for anxiolysis during dental implant surgery: A prospective study. *International Journal of Clinical and Experimental Hypnosis, 59*(2), 180–197. https://doi.org/10.1080/00207144.2011.546196

Elkins, G. (2017). Hypnotic relaxation therapy. In G. R. Elkins (Ed.), *Handbook of medical and psychological hypnosis: Foundations, applications, and professional issues* (pp. 83–97). Springer Publishing.

Epstein, S. J., & Deyoub, P. L. (1981). Hypnotherapy for fear of choking: Treatment implications of a case report. *International Journal of Clinical and Experimental Hypnosis, 29*(2), 117–127. https://doi.org/10.1080/00207148108409152

Flory, N., Salazar, G. M., & Lang, E. V. (2007). Hypnosis for acute distress management during medical procedures. *International Journal of Clinical and Experimental Hypnosis, 55*(3), 303–317. https://doi.org/10.1080/00207140701338670

Glaesmer, H., Geupel, H., & Haak, R. (2015). A controlled trial on the effect of hypnosis on dental anxiety in tooth removal patients. *Patient Education and Counseling, 98*(9), 1112–1115. https://doi.org/10.1016/j.pec.2015.05.007

Greenberg, P. E., Sisitsky, T., Kessler, R. C., Finkelstein, S. N., Berndt, E. R., Davidson, J. R., Ballenger, J. C., & Fyer, A. J. (1999). The economic burden of anxiety disorders in the 1990s. *The Journal of Clinical Psychiatry, 60*(7), 427–435. https://doi.org/10.4088/JCP.v60n0702

Grover, M. P., Jensen, M. P., Patterson, D. R., Gertz, K. J., & Day, M. A. (2018). The association between mindfulness and hypnotizability: Clinical and theoretical implications. *American Journal of Clinical Hypnosis, 61*(1), 4–17. https://doi.org/10.1080/00029157.2017.1419458

Hammond, D. C. (2010). Hypnosis in the treatment of anxiety- and stress-related disorders. *Expert Review of Neurotherapeutics, 10*(2), 263–273. https://doi.org/10.1586/ern.09.140

Hirsch, J. A. (2012). Virtual reality exposure therapy and hypnosis for flying phobia in a treatment-resistant patient: A case report. *American Journal of Clinical Hypnosis, 55*(2), 168–173. https://doi.org/10.1080/00029157.2011.639587

Hofmann, S. G., Sawyer, A. T., Witt, A. A., & Oh, D. (2010). The effect of mindfulness-based therapy on anxiety and depression: A meta-analytic review. *Journal of Consulting and Clinical Psychology, 78*(2), 169–183. https://doi.org/10.1037/a0018555

Huet, A., Lucas-Polomeni, M.-M., Robert, J.-C., Sixou, J.-L., & Wodey, E. (2011). Hypnosis and dental anesthesia in children: A prospective controlled study. *International Journal of Clinical and Experimental Hypnosis, 59*(4), 424–440. https://doi.org/10.1080/00207144.2011.594740

Kessler, R. C., Chiu, W. T., Demler, O., Merikangas, K. R., & Walters, E. E. (2005). Prevalence, severity, and comorbidity of 12-month DSM-IV disorders in the National Comorbidity Survey Replication. *Archives of General Psychiatry, 62*(6), 617–627. https://doi.org/10.1001/archpsyc.62.6.617

Lang, E. V., Berbaum, K. S., Pauker, S. G., Faintuch, S., Salazar, G. M., Lutgendorf, S., Laser, E., Logan, H., & Spiegel, D. (2008). Beneficial effects of hypnosis and adverse effects of empathic attention during percutaneous tumor treatment: When being nice does not suffice. *Journal of Vascular and Interventional Radiology, 19*(6), 897–905. https://doi.org/10.1016/j.jvir.2008.01.027

Milling, L. S., Gover, M. C., & Moriarty, C. L. (2018). The effectiveness of hypnosis as an intervention for obesity: A meta-analytic review. *Psychology of Consciousness: Theory, Research, and Practice, 5*(1), 29–45. https://doi.org/10.1037/cns0000139

Noble, S. (2002). The management of blood phobia and a hypersensitive gag reflex by hypnotherapy: A case report. *Dental Update, 29*(2), 70–74. https://doi.org/10.12968/denu.2002.29.2.70

Olendzki, N., & Elkins, G. (2017). Mindfulness and hypnosis. In G. R. Elkins (Ed.), *Handbook of medical and psychological hypnosis: Foundations, applications, and professional issues* (pp. 579–588). Springer Publishing.

Otani, A. (2016). Hypnosis and mindfulness: The twain finally meet. *American Journal of Clinical Hypnosis, 58*(4), 383–398. https://doi.org/10.1080/00029157.2015.1085364

Otani, A. (2020). The Mindfulness-Based Phase-Oriented Trauma Therapy (MB-POTT): Hypnosis-informed mindfulness approach to trauma. *American Journal of Clinical Hypnosis, 63*(2), 95–111. https://doi.org/10.1080/00029157.2020.1765726

Reid, D. B. (2016). A case study of hypnosis for phagophobia: It's no choking matter. *American Journal of Clinical Hypnosis, 58*(4), 357–367. https://doi.org/10.1080/00029157.2015.1048544

Reid, D. B. (2017). Treating panic disorder hypnotically. *American Journal of Clinical Hypnosis, 60*(2), 137–148. https://doi.org/10.1080/00029157.2017.1288608

Saadat, H., Drummond-Lewis, J., Maranets, I., Kaplan, D., Saadat, A., Wang, S. M., & Kain, Z. N. (2006). Hypnosis reduces preoperative anxiety in adult patients. *Anesthesia and Analgesia, 102*(5), 1394–1396. https://doi.org/10.1213/01.ane.0000204355.36015.54

Saadat, H., & Kain, Z. N. (2007). Hypnosis as a therapeutic tool in pediatrics. *Pediatrics, 120*(1), 179–181. https://doi.org/10.1542/peds.2007-1082

Schoenberger, N. E., Kirsch, I., Gearan, P., Montgomery, G., & Pastyrnak, S. L. (1997). Hypnotic enhancement of a cognitive behavioral treatment for public speaking anxiety. *Behavior Therapy, 28*(1), 127–140. https://doi.org/10.1016/S0005-7894(97)80038-X

Schupp, C. J., Berbaum, K., Berbaum, M., & Lang, E. V. (2005). Pain and anxiety during interventional radiologic procedures: Effect of patients' state of anxiety at baseline and modulation by nonpharmacologic analgesia adjuncts. *Journal of Vascular and Interventional Radiology, 16*(12), 1585–1592. https://doi.org/10.1097/01.RVI.0000185418.82287.72

Shenefelt, P. D. (2018). Mindfulness-based cognitive hypnotherapy and skin disorders. *American Journal of Clinical Hypnosis, 61*(1), 34–44. https://doi.org/10.1080/00029157.2017.1419457

Simon, E. P. (1999). Hypnosis using a communication device to increase magnetic resonance imaging tolerance with a claustrophobic patient. *Military Medicine, 164*(1), 71–72. https://doi.org/10.1093/milmed/164.1.71

Stanton, H. E. (1984). A comparison of the effects of an hypnotic procedure and music on anxiety level. *Australian Journal of Clinical and Experimental Hypnosis, 12*(2), 127–132.

Stanton, H. E. (1994). Reduction of performance anxiety in music students. *Australian Psychologist, 29*(2), 124–127. https://doi.org/10.1080/00050069408257335

Steggles, S. (1999). The use of cognitive-behavioral treatment including hypnosis for claustrophobia in cancer patients. *American Journal of Clinical Hypnosis, 41*(4), 319–326. https://doi.org/10.1080/00029157.1999.10404231

Valentine, K. E., Milling, L. S., Clark, L. J., & Moriarty, C. L. (2019). The efficacy of hypnosis as a treatment for anxiety: A meta-analysis. *International Journal of Clinical and Experimental Hypnosis, 67*(3), 336–363. https://doi.org/10.1080/00207144.2019.1613863

Whitehouse, W. G., Dinges, D. F., Orne, E. C., Keller, S. E., Bates, B. L., Bauer, N. K., Morahan, P., Haupt, B. A., Carlin, M. M., Bloom, P. B., Zaugg, L., & Orne, M. T. (1996). Psychosocial and immune effects of self-hypnosis training for stress management throughout the first semester of medical school. *Psychosomatic Medicine, 58*(3), 249–263. https://doi.org/10.1097/00006842-199605000-00009

Wojcikiewicz, A., & Orlick, T. (1987). The effects of posthypnotic suggestion and relaxation with suggestion on competitive fencing anxiety and performance. *International Journal of Sport Psychology, 18*(4), 303–313.

Yapko, M. D. (2011). *Mindfulness and hypnosis: The power of suggestion to transform experience.* W. W. Norton.

Yapko, M. D. (2014). *Essentials of hypnosis* (2nd ed.). Routledge. https://doi.org/10.4324/9781315747606

Zarren, J. L., & Eimer, B. N. (2002). *Brief cognitive hypnosis: Facilitating the change of dysfunctional behavior.* Springer.

3 HYPNOSIS AND DEPRESSION

MICHAEL D. YAPKO AND SHAWN R. CRISWELL

INTRODUCTION

Depression has been recognized as a disabling condition throughout history, chronicled in narratives of pain and suffering in both scientific and nonscientific literature. More than 300 million people worldwide are currently estimated to be suffering from depression, reflecting an increase of more than 18% between 2005 and 2015 (World Health Organization, 2017). The costs of depression on a variety of levels are huge: individuals suffer, marriages and families splinter, and societies endure the consequences of the destructive behaviors of people coping badly or not at all with their depression. Businesses bear the negative effects of employees too disabled to function properly, the economic costs of greater health care expenses for depressed patients are huge, and the tragedy of suicides and lives lost to despair is impossible to overstate (Yapko, 2016, 2019).

What is Depression? Issues of Diagnosis

Over the last half-century, there have been numerous attempts to characterize depression and identify its various subtypes. In the United States,

https://doi.org/10.1037/0000347-003
Evidence-Based Practice in Clinical Hypnosis, L. S. Milling (Editor)

the American Psychiatric Association created the *Diagnostic and Statistical Manual (DSM)* in 1952 to categorize mental health concerns, including depression. The *DSM* has gone through multiple editions with adaptations as to how they conceptualize and then create criteria for forming depression diagnoses. The current edition, the *DSM-5*, considers depressed mood (which can express as irritability) and/or loss of pleasure or interest as depression's essential features. The *DSM-5* also includes a frequency and persistence threshold where depression symptoms must have occurred most days, most of the time for at least 2 weeks in order to diagnose an episode of major depression. Other possible symptoms of depression include fatigue or loss of energy, changes in sleep (insomnia or hypersomnia), significant losses or gains in either weight or appetite, changes in psychomotor activity level including agitation or slowing down, suicidal thoughts or actions (or other preoccupation with death), cognitive problems in areas such as concentration or decision making, and feelings of worthlessness or excessive or inappropriate guilt. The *DSM-5* discusses how in many cultures patients with depression may present with various somatic complaints such as pain or gastrointestinal distress as their primary concern (American Psychiatric Association, 2013).

The range of possible *DSM-5* diagnoses that a person could have where depression plays a key role is impressively large. But, given its highly varied range of manifestations, how reliable is a diagnosis of depression? The answer is discouraging, for there are 227 possible and 170 likely symptom combinations that can all result in a *DSM-5* diagnosis of major depressive disorder (Zimmerman et al., 2015). Furthermore, in test–retest reliability studies of the *DSM-5* major depressive disorder diagnosis, the kappa coefficient (a statistic that quantifies interrater reliability that can range from 0 to 1.0) is only 0.28. Thus, it is considered "questionable" as a reliable diagnosis (Regier et al., 2013).

While using the *DSM-5* diagnostics may be essential for billing insurance or obtaining research funding, it seems apparent that simply selecting a specific *DSM-5* diagnosis according to a symptom profile is clinically not the most useful way to understand, much less treat, a client's depression. When assessing the client, it seems essential to screen for common symptoms of depression, such as sleep disturbance, and to determine if an adequate medical assessment has captured relevant information about the impact of medical conditions or substance use. It is, however, the personalized descriptions of the experience of depression in the client's own words that can provide the most salient specific targets for treatment. After all, the exact details of a depression experience can vary dramatically from person to person and even from episode to episode within the same person. Furthermore, understanding *how* someone generates depression is more important than speculating *why*, if we are to offer effective treatment. For us, the word "depression" refers to a multidimensional experience that is as unique as the person suffering its effects. Consequently, we strive to aim treatment, hypnotic and otherwise, at those subjective patterns that give rise to depression on an individual-by-individual basis.

Causes of Depression: A Growing Social Emphasis

There are many pathways into depression. Some of these are *biological* (e.g., diseases, medication side-effects, systemic inflammation), some are *psychological* (e.g., cognitive distortions, negative coping strategies, poor problem-solving skills), and others are *social* (e.g., poor attachment history, enduring early losses, domestic violence, poor social role modeling, poverty, discrimination).

It is our contention that despite the lion's share of research money still going to the study of biological treatments, especially medications, the evidence has grown to overwhelmingly support the position that the social and interpersonal dimension of depression is actually the greater influence on its onset and course. Depression is far more about one's circumstances—and reactions to them—than biology alone. Simply put, *depression is far more a social than a medical problem*; the sharp rise in the rate of depression during the first year of the COVID-19 pandemic clearly underscores this point and is buttressed by some recent neuroscientific studies that arrived at this same conclusion (Kumar et al., 2017; Menard et al., 2017; Yang et al., 2017; Yapko, 2009, 2019). Furthermore, there is recent evidence that adopting the prevailing biological perspective that depression is caused by a biochemical imbalance and "educating" the client to this misleading notion leads to demonstrably poorer treatment outcomes (Lebowitz et al., 2021; Schroder et al., 2020).

Given the degree to which we are neurologically "wired" to be social, how we build, maintain or sever our connections to others has a profound impact on our mood and outlook. Thus, it is little surprise how often other people become a basis for depression. Rejection, loneliness, betrayal, violence, discrimination, abuse, and lack of social and emotional support are the most obvious ways people can be the source of intense emotional distress, which can easily give rise to depression.

Relationships as Risk Factors for Depression and Targets of Treatment

It is part of the human condition to experience adversities and unpleasant emotions across the lifespan. Relationships necessarily involve challenges at times. Simply going through something difficult and even feeling deep despair, however, does not necessarily equate with developing depression.

This is encouraging because it reinforces the observation that adverse events alone don't cause and maintain depression. Rather, it is when people don't know how to respond effectively or how to access the resources they need when facing some challenge that they are at an elevated risk for developing depression. This is not meant to blame someone for succumbing to depression. After all, many social ills such as discrimination, poverty, and multigenerational trauma create situations that would be difficult or even impossible for anyone to manage. When treating depression and striving to prevent future episodes, it is therefore important to understand not only the difficulties that a person faces but especially the ways they perceive and strive to manage them.

Some attempts to escape discomfort related to life challenges can create even more problems, a phenomenon known in the depression literature as "stress generation" (Hammen, 1991). Substance abuse, procrastination, forming unhealthy relationships, isolating, giving up, compulsive behavior, and lashing out at others are just a few of the stress-generating actions people may take on an interpersonal dimension that can either create or worsen depression.

How a person thinks about themselves and their circumstances can also contribute to social distress and lead to depression. Consider someone's low tolerance for ambiguity: When a person doesn't recognize that a social situation is inherently ambiguous, they may go straight to interpreting the situation negatively and respond reflexively (Yapko, 2001b). For example, there are many possible reasons why a neighbor did not greet a person or why their friend yawned during a conversation. Interpreting that the neighbor doesn't like them or that the friend is bored by them are negative projections and are self-injurious. While it might be understandable to want an explanation because uncertainty is typically uncomfortable for humans, jumping to hurtful conclusions can contribute to stress-generating actions such as avoiding social contact with a friend or neighbor or even direct conflict that harms the relationship, perhaps irreparably and depressingly.

Social skills, persistence, problem-solving skills, flexibility, critical thinking skills, developing and maintaining healthy routines, foresight, impulse control, and skills to identify and self-regulate emotions are all essential skills for meeting the challenges of life. They hold great potential to not only reduce but even *prevent* depression's onset. Knowing how and when to apply the salient skills or mindsets for a specific situation can be challenging. There is no one-size-fits-all formula for living well. Instead, we strive to help our depressed clients respond to the unique characteristics of each context and identify what resources to draw upon to manage it effectively (Yapko, 2010). Giving up and developing apathy, the product of hopelessness, can be worsened if a client doesn't even know the first steps to take in order to succeed. A clinician needs to provide a clear road map of steps to take to achieve the goal *and* amplify positive expectations for success by expending the effort to try. Helping clients answer the vital question "Why bother?" while encouraging them to develop positive expectancy and take sensible, goal-directed actions are cornerstones of the effective treatment of depression. Hypnosis can play a pivotal role in helping accomplish these tasks of treatment (Yapko, 1992, 2001a, 2019, 2021).

Hypnosis as a Treatment Tool in Addressing Depression

Why employ hypnosis specifically in the treatment of depression? It's not because the mere act of performing hypnosis is innately therapeutic. Rather, it is what happens *during* hypnosis that has great therapeutic potential. When hypnosis is applied in a goal-oriented fashion:

> Hypnosis does many things that are immediately relevant to helping depressed individuals. Hypnosis: (1) helps people focus; (2) facilitates the acquisition of new skills; (3) encourages people to define themselves as more resourceful than previously realized (enhancing their self-image as a result); (4) makes transfer of information from one context to another easier and more efficient; (5) establishes helpful subjective associations more intensively; (6) provides learning to be more experiential and meaningful; and (7) defines people as active managers of their internal world. Hypnosis helps people sharpen key perceptual distinctions, create a safe distance from powerful feelings, proceed with new possibilities in deliberate behavioral sequence, rehearse new responses, develop undeveloped personal resources, and detach from a sense of victimhood. No one gets past depression without achieving all of these things and more. (Yapko, 2019, p. 454)

Hypnosis isn't so much about *making* positive change happen as it is about creating an active learning experience that *encourages* and *allows* positive changes to occur. There are some things that some people can't do intentionally yet somehow, they can do them when using hypnosis. One stunning example of this is how people can use hypnosis to allow themselves to undergo surgery without a general anesthetic. It can be equally life and health enhancing to use hypnosis to support amplification of positive affect, hopefulness for the future, increased flexibility in thinking, more consistent skillful social engagement, taking positive actions even when a person doesn't necessarily feel like it, noticing more of what's right and less of what's wrong, and so much more.

When a clinician is intervening, the clinician is not treating "the depression." Rather, they are treating a person. Thus, it seems essential to recognize that establishing a therapeutic alliance where the client understands and agrees with the overall approach and expects it to help them is the context in which everything else follows. The needs of the client are best met by addressing specific patterns and risk factors and teaching salient skills that empower the client. Creating a supportive atmosphere can encourage learning. People learn better when they are relaxed and engaged; these are compelling reasons to employ hypnosis in treatment when teaching skills in psychotherapy is so heavily emphasized.

Helping a client define their goals in ways that are specific and realistic can be helpful for getting the treatment of depression off to a good start. Defining treatment goals is an essential and often complex process, especially when a depressed person presents their problems in a vague and global way even while thinking that they are being clear and specific. Defining the problem as "depression" is simply not specific enough to create a good quality therapy intervention.

Once the goals have been identified in specific, concrete terms, the clinician can sort out the order, priority and pacing of addressing the goals. Each goal will have specific skills, mindsets and resources that need to be built, amplified or contextualized. Therapy techniques and approaches can be matched to the needs of the client. Hypnosis can then be used to catalyze the selected therapeutic approaches. The more a clinician is able to use the client's language, values, preferences and interests, the more likely they are to elicit positive experiential learning. The clinician's suggestions will need to be accepted and utilized by the client if they are to be helpful. After all, the suggestions will have no effect if the client can't find a way to make use of them.

There are many paths into depression and, fortunately, also many paths out of depression. Using hypnosis to treat depression provides many distinct advantages to the therapy process. These include the ability to: (a) develop the therapeutic alliance; (b) identify relevant and specific treatment goals; (c) select and personalize skills, mindsets, and empowering resources the client can more readily integrate; (d) build receptivity and positive expectations; (e) check in with the client during the hypnosis session to make sure that they are able to understand, contextualize and use the suggestions; and (f) structure home practice to further the client's ability to actively engage in effectively managing their lives.

REVIEW OF OUTCOME RESEARCH

The standard in the field of psychotherapy is to employ treatments with a proven value, a so-called evidence-based practice: "Evidence-based practice is the integration of the best available research with clinical expertise in the context of patient characteristics, culture and preferences" (American

Psychological Association, 2008). In the prior sections of this chapter, using our "clinical expertise," we described the merits of hypnosis in treating depression. We emphasized the need to individualize the treatment while keeping certain essential risk and resilience factors in mind. We mentioned the obvious, but often overlooked, point that no matter how brilliant a clinical intervention is, it only works for the client if they are able to accept and utilize it effectively. It is this individualization of treatment, and ongoing collaboration with the client to assess whether the treatment is specifically useful to that client, that allows us to attend to "the context of the patient characteristics, culture and preferences."

Research related to "patient characteristics, culture and preferences" is not well enough developed within the treatment of depression with hypnosis to provide clear guidance. Even when only including participants with higher levels of measured "hypnotizability," research results don't always indicate greater treatment effect size (Lucas, 1985).

Research Specifically Related to Treating Depression With Hypnosis

"The best available research" related specifically to treating depression with hypnosis comprises a limited number of meta-analytic and primary research studies. In large part, this is because hypnosis is not considered a therapy in its own right. Rather, it is a vehicle for delivering therapeutic ideas and experiences. So, when hypnosis is employed, there is a practical conundrum: how do we separate and measure the impact of the "hypnosis" versus the therapeutic suggestions offered in hypnosis? The situation is further complicated by the different ways that different studies define "depression." Some studies in the field of hypnosis measure depression level as a secondary outcome when the treatment is focused on other areas (e.g., pain). However, we focused on studies where the hypnotic treatment was specifically targeting depression, though other associated conditions may have been involved.

We are able to draw some general conclusions from the empirical research related to treating depression with hypnosis. "Effect size" is a type of measure that seeks to describe the magnitude of the effects in a study rather than limit the conclusions as to whether the results are statistically significant. For psychological treatment, effect sizes that are at least "moderate" are generally considered to be clinically significant. Treating depression with hypnosis is at least at the level of moderate effectiveness. This compares favorably to the impact of other, more well-funded and studied psychological treatments, such as *cognitive-behavioral therapy* (CBT), *behavioral activation therapy* (BA), and *interpersonal therapy* (IPT), which are also clinically significant at least moderately (Cuijpers, Karyotaki, de Wit, & Ebert, 2020; Cuijpers, Karyotaki,

Eckshtain, et al., 2020). Hypnosis is typically used within the context of psychological treatments for depression. Research that compares psychological treatment without hypnosis to that same treatment *with* hypnosis shows that hypnosis enhances the treatment effects (Alladin & Alibhai, 2007; Kirsch et al., 1995; Ramondo et al., 2021). This further supports the use of hypnosis in the treatment of depression.

Study Details

There have been two recent meta-analytic studies that specifically and exclusively examined the use of hypnosis in the treatment of depression. They found that there was a moderate effect for treatment. Shih et al. (2009) reported an effect size of 0.57 where $p < .001$ (CI = 0.32 to 0.81) from the six studies included in their calculations. Milling et al. (2019) obtained a mean weighted effect size at the end of treatment of 0.71 with $p \le .001$ (CI = 0.51 to 0.91) for depression symptoms in adults in the 13 studies they examined. They also reported a mean weighted effect size of 0.52 with $p \le .01$ (CI = 0.17 to 0.87) for the longest term follow-ups in four studies.

The individual studies included within the meta-analytic studies and the two additional studies related to treating depression with hypnosis that were controlled (Beevi et al., 2019; Chiu et al., 2018) as well as a relevant benchmarked primary care setting study (Dobbin et al., 2009) showed that clinically significant results can be attained in different outpatient settings, with different populations and with different treatment configurations. Though many of the studies occurred in the United States (Butler et al., 2008; Lucas, 1985; Sudweeks, 1998; Swenson, 1985; Van Sky, 1983) several studies took place in other countries (Beevi et al., 2019; Chiu et al., 2018; de Klerk et al., 2004; Dobbin et al., 2009; González-Ramírez et al., 2017; Guse et al., 2006; Liossi & White, 2001; Suzuki, 2003; Wu et al., 2005). Some of the hypnosis treatment was provided in group settings (Butler et al., 2008; Sudweeks, 1998). Other hypnotic sessions were delivered through audio recordings (Dobbin et al., 2009; Van Sky, 1983; Wu et al., 2005).

Many treatments can have a positive effect on depression symptoms. It makes clinical sense to use this knowledge to match the type of treatment to the needs of the specific client. Hypnosis can be added to any of the treatments and may serve to enhance their benefits. For example, there are studies using CBT—a well-researched method for treating depression—that demonstrate that combining it with hypnosis seems to be more effective than using it without hypnosis. Kirsch et al. (1995) conducted a meta-analysis of 18 studies comparing CBT with CBT enhanced by hypnosis. These researchers concluded "the adjunctive use of clinical hypnosis can help make CBT a more efficacious and enduring treatment, with 66% of participants at post treatment, and 72% at follow-up, experiencing better outcomes than their CBT counterparts" (p. 26). Results showed that CBT combined with hypnosis was superior to CBT without hypnosis in relieving depression.

In sum, the empirical research base suggests that treating depression with hypnosis is effective. Furthermore, the research suggests that adding hypnosis to other psychological treatments enhances the effectiveness of those depression treatments.

Using Hypnosis to Treat Depression—Focusing on the Social Side of Depression

We have provided information about a range of possible approaches for treating clients who present with depression. In the remainder of this chapter, we will provide a more in-depth examination of the use of hypnosis to treat the social side of depression, the area of focus for the case example and hypnosis protocol that we include.

The clinical literature identifies a number of interpersonal patterns that are closely associated with depression. These include (a) an internal orientation that limits one's ability to "read" other people or situations accurately; (b) poorly defined interpersonal boundaries that fail to establish clear self-definition and "rules" for managing interactions in healthy and effective ways; (c) negative ruminations about other's perceptions of them; (d) excessive approval-seeking; (e) excessive and/or inappropriate guilt driven by an unrealistic sense of responsibility for others' feelings; and (f) conflict avoidance. ITP is a well-validated treatment approach that addresses these and other relational issues and patterns (Greenberger & Padesky, 2016; Wilhelm & May, 2017; Weissman et al., 2018; Yapko, 2009).

In viewing depression as *process driven* (i.e., a product of ongoing patterns underlying one's perceptions and responses to life events) rather than *event driven* (i.e., caused by a significant, usually painful, event), our approach as described earlier is to address the ways an individual manages those areas of their life that give rise to their depressed feelings (Yapko, 2021). In the following case example, there are specific patterns evident in the client's way of self-organizing her subjective experience that make her substantially more vulnerable to depression. In fact, all six of the patterns described above are evident in this client's presentation, making it abundantly clear that the appropriate targets for treatment fall in the interpersonal category.

CASE EXAMPLE

The client in this case presentation is a psychotherapist participating in an intensive, multiphase clinical hypnosis and strategic psychotherapy training program taught by the senior author. We have called her Mary, not her real name, and altered any other identifying details as well to preserve her anonymity.

There were approximately two dozen other professionals attending the course. Mary volunteered to serve as a demonstration subject in the course, putting her name on a slip of paper as did several other volunteers, leaving it to the fate of a random draw as to who would be the instructor's partner in the process. A number of self-selection criteria were suggested to potential volunteers to help make sure they were appropriate in the problem they selected to address and that they understood how the intervention process would unfold. Mary's name was chosen, she was offered the chance to reconsider whether she still wanted to participate, and Mary affirmed that she wanted to proceed.

The Interview

(Note: The interview and session transcripts have been lightly edited for space, clarity, and readability. The therapist is identified as "T" and the client is identified as "C" throughout the interview transcript.)

T: "What would you like help with?"

C: "I'll try to put this together in the best way that I can. I've made progress on this issue, but not enough and I want to make more. The issue: I have a really hard time setting limits and keeping them. That includes limits on myself sometimes, and especially in my close relationships, but in my relationships in general. But, more specifically, just recently I've had a difficult period with my younger son. I am his mom; my head says, 'This is what I need to do,' but my desire for harmony and to be loved swishes in like a flood. In the past it has altered some of my decisions and has affected lots of my relationships in many, many situations. I don't know if I'm making myself clear or not."

T: "I've got questions, naturally. Let's talk this out. Let's get your definition of terms straight first. What are we talking about when you use the phrase 'setting limits?' What exactly do you mean by that?"

C: "Well, like what just happened here when you asked whether I could be recorded is a perfect example . . . I was conflicted. It's not that important.

I mean, I'm getting up in front of 20 people to talk about something very personal, and I made the choice to put my name in the hat or in the box to possibly be drawn as a demonstration subject. So, it's a mix of feelings."

T: "Generally, do you know how you feel at a given time?"

C: "Not all the time. That's part of the problem. Other times my feelings of wanting to keep harmony override my other feelings, whatever they are."

T: "It presupposes that you first know what those feelings are and then you start to override them for the sake of approval. Is that right?"

C: "Correct."

T: "That was the question I was asking you: Do you know how you feel about things before you start the process of overriding those feelings?"

C: "Yes. Most of the time."

T: "So, you would say generally you're tuned in pretty well to how you're feeling about things?"

C: "Yes. Most of the time. I think I am now."

T: "And then what you'll do is talk yourself out of that feeling, or try to talk yourself out of that feeling, in order to please somebody because you think that will make you more likable or more lovable or more acceptable? Am I understanding the sequence you follow correctly?"

C: "Yes, and I can see that I've made some progress on this issue. I've moved in a direction that I like. Just recently I made several different decisions that were kind of big that I knew would lead people to have some negative reactions towards me. But I made those decisions anyway and so far I've stuck with all of them. So that's how I know I've made some progress."

T: "Did you know what you wanted to do and then had to override your fear of negative reactions to actually do it?"

C: "One of the situations was irreversible in that I was resigning from a committee I was on. Another one of the situations would also be too late to change. It was a situation with some office mates and I didn't like what was going on regarding some waiting room redecorations we were planning. I didn't like the process of how they were going about it, so I chose to disengage from the process. Now it's being done without me, and I'm being pleasantly cordial about it. So, it's over and I can't go back on either decision."

T: "The question I asked was, in those successful instances of making what could be an unpopular decision, did you know how you felt in terms of fear of disapproval and then start to override that feeling to make the tough decision?"

C: "Yes, I started the override of how I really felt in order to get along with my colleagues."

T: "And then you corrected for it somehow and still took the position that could be unpopular. How did you do that?"

C: "How I do a lot of things, by talking with intimates that help me sort of process it. It's through support from friends."

T: "They helped you clarify your position?"

C: "And why I took the original position and why I would want to stay there."

T: "Okay. So, by talking it through with your friends, you were able to hold to the original feeling that you had that helped you dissipate the fear of disapproval that might have led you to override your feelings?"

C: "Yes."

T: "What was it about talking with them that allowed you to do that?"

C: "It's the validation of my position, reminding me of the validity of my original position."

T: "So, they reinforced that your original position was valid."

C: "It made sense. It was what I really wanted. I wasn't off the mark."

T: "Did you already know that? Or did you need them to tell you that it was a sensible position to take?"

C: "I knew it was, yeah."

T: "But you wanted reinforcement?"

C: "I hate that I wanted that reinforcement, but yeah. I'm old enough that I should be able to reinforce myself."

T: "But there's also a value in reality testing, isn't there? So, let me ask a different question now about this. How do you know when you need to set a limit?"

C: "Sometimes I'll start to get anxious or I'll get angry feelings in my body. My breathing slows down and it gets a little bit shallower. I think about the consequences of my saying yes and immediately I know that I'm going to be angry or unhappy if I do. So sometimes I know by going forward in my thinking. I've been trying to do this in my relationship with food as well, by going forward and thinking about how I will feel if I eat something. If I think past saying yes in some situation, then I can then go back and see that no is the better response, if that makes any sense."

T: "Well, it does make sense, but it only tells me the latter half of the sequence. Now let me ask about the first part of the sequence. Your answer might be that you don't know. The question I'm really asking is how you know when you need to set a limit. You've told me about the emotional response and about the strategy of jumping ahead and thinking about how you think you're going to feel if you say yes or no, but I'm back a step. How do you know when you even have to confront this issue of whether to set a limit or not?"

C: "Well, the first thing that comes to mind right now is when I don't feel safe in some situation. I don't know if that answers your question. I start to feel like I'm in, I'm in an area—wow, I'm really having a hard time with trying to answer this. I guess maybe it would help to go to something specific, but it's like, I have thoughts that 'This isn't right. It doesn't make sense and it doesn't feel good. It just doesn't feel good.' Take the situation with my colleagues recently over this waiting room decorating thing. I was very aware that I did not want to help process the waiting room plans because I could tell the way the other people, who I don't know very well, were going about it. It didn't feel safe, and so I didn't want to open myself up in that situation. And I feel like my instincts were good. I really think my instincts are very good. I feel good about my instincts most of the time."

T: "That part doesn't seem to be the difficult part, being aware of how you feel or being aware of what your instincts are telling you. The part that you're really describing to me, the part that's more difficult is when it goes from within yourself to between you and the other person. How do you know, when you do set a limit, whether it should be unyielding or flexible?"

C: "I don't think I've ever set an unyielding limit my life. So, I couldn't even tell you—"

T: "Take it outside yourself for a second. How do you observe other people manage this who also want to be loved? Do any of them seem to manage it better than you?"

C: "I have a friend, also a mother, who I think demonstrates boundaries much better than I do in situations where I failed."

T: "It's a woman you know? How does she do her boundaries?"

C: "She's so totally different from me. She just says no and then sticks to it because it's the right thing to do."

T: "But what does she do with her desire for love and approval?"

C: "I don't know."

T: "You haven't asked her that?"

C: "Not specifically. Okay."

T: "There's a good homework assignment for you. It's truly one of the best ways to learn, seeing people who are really good at something and then grilling them to learn how they do what they do. I think that would be most instructive for you to do that with people with good boundaries. It would help take a lot of pressure off of you for you to know your desire for approval and love is normal but you haven't yet learned how to manage it very well. It's not an addiction, it's a basic human need. If I were to ask everybody in here, 'How many of you want love and approval?' do you think there is anyone who isn't going to raise their hand? Wanting love is a given; the part that's negotiable, though, is how far you are willing to go to get it."

C: "Right. And that's really what we're talking about, right? Yeah."

T: "So, in your system, you say you know you need to set a limit when you feel unsafe, you feel anxious, or you feel angry. These are signs you use that suggest a need for limit setting. How, then, do you decide whether to actually say something or not?"

C: "Well, life and wisdom have taught me to wait. Then the emotional intensity goes down, and I can think about it more clearly and not be so reactive. I think about it, I'll make a decision, and then I try to act on it pretty quickly, like within a day or two."

T: "When you're thinking about it, is that when you're most likely to try to override your feelings and then give in? Or does thinking about it more likely result in you saying, 'I'm not doing that?'"

C: "No. Usually that first initial thinking about it might be when I talk to a loved one about the situation where I kind of just really try to integrate my mind and my gut about what I want to do. It's typically a little bit later, after the limits have been set, that I start to want to override it."

T: "When you've made a decision, how do you then start to second guess that decision?"

C: "I have thoughts come in. I start second guessing myself, thinking that maybe, just maybe, I was being too rigid. Or maybe I'm not being open enough. Or maybe I really haven't looked at it carefully enough from the other party's point of view. Or maybe I'm not being a good team player. Those are the ways I start questioning and doubting myself."

T: "Have you ever started to question yourself in that way and then stopped the questioning?"

C: "Yes."

T: "How did you do that?"

C: "I'm usually trying to redirect my attention and it depends on the circumstances. But I try to affirm that this is a good decision. This is a new behavior for me in some ways and so it's a little uncomfortable, but I also tell myself that I'm good enough and that this is also a self-respect issue. I try to give myself these cognitions, I guess."

T: "Can it be a good decision when it irritates the hell out of somebody else?"

C: "Yes, for sure, because it's the right decision for me in my behavior with them. And so even though they might be angry or hurt, I feel like somewhere deep inside I just know that it's right. I have a specific situation going on with my son right now about giving him money. It's extremely painful and shouldn't have happened. But not giving in I know is the right thing to do. It's right for him, too, it's the more loving thing for a mother to do at this juncture even though he's very angry with me. And I should have done it better, but I'm not going to beat myself up over how I handled it. I have regrets; we all have regrets. I didn't say no to him more often earlier in his life. It didn't serve him or me to have this issue at all. And it didn't serve me. I think that answers your question in terms of—"

T: "Recognizing that you can be right and still irritate somebody else."

C: "Yes. And even if I don't happen to be right, I have to just be comfortable that this was a good choice. It's okay for me to say no sometimes when I don't want to say yes. A recent example was declining the simple invitation to a social event even though I didn't have other plans. I just didn't want to go but saying no to that kind of thing would never have occurred to me many years ago—"

T: "Is there anything else about this that you think I should know?"

C: "No. But as I'm talking with you, I'm realizing that there's just something about all this . . . it feels like I get flooded with feelings. I would like for the flood to become more self-manageable. I mean, I don't mind going to my loved ones for support. I love going to my loved ones, and they don't seem to mind that I do, but I would like to be able to be a little more self-sufficient. I want it to be more thoughtful, not impulsive, when I set a limit. It's very important to me to be respectful of others and be cordial and not have to clean up a mess from how I reacted. There was a time in my life where I had a little temper, and it's nice to not have that, at least on the outside, anymore. I like to be peaceful with people, and it would be nice to just be able to kind of process it through by myself without always needing to go to others."

T: "Understood. Would you like to begin our hypnosis session now?"

C: "Yes, that would be good."

HYPNOSIS PROTOCOL

This section presents a full transcript of the hypnosis intervention with the client.

Induction (Conversational)

T: *"You can arrange yourself in whatever way is comfortable for you. . . .
Once you've settled into a position you feel good in, you can let your
eyes close. . . . That's right. . . . Given that you're quite experienced with
developing comfort . . . it really doesn't take a lot of time or effort to
focus yourself. . . . Of course, you know as well as I do that each person
has their own pace. . . . Some people can settle in really quickly. . . . Some
take a while. . . . Most people are somewhere in between . . . but given
that you already know a lot about how to focus yourself . . . and even
from your experience during the group hypnosis earlier this morning . . .
that you were generous enough to share . . . about the heaviness of
your head and the comfort of your body . . . highlights your hypnotic
abilities . . ."*

Building a Response Set

T: *"Now having a heavy head doesn't pose any great therapeutic advantages, but it really does speak to your ability to get that comfortable . . . to get that absorbed. . . . And it's that capacity of yours I'm particularly interested in right now . . . certainly you know as well as I do how valuable it is to develop that quality of absorption. . . . And initially it's much more general . . . not yet specific . . . what the general indicators are that you're evolving a deepening focus . . . your breathing slowing down . . . your body getting more and more comfortable . . . your thoughts getting more focused. . . . And then as you start to evolve a deeper quality of comfort . . . you'll likely notice other subtle shifts taking place in your awareness. . . . Of course, it isn't really going to be something that I can know from the outside . . . the way that you can know it from the inside . . . such as the sensations of your hands resting on your thigh. . . . Well, those are your fingertips. . . . It is the fabric of your pants that you're feeling . . . and how can I possibly share in that experience of yours? . . . And what you're feeling at a given moment . . . you know better than anyone else possibly could . . ."*

Therapeutic Theme: Recognizing and Honoring Your Uniqueness

T: *"But it's an interesting thing how each person comes to evolve a quality of self-awareness . . . some more so, some less so. . . . It's true that it's one of the great tasks we all have in life is to develop a sense of your own uniqueness. . . . And isn't that one of the great paradoxes of life, the uniqueness of each person . . . that we all have in common . . . you're unique and I'm unique . . . just like everyone else . . . but there's something comforting about knowing that just like everybody else, you're unique . . . the enjoyable paradox of wondering who you are. . . . and discovering things about yourself all the time. . . . It's so very clear that each unique person is ultimately alone . . . and no matter who they are . . . no matter how much I might care for you . . . if you break your leg . . . you're going to have be the one to wear the cast . . ."*

Therapeutic Theme: The Limits of Responsibility

T: *"So, it raises a pretty interesting question. . . . How responsible am I really for your hypnotic experience? . . . How responsible am I really for what you learn or don't learn . . . or what you experience and what you don't experience? . . . And I wonder just what I might say if you told me that your hypnotic experience is entirely generated by me . . . but of course there's little risk of that happening . . . since you're already quite aware that even though there's a lot that I can say . . . a lot that I can offer you that can make quite a difference in your way of reacting to challenging situations . . . it's still your choice as to what you focus on . . . and what you absorb . . . what you hear . . . and what you allow. . . . And in that respect, isn't it true that each person has to define their own awareness, their own experience? . . . I can't really decide for you just when you might want to adjust your physical position to be more comfortable. . . . I can't really decide for you just when your body feels light enough . . . or detached enough . . . to turn your attention elsewhere . . ."*

Therapeutic Theme: People's Preferences or Requests Aren't Mandates

T: *"And so as much as I might want to do hypnosis correctly . . . you know and I know there are lots of different factors to take into account . . . in you determining what's worth focusing on . . . what's worth accepting and using. . . . And in all the years to come there will be a lot of people you'll encounter who are more than willing to try to decide for you . . . about all kinds of things big and small . . . there will be plenty of opportunities when you're with somebody for them to suggest something from the menu that you'd prefer not to have . . . whether it's a restaurant menu . . . or a relationship menu . . . or a financial menu of ways to give them money . . . or a sexual menu . . . or an insurance menu. . . . But it's all the same. . . . I can't really look at you from the outside and decide that you would prefer half a cup of decaf coffee, much less whether you want cream in it. . . . But there are plenty of people in the world who would be happy to tell you what the correct way is to drink coffee. . . . People who would willingly criticize you for drinking your coffee wrong. . . . Telling you that you should put this in your coffee, not that. . . . It's such an interesting and curious thing how wonderfully tolerant and even affectionate other people can be when you're doing things their way . . . according to their wishes or beliefs . . . with little regard for yours . . . but there's something much deeper for you to start to focus on and absorb now. . . . It has a lot to do with simple choices . . . and also the not so simple choices. . . . The simple choices about what coffee to drink . . . when you know whether you want cream and sugar or not. . . . There's something about that very superficial example that has deeper implications. . . . How do you know how you prefer your coffee? . . . How do you decide that's the right choice for you? . . . And when I asked you earlier do you know what you feel? . . . You were pretty quick to say that you do . . . and now there's a new, next step evolving within you at this very moment. . . . Going from knowing what you feel to recognizing someone else's attempts to have you do things their way . . . for their benefit . . . your getting in line with them supports them. . . . Because it's in that moment of not being sure whether it's okay to drink your coffee your way . . . to want or not want cream or sugar . . . you have the chance to acknowledge your own preferences . . . and honor them. . . . And how quickly that recognition can come to mind . . . that so many interactions you have are about coffee in a way. . . . Somebody asks how you feel about something . . . and you're immediately aware of how you feel or what you prefer. . . . And then the next thought you can have is, "It's just a cup of coffee," metaphorically speaking. . . . So, whether it's someone asking for your time, they're just offering you a cup of coffee . . . someone asking for your money . . . is just asking for a free cup of coffee . . . someone asking for anything from you . . . your support, your expertise, is offering you a chance to give . . . and how different for you to focus on what they want from you and how they go about asking for it instead of how it feels to be asked . . ."*

Therapeutic Theme: Managing Others' Reactions to Your Limit Setting

T: *"So, if you decide to say yes to a request . . . it's because you choose it . . . and if you decide to say no, it's out of an awareness that you don't want the cream and sugar they're promoting . . . and when you say no, there will be the inevitable reaction of someone not getting what they want . . . and how good it can feel to know that you recognize and honor your own wishes and preferences . . . and you can hope they have the maturity to do the same . . . and you can shift your focus to them . . . and discover about them whether they can graciously accept your choices . . . or whether they strive to push against your preferences for their gain at your expense. . . . What a calming difference in you to shift from analyzing what it says about you to instead focusing on what it says about them . . . in the way they react to the limits you set by expressing your preferences. . . . How great the relief is that you can experience when you no longer find yourself questioning and second-guessing yourself . . . when you are clear about how you like your coffee . . . and your life . . ."*

Therapeutic Theme: Revisiting the Issue of Limits of Responsibility Through Metaphor

T: "It's a curious thing that happens when you're really not clear about where the limits of your responsibility to others begins and ends. . . . Well, I can tell you about a distressed woman who came to see me. . . . She was in her late fifties and had a daughter in her mid-thirties. . . . And she presented the problem to me that her daughter was getting married . . . to a musician who had tattoos all over and a nose ring . . . which she found utterly horrifying . . . and she asked me with tears in her eyes, "Where did I go wrong in raising my daughter? Why is she doing this to me?" . . . Now, if her daughter was 12, I might have entertained that question. . . . But her daughter was 34! . . . And I really wanted to tell her . . . and I did. . . . "Your daughter's 34. She gets to marry anybody she chooses. And it's not about you. . . . It's about the choices she makes that she's going to have to live with." . . . And it was interesting how, when I said that to her, she had no idea what I was talking about because it was her daughter . . . and in her view, a mother is responsible for her daughter and her daughter's choices . . . whether they be career choices, financial choices, or whatever choices . . . which I thought was interesting . . . then I asked her what her daughter had for breakfast that morning. . . . She confessed that she didn't know. . . . And I had to ask what kind of mother doesn't know what her daughter's eating for breakfast? . . . And when I asked her what's in her daughter's refrigerator, she confessed that she didn't know. . . . And I wondered what kind of mother doesn't know what's in her daughter's refrigerator. . . . And I asked her where her daughter went on a recent vacation and she said Hawaii. . . . Then I asked, "Well, what did she do while she was there?" . . . She didn't know. . . . I had to ask, what kind of mother lets her daughter go to Hawaii without knowing where she's going and what she's doing? She got really annoyed after a while before she said, "For God's sake, she's 34!" . . . I had to ask her to repeat that. . . . And it took her a while, but it finally became abundantly clear to her that no adult can be responsible for the choices that another adult makes. . . . So the natural reflex is to look for blame when someone makes a bad decision . . . sometimes it's blaming others for our own bad choices . . . for example, if this hypnosis session isn't perfect, I'm going to blame you and be deeply disappointed because you shouldn't have let me say that . . . you shouldn't have forced me to suggest these things *to you. . . . And sometimes the reflex is to blame ourselves. . . . It's my fault you squandered your money . . . it's my fault you were out driving while intoxicated. . . . When she eventually got the point that her daughter's choosing to marry a musician with tattoos and a nose ring . . . she finally reached a point in the session where she said so calmly, "Well, it's her marriage and I wish them well." . . . She finally got the point that no adult is responsible for the choice another adult makes. . . . It means you can hate someone's choices, but accept them graciously nonetheless . . . you can regret someone's choices but be clear that they made those choices. . . . You may even want to ask, "Is that really the best choice you could come up with?" . . . Those are usually just "inside words," though. . . . But if you actually asked someone that question . . . a lot of times people will say yes! And isn't that part of what you've learned in doing therapy? People make choices then suffer the consequences . . . and then you try and teach them new ways, better ways of making choices. . . . But you know as well as I do that there are some people who will fall in a rut and work hard to climb out of it . . . and others who will fall in a rut and start to decorate it. . . . People make choices all the time. . . . And as you grow ever clearer that other people make their choices and have to live with the consequences of those choices. . . . Once you're clear on that you can sit back and wait for the emotional flood to come only to discover it's a "no-show." . . . What a difference! That's right . . . the flood that never arrived . . . because it's so clear that other people choose . . . whether it's musicians with tattoos and nose rings . . . or people who live in places you wouldn't live . . . or take drugs you wouldn't take . . . or go to movies you wouldn't see . . . eat stuff you wouldn't eat . . . buy stuff you wouldn't buy . . ."*

Therapeutic Theme: People Want What They Want, but Demands Aren't Mandates

T: *"People get to make their own choices . . . and they get to ask for what they want. . . . What you're becoming more immediately aware of is that someone can place a demand on you. . . . Someone can want your time, your money, your expertise, your support. . . . If you have it, whatever it is . . . somebody out there wants it. . . . So, what else is new? It's no different than when you were young and single and dating . . . it wasn't real tough to figure out what the boys in high school wanted from you, was it? . . . Gee, who would have guessed they'd say things and do things to get what they want? . . . Surprise! You have a body and somebody wants it. . . . You have time*

and somebody wants it. . . . You have money or expertise and some-
body wants it. . . . And now you can become aware so quickly that
somebody wants something from you . . . and you get to decide
whether you feel like sharing or donating . . . or whether the answer is
"pass." And when you say no, then you get to grab your popcorn . . .
metaphorically speaking . . . and watch the show. . . . What do they
say or do to get you to reconsider? . . . Do they try and make you
feel guilty? . . . Pack your bags, we're going on a guilt trip. . . . Well,
it'd be nice to have something to say right there in that moment . . .
to brush off the guilt trip. . . . Someone else uses threats to get what
they want. . . . It would be nice to have something to say in that
moment . . . instead of wondering and doubting and second guessing
yourself. . . . Now, there's a very different sequence evolving out of
this for you. . . . Someone can ask you for anything that they think
you have. . . . So what? Let them ask—it's just what people do. . . .
If you have it, somebody wants it. . . . But what a difference to have
that sense that it's no longer up to you to compensate for someone
else's bad choices, whether relatives or friends or colleagues. . . .
You're discovering the power that comes from knowing you have the
ability to step back and watch the show. . . . When you say no, just
what is this person willing to do to get what they want? Enjoy the
show. . . . It'll teach you a lot about that person and what they're
willing to do to hurt someone else, you perhaps, simply to get what
they want. . . . Only for you, not anymore . . ."

C: "They can ask."

T: *"Yes, they can ask, but you're going to learn something when you*
discover whether they have good enough boundaries to accept your
answer graciously. . . . And as you discover, not everyone has great
boundaries."

C: "They can ask."

Therapeutic Strategy: Affective Reassociation

T: *"Yes, and you can answer . . . but your days of asking why a daughter*
marries a musician are pretty much over. . . . Now, I'm not suggesting
that you go out and get a tattoo . . . but if you were to get one,
it would be a good phrase to put somewhere on your backside. . . .
That might be just the right thing to show someone when they don't
graciously accept the choice you've made. . . . This is one of the nice
things about a playful imagination . . . you can imagine it's there

and when you say no and they don't react well . . . the other person will just wonder about the smile on your face that they really don't understand. . . . We'll just keep that between us! Now, I've talked about a lot of different things . . . much more than just tattoos, but when you find yourself thinking, no, it's just another cup of coffee with someone else's instructions on how to drink it. . . . Well, you know, the rest . . ."

Checking-In for Feedback

T: *"And so, in just a moment, I'd like to ask you to describe out loud what you're aware of at this point. . . . And you can describe it easily . . . still continuing to be focused. . . . And if you would describe what you're aware of right now . . ."*

C: "I am aware that I have a new, a new step. . . . I can't quite articulate it, but it's there. . . . And that I don't have to be flooded, that I can "pass" on the flood. . . . And that I'm truly not responsible for even a 21-year-old's choices or his feelings about my choices that were really clear. . . . They don't really change for this person . . ."

T: *"What age does somebody learn to respect the choices that others make? Twenty-one sounds about right, don't you think?"*

C: "Yes."

Posthypnotic Suggestions

T: *"And the same goes for you respecting the choices that you make for yourself. Sixty sounds about right, don't you think? . . . And I can articulate the next step . . . it's going from being aware that someone is making a demand, whether it's for your time or your money or anything else you have . . . to an immediate awareness as to whether you want to meet that demand or not. . . . Sometimes you'll choose to say no, sometimes you'll say, yes, it's okay, because you've got some to spare, and it doesn't hurt you or the other person. . . . The times to really know yourself are the times when the answer is no. . . . Five minutes from now and 5 days from now, it's still going to be no. . . . You can say how you feel without second guessing. . . . And you can tattoo anything on your backside you want to in your imagination . . . and decide to show it at just the right moment because that's your answer, metaphorically speaking. . . . After all, I'd hate for you to get arrested for mooning someone! . . . So, with a sense of renewed clarity,*

you can realize that people can ask you for anything they want. . . .
And how clearly now you can decide to answer . . . and then sit back
and watch the show . . . that reveals so much of who they are . . ."

Closure and Disengagement

T: *"Take whatever time you want to now . . . to process your thoughts*
and feelings . . . in order to bring this experience to a comfortable
close . . . you can integrate all these different ideas at a deep level
within you . . . and when you feel like you are ready to . . . you can
start the process of slowly re-orienting yourself at a gradual, com-
fortable rate . . . fully re-orienting now . . . and letting your eyes open
whenever you're ready."

Goals of the Session

The need to set effective limits in one's relationships, defining what you
will and won't accept in your relationships with others, is ever present. The
process of setting limits, though, is complex with multiple steps involved. The
inability to set limits well can arise for any number of reasons. After all, "setting
limits" is a global phrase that represents a number of specific skills one would
have to have in order to do so successfully. Table 3.1 identifies 10 key skills
needed to set limits effectively in order to reach the final point of feeling good
about how one has handled a difficult interaction.

Discussion of the Session

A review of the hypnosis session transcript will reveal how each of the skills
contained in Table 3.1 were addressed either directly or indirectly in Mary's

TABLE 3.1. Skills Comprising the Ability to Set Limits Effectively

1. Ability to recognize one's needs (Self-definition)
2. Acceptance of personal limits as valid (Self-acceptance of values, preferences)
3. Empathy for the other person's wishes or demands (Understanding what they want and why they want it)
4. Goal orientation—a sense of purposefulness (Why set a limit?)
5. Recognition of contextual cues (What is appropriate/reasonable in this situation?)
6. Limits defining assertiveness (As opposed to either passive or aggressive)
7. Ability to communicate needs congruently (Having the words to express the boundary)
8. Ability to compartmentalize fear/anxiety (Set aside the fear of rejection)
9. Ability to tolerate other person's response (Manage the conflict or manipulative tactics)
10. Feelings of confidence (Positive self-appraisal for managing the interaction well)

session. From the very start of the interview, it was important to determine whether Mary even knows what her values and preferences are, whether she knows when a demand is being made on her, whether she has a means of evaluating whether the demand is one she wants to fulfill, and whether she recognizes whatever manipulative tactics are being used to get compliance from her. Ultimately, for Mary, as seems to be true for most people, the breakdown in setting limits effectively is in the desire to avoid conflict. The focus is so heavily on internal feelings (e.g., fear of rejection or worse) that there is little capacity to keep the focus on key external variables (e.g., Why is this person making unreasonable demands of me? Why are they willing to hurt me for some personal gain? Is it my responsibility to meet their demand?). A significant portion of the hypnosis session built on her self-awareness to help her develop greater awareness for both circumstances and the other person before responding to any specific demand. This would greatly reduce the emotional flooding she experienced, reduce her ruminations and sense of guilt in disappointing someone and her fear of their anger or rejection, and help her feel more decisive and in charge.

Hypnosis is an especially effective vehicle for associating people to their resources, either existing ones not being employed or new ones first being developed. Mary's focus was shifted from her internal orientation (i.e., how the interaction made her feel) to a greater external orientation in order to determine what would be an effective response she could feel good about having made. Hypnosis as a vehicle of empowerment is evident and given the helplessness and hopelessness so typical of depression, encouraging a sense of empowerment is vital to recovery.

Follow-Up Feedback, 8 Weeks Later (Edited)

Approximately 8 weeks after our session, Mary was asked to provide some feedback about it. She wrote the following:

> I have experienced several opportunities since [our session] to receive requests of all kinds and shapes. It has been nothing short of remarkable the shift that I have experienced. I have a huge 60th birthday gift from you. . . . A new view from a different perspective. My eye prescription has changed for the better!! . . . The flooding has gone. My feelings of sadness around my son are there, but it is not a flood. Recently, like within the past week, [my son] told me that he wanted to move back in with me. In the past, I have always told him that "he was always welcome to come home," and he has at times. This time, he was very upset because THIS time I told him that he could come WITH stipulations only. I made these conditions very clear . . . [There was] perhaps a moment of second guessing [but] no flood. I did not go to anyone for their opinion. My point is that it was clear to me that I know what is right and I did it. I drank my coffee the way that is best for me and for him I believe as well. My heart aches a bit for him and as a mother

I am worried for him. I had a conversation with him at length a few days ago when I clarified my conditions. I texted an empathic response to his reaction to my conditions. I am on course . . . I am going through some problems in a personal relationship and the skills are working there as well. My tattoo is smiling! . . .

Of course, my work has improved from this experience and from all the learning. Thank you.

Looking forward to our time together.

Warmest regards,
[Mary]

Follow-Up Feedback, 8 Years Later

Note: Once I decided to use this session as a teaching opportunity in this chapter, I contacted Mary to ask if she would care to provide any additional feedback about the longer-term effects of our session. She provided the following narrative, edited for readability.

It has been 8 years since my single hypnosis session with you. I'd had years of psychotherapy prior to this session and knew that I suffered depression. But as obvious as it seems in retrospect, I didn't recognize the connection between my relationship skill deficits and the depression and anxiety I experienced. I felt easily manipulated, guilty, fearful of rejection, and too much self-doubt.

The session informed me about the central issue of responsibility and how my boundaries and overall interactions were affected by how I viewed and managed it. Cognitively I understood that I was overly responsible for others, which gave rise to frequent and debilitating feelings of guilt. I was, therefore, underresponsible for myself, consistently putting others' demands—even unreasonable ones—ahead of my own best interests. I had little or no sense of how to protect myself when others made their requests or demands of me or how to manage their negative reactions if I refused them.

In this session, especially during hypnosis, you taught me about how to reframe peoples' demands as simple statements of their wishes that I could choose to fulfill—or not—depending on the consequences for me. This powerful lesson has been with me ever since and is now completely integrated within me. I've even taught it to my colleagues, clients, and others. The concepts of self-awareness, self-acceptance and self-protection that you instilled in me during the session, which I remembered even without re-listening to the recording of our session, were so very helpful. The suggestions about how I prefer my coffee despite others questioning it, the subjective ways I would experience the session as it unfolds (such as the sensory experience of my hands resting on and touching the fabric of my pants), and that healing was each individual's responsibility (i.e., "if you break your leg you have to wear the cast") were all memorable, practical and very helpful to me.

The concept of people making requests that I had perceived as non-negotiable demands was critically important to me and gave rise to my finding the "space" to take control in how I responded. This was an *enormous* change for me and is always present in my life now. I have much more awareness of my ability to choose how to respond without being drowned in that flood of affect I used to have. Now when a great deal of emotion is present, I am able to more deliberately detach from and observe it. As a direct result, my decision making is much more effective. I am able to make more decisions without feeling I have to reach out to intimates, even though I still do at times just to "reality-test." As a consequence, in the years since our session, life has been much more even and less filled with emotional upsets. I feel the session helped in so many ways, for which I am grateful.

CONCLUSION

Depression has too often been characterized as a disease or mental illness, minimizing or ignoring the substantial evidence that so many of depression's points of origin begin in and then manifest themselves in the interpersonal arena of the individual's life. No amount of medication can teach people social skills or build them a support network. We strongly believe there will never be a purely biological cure for depression any more than there will be one for other socially based problems such as racism or poverty.

This chapter has focused on this all-important social dimension of depression, highlighting the role hypnosis can play in helping to empower all those depressed people who feel disempowered. No one recovers from depression when helplessness defines their approach to life's challenges. Someone may have been genuinely victimized, but hypnosis can help empower them to take control of their life back. Hypnosis as a vehicle for teaching critically important social and problem-solving skills and effective self-regulation strategies holds great potential as a tool of treatment. We enthusiastically encourage its integration into goal-oriented, multidimensional treatments.

REFERENCES

Alladin, A., & Alibhai, A. (2007). Cognitive hypnotherapy for depression: An empirical investigation. *International Journal of Clinical and Experimental Hypnosis, 55*(2), 147–166. https://doi.org/10.1080/00207140601177897

American Psychiatric Association. (2013). *Diagnostic and statistical manual of mental disorders* (5th ed.). https://doi.org/10.1176/appi.books.9780890425596

American Psychological Association. (2008). *Evidence-based practice in psychology.* https://www.apa.org/practice/resources/evidence

Beevi, Z., Low, W. Y., & Hassan, J. (2019). The effectiveness of hypnosis intervention in alleviating postpartum psychological symptoms. *American Journal of Clinical Hypnosis, 61*(4), 409–425. https://doi.org/10.1080/00029157.2018.1538870

Butler, L. D., Waelde, L. C., Hastings, T. A., Chen, X. H., Symons, B., Marshall, J., Kaufman, A., Nagy, T. F., Blasey, C. M., Seibert, E. O., & Spiegel, D. (2008). Meditation with yoga, group therapy with hypnosis, and psychoeducation for long-term depressed mood: A randomized pilot trial. *Journal of Clinical Psychology, 64*(7), 806–820. https://doi.org/10.1002/jclp.20496

Chiu, L., Lee, H. W., & Lam, W. K. (2018). The effectiveness of hypnotherapy in the treatment of Chinese psychiatric patients. *International Journal of Clinical and Experimental Hypnosis, 66*(3), 315–330. https://doi.org/10.1080/00207144.2018.1461472

Cuijpers, P., Karyotaki, E., de Wit, L., & Ebert, D. D. (2020). The effects of fifteen evidence-supported therapies for adult depression: A meta-analytic review. *Psychotherapy Research, 30*(3), 279–293. https://doi.org/10.1080/10503307.2019.1649732

Cuijpers, P., Karyotaki, E., Eckshtain, D., Ng, M. Y., Corteselli, K. A., Noma, H., Quero, S., & Weisz, J. R. (2020). Psychotherapy for depression across different age groups: A systematic review and meta-analysis. *JAMA Psychiatry, 77*(7), 694–702. https://doi.org/10.1001/jamapsychiatry.2020.0164

de Klerk, J. E., du Plessis, W. F., Steyn, H. S., & Botha, M. (2004). Hypnotherapeutic ego strengthening with male South African coronary artery bypass patients. *American Journal of Clinical Hypnosis, 47*(2), 79–92. https://doi.org/10.1080/00029157.2004.10403627

Dobbin, A., Maxwell, M., & Elton, R. (2009). A benchmarked feasibility study of a self-hypnosis treatment for depression in primary care. *International Journal of Clinical and Experimental Hypnosis, 57*(3), 293–318. https://doi.org/10.1080/00207140902881221

González-Ramírez, E., Carrillo-Montoya, T., García-Vega, M., Hart, C., Zavala-Norzagaray, A., & Ley-Quiñónez, C. (2017). Effectiveness of hypnosis and Gestalt therapy as depression treatments. *Clínica y Salud, 28*(1), 33–37. https://doi.org/10.1016/j.clysa.2016.11.001

Greenberger, D., & Padesky, C. (2016). *Mind over mood: Change how you feel by changing how you think* (2nd ed.). Guilford Press.

Guse, T., Wissing, M., & Hartman, W. (2006). The effect of a prenatal hypnotherapeutic programme on postnatal maternal psychological well-being. *Journal of Reproductive and Infant Psychology, 24*(2), 163–177. https://doi.org/10.1080/02646830600644070

Hammen, C. (1991). Generation of stress in the course of unipolar depression. *Journal of Abnormal Psychology, 100*(4), 555–561. https://doi.org/10.1037/0021-843X.100.4.555

Kirsch, I., Montgomery, G., & Sapirstein, G. (1995). Hypnosis as an adjunct to cognitive-behavioral psychotherapy: A meta-analysis. *Journal of Consulting and Clinical Psychology, 63*(2), 214–220. https://doi.org/10.1037/0022-006X.63.2.214

Kumar, P., Waiter, G. D., Dubois, M., Milders, M., Reid, I., & Steele, J. D. (2017). Increased neural response to social rejection in major depression. *Depression and Anxiety, 34*(11), 1049–1056. https://doi.org/10.1002/da.22665

Lebowitz, M. S., Dolev-Amit, T., & Zilcha-Mano, S. (2021). Relationships of biomedical beliefs about depression to treatment-related expectancies in a treatment-seeking sample. *Psychotherapy, 58*(3), 366–371. https://doi.org/10.1037/pst0000320

Liossi, C., & White, P. (2001). Efficacy of clinical hypnosis in the enhancement of quality of life of terminally ill cancer patients. *Contemporary Hypnosis, 18*(3), 145–160. https://doi.org/10.1002/ch.228

Lucas, S. (1985). *The effect of hypnotically induced mood elevation as an adjunct to cognitive treatment of depression* [Unpublished doctoral dissertation]. North Texas State University.

Menard, C., Pfau, M. L., Hodes, G. E., Kana, V., Wang, V. X., Bouchard, S., Takahashi, A., Flanigan, M. E., Aleyasin, H., LeClair, K. B., Janssen, W. G., Labonté, B., Parise, E. M., Lorsch, Z. S., Golden, S. A., Heshmati, M., Tamminga, C., Turecki, G., Campbell, M., . . . Russo, S. J. (2017). Social stress induces neurovascular pathology promoting depression. *Nature Neuroscience, 20*(12), 1752–1760. https://doi.org/10.1038/s41593-017-0010-3

Milling, L. S., Valentine, K. E., McCarley, H. S., & LoStimolo, L. M. (2019). A meta-analysis of hypnotic interventions for depression symptoms: High hopes for hypnosis? *American Journal of Clinical Hypnosis, 61*(3), 227–243. https://doi.org/10.1080/00029157.2018.1489777

Ramondo, N., Gignac, G., Pestell, C., & Byrne, S. (2021). Clinical hypnosis as an adjunct to cognitive behavior therapy: An updated meta-analysis. *International Journal of Clinical and Experimental Hypnosis, 69*(2),169–202. https://doi.org/10.1080/00207144.2021.1877549

Regier, D. A., Narrow, W. E., Clarke, D. E., Kraemer, H. C., Kuramoto, S. J., Kuhl, E. A., & Kupfer, D. J. (2013). DSM-5 field trials in the United States and Canada, part II: Test–retest reliability of selected categorical diagnoses. *The American Journal of Psychiatry, 170*(1), 59–70. https://doi.org/10.1176/appi.ajp.2012.12070999

Schroder, H. S., Duda, J. M., Christensen, K., Beard, C., & Björgvinsson, T. (2020). Stressors and chemical imbalances: Beliefs about the causes of depression in an acute psychiatric treatment sample. *Journal of Affective Disorders, 276*, 537–545. https://doi.org/10.1016/j.jad.2020.07.061

Shih, M., Yang, Y. H., & Koo, M. (2009). A meta-analysis of hypnosis in the treatment of depressive symptoms: A brief communication. *International Journal of Clinical and Experimental Hypnosis, 57*(4), 431–442. https://doi.org/10.1080/00207140903099039

Sudweeks, C. (1998). *Effects of cognitive group hypnotherapy in the alteration of depressogenic schemas* [Unpublished doctoral dissertation]. Washington State University.

Suzuki, T. (2003). The effects of hypnosis on emotional responses of depressed students in frustrating situations [Published in Japanese]. *Shinrigaku Kenkyu (Japanese Journal of Psychology), 73*(6), 457–463.

Swenson, C. (1985). *The relationship between mood elevation and attribution change in the reduction of depression* [Unpublished doctoral dissertation]. North Texas State University.

Van Sky, J. (1983). *Effects of a self-administered hypnotic cognitive treatment on depression* [Unpublished doctoral dissertation]. United States International University.

Weissman, M., Markowitz, J., & Klerman, G. (2018). *The guide to interpersonal psychotherapy: Updated and expanded edition.* Oxford University Press.

Wilhelm, K., & May, R. (2017). Interpersonal therapy in the general practice setting. *Medicine Today, 18*(8), 41–49.

World Health Organization. (2017, March 30). *Depression: Let's talk* [News release]. https://www.who.int/news/item/30-03-2017--depression-let-s-talk-says-who-as-depression-tops-list-of-causes-of-ill-health

Wu, W., Lin, S., Wu, G., & Li, L. (2005). Influence of preoperative supportive psychotherapy on the postoperative mental state and sexual life in patients with uterine cervix cancer [Published in Chinese]. *Zhongguo Linchuang Kangfu (Chinese Journal of Clinical Rehabilitation)*, *9*(16), 42–43.

Yang, J., Yin, P., Wei, D., Wang, K., Li, Y., & Qiu, J. (2017). Effects of parental emotional warmth on the relationship between regional gray matter volume and depression-related personality traits. *Social Neuroscience*, *12*(3), 337–348. https://doi.org/10.1080/17470919.2016.1174150

Yapko, M. D. (1992). *Hypnosis and the treatment of depressions: Strategies for change.* Brunner/Mazel.

Yapko, M. D. (2001a). *Treating depression with hypnosis: Integrating cognitive-behavioral and strategic approaches.* Routledge.

Yapko, M. D. (2001b). Hypnotic intervention for ambiguity as a depressive risk factor. *American Journal of Clinical Hypnosis*, *44*(2), 109–117. https://doi.org/10.1080/00029157.2001.10403466

Yapko, M. D. (2009). *Depression is contagious: How the most common mood disorder is spreading around the world and how to stop it.* Simon & Schuster.

Yapko, M. D. (2010). Hypnotically catalyzing experiential learning across treatments for depression: Actions can speak louder than moods. *International Journal of Clinical and Experimental Hypnosis*, *58*(2), 186–201. https://doi.org/10.1080/00207140903523228

Yapko, M. D. (2016). *Keys to unlocking depression.* Yapko Publications.

Yapko, M. D. (2019). *Trancework: An introduction to the practice of clinical hypnosis* (5th ed.). Routledge.

Yapko, M. D. (2021). *Process-oriented hypnosis: Focusing on the forest, not the trees.* W. W. Norton.

Zimmerman, M., Ellison, W., Young, D., Chelminski, I., & Dalrymple, K. (2015). How many different ways do patients meet the diagnostic criteria for major depressive disorder? *Comprehensive Psychiatry*, *56*, 29–34. https://doi.org/10.1016/j.comppsych.2014.09.007

4 HYPNOSIS FOR ACUTE AND PROCEDURAL PAIN

LEONARD S. MILLING

INTRODUCTION

Although pain serves as an adaptive warning signal to protect the individual from physical harm, it can also be the source of tremendous distress and dysfunction. Pain ranks among the most prevalent of medical complaints. A recent survey showed that approximately 126 million adults in the United States had experienced some form of pain in the previous 3 months, with more than 23 million (10%) reporting a lot of pain (Nahin, 2015). According to the Institute of Medicine (2011), pain is one of the most common reasons for seeing a physician or taking medications. For example, during physician office visits, drugs for pain relief are one of the most frequently prescribed medications (Cherry et al., 2003). Similarly, pain is one of the most common reasons why people are seen in the emergency department, accounting for more than 40% of emergency room visits annually (Pletcher et al., 2008).

The personal and societal costs of pain are staggering. Pain can cause immense suffering. For instance, a survey of 250 adults who had recently undergone surgical procedures showed that 82% experienced acute pain after surgery, with 71% reporting moderate, severe, or extremely severe

https://doi.org/10.1037/0000347-004
Evidence-Based Practice in Clinical Hypnosis, L. S. Milling (Editor)

pain (Apfelbaum et al., 2003). Likewise, studies of women undergoing child-birth for the first time have reported that 60% of new mothers rated the pain as severe or extremely severe (Melzack et al., 1981, 1984). Pain can have serious personal consequences including anxiety and depression, as well as reduced quality of life, disturbed sleep, reduced mobility and loss of strength, impaired immune functioning and increased susceptibility to disease (Brennan et al., 2007). Moreover, acute pain increases the risk for developing chronic pain (Sinatra, 2010).

Pain also produces tremendous costs to society. The Institute of Medicine (2011) estimated the annual economic costs of pain in the United States to be at least $560 billion to $635 billion, including the costs of health care ($261 billion to $300 billion) and lost productivity ($297 billion to $336 billion). According to the Institute of Medicine, these estimates exceed the annual costs associated with heart disease, cancer, and diabetes. Indeed, in 2008, federal and state programs (e.g., Medicare, Medicaid, the Department of Veteran Affairs, TRICARE, workers' compensation) paid out $99 billion for medical expenses related to pain.

Pain can be described as acute or chronic. *Acute pain* tends to develop sud-denly, is typically time-limited, and usually can be linked to a specific injury, illness, or event (Institute of Medicine, 2011). Common forms of acute pain include burn wound care, childbirth, postsurgical pain, and invasive medical procedures (e.g., bone marrow aspirations, lumbar punctures). In contrast, *chronic pain* is generally considered to be pain lasting 3 to 6 months beyond the time associated with normal healing (Merskey & Bogduk, 1994). Common forms of chronic pain include fibromyalgia, irritable bowel syndrome, migraines, arthritis, low back pain, and temporomandibular joint disorder. This chapter addresses the use of hypnosis for relieving acute pain, including the pain caused by invasive medical procedures

REVIEW OF OUTCOME RESEARCH

Acute pain is perhaps the most thoroughly investigated application of clin-ical hypnosis. This section of the chapter reviews randomized controlled studies in which the primary focus is the use of hypnosis to alleviate acute and procedural clinical pain. Methodologically, *randomized controlled trials* are widely considered the gold standard for evaluating the effectiveness of an intervention. Incorporating both a treatment group and a control group (e.g., standard care, attention, wait list, or no-treatment control) that are treated identically aside from the intervention being evaluated maximizes the likelihood that any differences between the groups in outcome can be attributed to the intervention. Randomly assigning participants to the treatment and control groups minimizes the possibility there will be systematic differences between participants in the two groups at the outset of a study that could affect the results (e.g., attitudes towards hypnosis). The review of the research literature also appraises characteristics of interventions and patients that appear to be associated with outcome so as to identify the circumstances in which hypnosis seems to be most efficacious.

Burn Wound Care

The procedures associated with burn wound care are often described by patients as excruciating (Perry et al., 1981). Serious burns may require hospitalization for an extended period of time and can involve twice daily dressing changes, debridement, physical therapy, and skin grafts. Debridement involves the removal of unhealthy tissue and debris from a burn wound. Necrotic tissue can be removed surgically, with topical medications, or in a medical whirlpool.

Patterson et al. (1992) conducted one of the first randomized controlled trials of the efficacy of hypnosis for relieving the pain associated with burn wound care. Participants were 33 adult burn patients who were randomly assigned to hypnosis, attention control, or standard care control conditions. The hypnosis intervention was based on rapid induction analgesia (Barber, 1977) and involved a 25-minute, live, individual session prior to the second dressing change during which patients were given suggestions for relaxation and comfort plus a posthypnotic suggestion to experience these feelings during the dressing change when touched by a nurse on the forehead or shoulder. Patients receiving hypnosis retrospectively reported significantly less pain during dressing changes than those assigned to the attention control and standard care control groups.

In a follow-up study, Patterson and Ptacek (1997) randomized 61 adult burn patients to either a hypnosis or attention control condition. Once again, the hypnosis intervention was based on rapid induction analgesia and involved a 25-minute, live, individual session prior to the third dressing change during which patients were administered suggestions for relaxation, plus a posthypnotic suggestion for comfort during the dressing change when touched on the forehead or shoulder by a nurse. Nurses' retrospective ratings of pain experienced by patients in the hypnosis group during dressing changes were significantly lower than patients assigned to the attention control group. Differences in patients' self-reports of pain followed the same pattern and approached but did not achieve statistical significance.

In a third study of rapid induction analgesia, Wright and Drummond (2000) randomly assigned a mixed sample of 30 adult and adolescent burn patients to hypnosis or standard care control conditions. The 15-minute hypnosis intervention was delivered live during actual dressing changes and included suggestions to reduce pain, tension, and anxiety. Compared with controls, patients receiving the hypnosis intervention reported significantly lower ratings of pain intensity and unpleasantness during dressing changes both during and after the procedure.

Harandi et al. (2004) investigated the pain-reducing effects of hypnosis during physiotherapy (i.e., a procedure similar to physical therapy). Participants consisted of a mixed sample of 44 adult and adolescent female burn patients who were randomized to hypnosis or standard care control conditions. The hypnosis intervention was delivered in live individual sessions prior to physiotherapy and consisted of rapid induction analgesia, plus direct suggestions for pain reduction. Patients receiving hypnosis reported significantly less pain and anxiety during physiotherapy than those in the standard care control condition.

Finally, Chester et al. (2018) evaluated the efficacy of hypnosis for reducing the pain experienced by child and adolescent burn patients during dressing changes. Sixty-two youngsters between the ages of 4 and 16 were randomly assigned to hypnosis or standard care control conditions. The hypnosis intervention was delivered live during dressing changes and consisted of suggestions to imagine being in a favorite place, plus glove anesthesia suggestions designed to reduce unpleasant sensations and to dissociate from the pain. Results generally showed no difference between the hypnosis and standard care conditions in child self-reports and parent ratings of pain intensity during dressing changes.

All in all, the findings of these investigations suggest the promise of hypnosis interventions based on rapid induction analgesia for relieving the pain experienced by adult and adolescent burn patients during dressing changes (Patterson et al., 1992; Patterson & Ptacek, 1997; Wright & Drummond, 2000) and physiotherapy (Harandi et al., 2004). These results are especially noteworthy because in at least three of these studies, the hypnosis intervention was brief (i.e., a single session of 25 minutes or less), yet effective.

Cancer Pain

Spiegel and Bloom (1983) studied the therapeutic effects of hypnosis for women diagnosed with metastatic breast cancer. This is an advanced breast cancer that has metastasized, or spread, to other locations in the body and can cause pain in the affected organs. Participants were 86 women with metastatic breast cancer who were randomly assigned to either a treatment or standard care control condition. Patients in the treatment condition then joined one of two support groups that met for 90 minutes each week for a period of 1 year. In one of these two support groups, patients received hypnotic suggestions to filter the hurt out of the pain by replacing it with icy, cold or warm, tingling sensations. Patients were given instructions to use these suggestions outside of the group setting. Over time, self-reports of pain were significantly lower in the hypnosis support group compared with the support group that did not receive hypnosis and the standard care control condition.

In an ambitious study, Syrjala et al. (1992) investigated the benefits of hypnosis for cancer patients undergoing bone marrow transplantation. Preparation for a bone marrow transplant typically consists of a high dose of chemotherapy or radiation (or both). These procedures can lead to oral mucositis (i.e., sores inside the mouth and throat that cause pain), as well as nausea and emesis. Participants were 67 adult cancer patients diagnosed with leukemia, lymphoma, or Hodgkin's disease undergoing their first bone marrow transplant. These individuals were randomized to hypnosis, cognitive-behavioral, attention control, or standard care control conditions.

The hypnosis intervention consisted of two 90-minute, live, individual outpatient training sessions plus ten 30-minute inpatient booster sessions held twice weekly that included suggestions for relaxation and imagery tailored to each patient's preferences that were designed to reduce pain and nausea. Recordings of suggestions were given to patients for practice between sessions. Similarly, the cognitive-behavioral intervention consisted of two 90-minute outpatient sessions, ten 30-minute inpatient sessions, plus recordings of sessions for practice. The cognitive-behavioral intervention included training in progressive muscle relaxation, autogenic relaxation, as well as cognitive restructuring (i.e., attention redirection, coping self-statements).

According to the authors, it was not possible to include the standard care group in the inferential statistical analyses. However, the hypnosis group reduced oral pain significantly more than the cognitive-behavioral and attention control groups. In contrast, there was no difference between the three groups in reports of nausea or frequency of emesis. These results indicate hypnosis was more effective than a control condition or an alternative psychological intervention in relieving the pain associated with bone marrow transplantation, although it should be noted the omission of guided imagery from the cognitive-behavioral treatment may have limited its impact.

Generally, the findings of these two investigations suggest hypnosis shows promise for relieving the pain produced by cancer and its treatment.

Labor Pain

Labor pain is primarily experienced during contractions in the first and second stages of labor and is often described by women as the most intense pain ever experienced (Niven & Murphy-Black, 2000). Through the years, a number of controlled trials have evaluated the efficacy of hypnosis for relieving labor pain, but many of these investigations did not utilize random assignment to condition (e.g., Beevi et al., 2017; Guthrie et al., 1984; Mairs, 1995). Very few randomized controlled studies have addressed the application of clinical hypnosis to childbirth.

Freeman et al. (1986) examined the effectiveness of self-hypnosis for managing the pain associated with labor and delivery. Participants were 82 women undergoing their first labor who were randomly assigned to either hypnosis or standard care control (i.e., childbirth education classes) conditions. Individuals in the hypnosis group were seen for weekly individual sessions starting at 32 weeks gestation during which they were given suggestions for relaxation and pain relief. Patients were taught how to imagine warmth or anesthesia in one hand and to transfer it to the abdomen. There were no differences between the hypnosis and control groups in self-reports of pain or use of epidural analgesia during childbirth.

In an impressive study, Harmon et al. (1990) randomized 60 women to hypnosis or standard care control (i.e., childbirth education classes) conditions. Participants in the hypnosis condition were given a recording containing suggestions for relaxation, enjoyment of childbirth, numbness in the dominant hand that could be transferred to any body part during labor, as well as feelings of postpartum well-being. Participants were instructed to listen to their recording daily. They also attended six 1-hour, live, group sessions where they listened to their recording and practiced using hypnosis to reduce the pain associated with an ischemic pain task.

Compared with the control group, the hypnosis group experienced less pain and used less medication during childbirth, as well as had shorter Stage 1 labors, higher Apgar scores at 1 and 5 minutes, and more spontaneous deliveries. The results of this study contradict those of Freeman et al. (1986) and highlight the importance of practice sessions (i.e., listening to the hypnosis recording on a daily basis), as well as an opportunity to experience hypnotic analgesia (i.e., with the ischemic pain task) prior to using it during labor.

Dental Procedures

Investigations of the use of hypnosis to relieve dental pain have involved a variety of dental conditions and procedures. Enqvist and Fischer (1997) evaluated the therapeutic benefits of hypnosis for patients undergoing surgical removal of a molar tooth. Sixty-nine patients were randomly assigned to hypnosis or standard care control conditions. Patients in the hypnosis group were instructed to listen to a 20-minute recording each day during the week before surgery that included suggestions to find a safe place, as well as for relaxation, reduced pain, control of bleeding, coagulation, and healing. There was no difference between the hypnosis and control groups in pain reported after oral surgery.

Eitner et al. (2010) studied the impact of hypnosis on dentin hypersensitivity. This condition occurs when dentin is exposed as a result of losing the protective layer of enamel. Eighty-two patients were randomized to hypnosis, fluoridation, desensitizer medication, or standard care control groups. The hypnosis intervention was delivered 1 day before the first sensitivity assessment and consisted of 10 to 15 minutes of suggestions that uncomfortable areas in the mouth would be covered with a protective coating so they would feel insulated like wearing a winter coat. Patients were then seen 1 day, 1 week, and 1 month after intervention during which a cold stimulus was applied to sensitive teeth. Patients receiving hypnosis reported significantly less pain than those in the standard care control condition. However, the difference between the hypnosis, fluoridation, and desensitizer treatment groups was not significant.

Ramírez-Carrasco et al. (2017) evaluated the effectiveness of hypnosis for reducing the behavioral distress experienced by children while receiving a dental anesthetic. Observational measures of behavioral distress are said to measure a combination of pain and anxiety. Forty children between the ages of 5 and 9 years were randomly assigned to hypnosis or standard care control conditions. While seated in the examination chair, youngsters in the hypnosis condition listened to an audio recording in which they were given suggestions to imagine being in a special garden with a fountain containing water that would make their mouth numb and relaxed. At this point, patients received the anesthetic injection. Results showed no difference between the hypnosis and control conditions in behavioral distress observed during the injection.

In another study of children receiving a dental anesthetic, Huet et al. (2011) randomly assigned 30 patients aged 7 to 12 to hypnosis or standard care control conditions. The hypnosis intervention was delivered live by a clinician to patients while receiving the anesthetic injection and consisted of suggestions and stories about things of interest to the child. Child self-reports of pain and observer ratings of anxiety during the dental procedure were significantly lower in the hypnosis group than in the standard care group.

All in all, the findings of these studies provide mixed support for the use of hypnosis to relieve dental pain. However, it should be noted that hypnosis was effective in reducing pain when it was provided live by a clinician either before or during the dental procedure (Eitner et al., 2010; Huet et al., 2011), but not when it was delivered solely via audio recording (Enqvist & Fischer, 1997; Ramírez-Carrasco et al., 2017).

Radiological Procedures

A number of studies have evaluated the use of hypnosis during radiological procedures and radiotherapy. Lang et al. (1996) examined the efficacy of hypnosis for relieving pain during a range of radiologic procedures (e.g., diagnostic arteriograms, transcatheter revascularizations). Thirty adult patients were randomly assigned to hypnosis or standard care control conditions. The hypnosis intervention was delivered live during the radiologic procedure and consisted of suggestions for relaxation, transformation of unpleasant sensations, and to imagine a nature scene or some other pleasant setting. Patients in the hypnosis condition reported significantly less pain and used less self-administered analgesic medication during the medical procedure than did patients in the control condition.

In a second study, Lang et al. (2000) randomized 241 adult patients referred for percutaneous transcatheter peripheral vascular and renal procedures to hypnosis, attention control, or standard care control conditions. The hypnosis intervention was delivered live during the medical procedure and consisted of suggestions for relaxation or for the sensation of floating, as well as to engage in imagery of a safe and pleasant experience. Results showed that pain increased with procedure time significantly more in the standard care and attention control conditions than in the hypnosis condition.

In a third study in this series, Lang et al. (2008) randomly assigned 201 patients referred for percutaneous tumor treatments via transcatheter embolization or radiofrequency ablation to hypnosis, attention control, or standard care control conditions. Once again, the hypnosis intervention was delivered live during the radiologic procedure and included suggestions for a sensation of floating, to experience a pleasant setting, and to transform discomfort into a sensation of warmth, coolness, or tingling. Patients assigned to the hypnosis condition reported significantly less pain and anxiety than those in the attention and standard care control conditions at several points during the medical procedure and used significantly less self-administered analgesic medication.

Together, the results of these three studies suggest hypnosis can be effective for reducing the pain and anxiety experienced by patients undergoing a variety of radiologic procedures, including peripheral vascular and renal procedures (Lang et al., 2000), as well as more invasive percutaneous tumor treatments (Lang et al., 2008).

Biopsies

Two randomized controlled trials evaluated the efficacy of hypnosis for managing the discomfort associated with breast biopsy. This procedure is related to the radiological procedures described in the previous section because X-ray or ultrasound is often used to make sure the tip of the biopsy needle has reached the suspicious tissue.

Lang et al. (2006) randomly assigned 236 women undergoing outpatient large core needle breast biopsy to hypnosis, attention control, or standard care control conditions. The hypnosis intervention was delivered live during the biopsy and included suggestions for the sensation of floating, to experience a pleasant setting, and to transform discomfort into sensations of warmth, coolness, or tingling. Self-reports of anxiety were significantly lower in the hypnosis condition than in the attention control and standard care control conditions. In contrast, self-reports of pain were lower in the hypnosis and attention control conditions than in the standard care condition, but the difference between the hypnosis and attention control groups was not significant.

Sánchez-Jáuregui et al. (2019) randomized 170 women undergoing breast biopsy to hypnosis plus music, music only, or standard care control conditions. Prior to and during the biopsy, patients in the hypnosis condition listened to an audio recording with a music background that contained suggestions to reduce pain and anxiety, whereas patients in the music only condition listened to the background music without suggestion. After the biopsy, patients receiving the hypnosis intervention reported significantly less anxiety and stress, but not less pain than those in the control condition. There was no difference between the hypnosis condition and the music only conditions in anxiety or stress.

The findings of these two studies suggest that hypnosis may be useful for reducing the anxiety associated with breast biopsy, but not necessarily the pain produced by this medical procedure.

Postsurgical Pain

Common complications during recovery from surgery include pain, nausea and vomiting, fatigue, and emotional distress. Montgomery and his colleagues (2002, 2007) conducted a series of studies of the efficacy of hypnosis for reducing the complications of breast surgery. Montgomery et al. (2002)

randomly assigned 20 women undergoing excisional breast biopsy to hypnosis or standard care control conditions. A 10-minute, live, individual hypnosis intervention was delivered just before surgery and included suggestions for relaxation, pain reduction, and to imagine a special place, as well as instructions for how the patient could use hypnosis on her own (i.e., self-hypnosis). Patients receiving hypnosis reported significantly less pain and emotional distress after surgery than the control group.

In a second study in this series, Montgomery et al. (2007) randomized 200 women undergoing excisional breast biopsy or lumpectomy to hypnosis or attention control conditions. A live, individual hypnosis intervention was delivered prior to surgery and lasted 15 minutes. It included suggestions for relaxation, pleasant visual imagery, reduced pain, nausea, and fatigue, as well as instructions for how patients could use hypnosis on their own. Results showed that after surgery, patients in the hypnosis group reported significantly less pain, nausea, fatigue, discomfort, and emotional upset than those in the control group. Moreover, patients receiving hypnosis used significantly less perioperative analgesic and sedative medications during the surgery process.

In an unpublished doctoral dissertation, Brooks (2002) investigated the impact of hypnosis on patients undergoing breast reduction surgery. Participants were 18 women who were randomly assigned to hypnosis, attention control, or standard care control conditions. The hypnosis intervention consisted of eight 30-minute weekly individual sessions in which patients were given suggestions for reduced pain, adjustment to body image changes, and rapid healing. Patients were given recordings that revisited the content of weekly sessions and were instructed to practice with them on a daily basis.

Following surgery, the difference between the hypnosis, attention control, and standard care control conditions in self-reports of pain was not statistically significant. However, this may have been due to the low statistical power produced by having only six participants in each of the three conditions. *Statistical power* is the probability of detecting a statistically significant treatment effect when the effect actually exists. Statistical power is affected by the number of participants in a study; as the number of participants increases, statistical power also increases.

Two studies investigated the use of hypnosis to manage the side effects associated with surgery to remove the gallbladder (i.e., cholecystectomies). In an unpublished doctoral dissertation, Taenzer (1983) randomized 40 adult patients undergoing gallbladder surgery to hypnotic, nonhypnotic suggestion, relaxation, or standard care control conditions. About 2 weeks prior to surgery, patients receiving one of the three interventions participated in a live, individual preparation session where they were taught how to use the techniques on their own.

The hypnotic intervention consisted of a hypnotic induction plus suggestions for relaxation, pain reduction, and pleasant imagery. The nonhypnotic intervention included only suggestions for pain reduction and pleasant imagery, whereas the relaxation intervention included only an induction and suggestions for relaxation (with no mention of hypnosis in either of these two conditions). At the end of the preparation session, patients were given a recording of the intervention for home practice each day. Results failed to show a difference between the four conditions in postoperative pain or emotional distress, although this may have been due to the limited statistical power associated with having only a total of 40 participants in a study with four experimental conditions.

More recently, Joudi et al. (2016) randomly assigned 120 adult patients undergoing laparoscopic gallbladder surgery to hypnosis or standard care control conditions. Immediately prior to surgery, patients in the hypnosis condition listened to an audio recording providing suggestions for pleasant imagery (i.e., walking in a beautiful garden), plus posthypnotic suggestions to revisit this imagery, plus reduced pain, nausea, or distress during recovery from surgery. Patients receiving hypnosis reported significantly less pain and consumed significantly less analgesic medication following surgery compared with those in the control condition. There was no difference between the two groups in postsurgical nausea and vomiting.

Radial keratotomy is a type of eye surgery to correct nearsightedness. It can be performed on an outpatient basis with local anesthetic, but patient movement during the procedure can affect outcome. John and Parrino (1983) randomly assigned 59 patients undergoing radial keratotomy to hypnosis and standard care control conditions. Just prior to the procedure, the surgeon read a 4-minute script containing suggestions for relaxation. However, the intervention was described in the consent form as "relaxation therapy," and it is not clear patients understood they were receiving hypnosis. There was no difference between the hypnosis and control conditions in the amount of movement during surgery or pain reported after the procedure.

Septorhinoplasty is a surgical procedure performed to change the shape of the nose (i.e., rhinoplasty) and to correct a crooked or deviated septum (i.e., septoplasty). Ozgunay et al. (2019) randomized 22 adult patients undergoing septorhinoplasty to hypnosis or standard care control conditions. The hypnosis intervention consisted of two 40-minute, live, individual sessions delivered prior to the day of surgery and one 20-minute session in the hospital before surgery and included suggestions for relaxation, pleasant imagery, numbness in the nose, as well as training in self-hypnosis. Use of analgesic medications during surgery and postoperative self-reports of pain were significantly lower in the hypnosis condition than in the control condition.

Finally, Lambert (1996) randomly assigned 52 pediatric patients aged 7 to 19 years undergoing a variety of surgical procedures to hypnosis or standard care control conditions. The hypnosis intervention consisted of a 30-minute, live, individual preparation session one week before surgery and included suggestions for relaxation, pleasant imagery, and minimal pain. Children receiving hypnosis rated their postoperative pain as significantly lower compared with youngsters in the control group, although there was no difference in self-reports of anxiety or in the amount of oral analgesic medication consumed.

Generally, investigations of the use of hypnosis to manage the complications associated with surgery show it is effective for reducing postsurgical pain. The few exceptions are doctoral dissertations in which the small number of participants may have reduced statistical power to the point where differences between the hypnosis and control conditions could not be detected (Brooks, 2002; Taenzer, 1983), as well as a study where the intervention was minimal and not clearly described as hypnosis (John & Parrino, 1983).

Bone Marrow Aspirations

In a bone marrow aspiration (BMA), a large-gauge syringe is inserted into the patient's hipbone and marrow is suctioned out. Snow et al. (2012) randomly assigned 80 adult patients undergoing BMAs to hypnosis or standard care control conditions. The hypnosis intervention was provided live during the medical procedure and included suggestions for relaxation, visualization of a beach scene, numbness, and reduced pain. Patients in the hypnosis condition reported significantly less anxiety, but not less pain, during the BMA than those in the control condition.

Katz et al. (1987) randomized 36 children between the ages of 6 and 11 years undergoing BMAs to hypnosis or attention control conditions. The hypnosis intervention lasted 20 minutes and was provided in a live, individual preparation session prior to the BMA. It included suggestions for imagery to reduce or reframe pain, distraction, relaxation, ego-strengthening, as well as a posthypnotic suggestion to reenter hypnosis when touched on the shoulder by the therapist during the actual BMA. However, suggestions were not delivered live during the actual medical procedure. Results showed no difference between the hypnosis and control conditions in self-reports of pain and observer ratings of behavioral distress.

Kuttner et al. (1988) compared the effects of hypnosis, distraction, and standard care in relieving the discomfort experienced by children undergoing BMAs. Forty-eight children aged 3 to 10 years were randomly assigned to one of the three aforementioned conditions. The hypnosis intervention was delivered live during the BMA and included imaginative stories tailored to the child's interests, as well as suggestions for pain reduction, time distortion, and ego-strengthening. In the distraction condition, the child was shown toys, puppets, and pop-up books and asked to select the distractor they wanted in the room during the procedure.

During the first posttreatment BMA, older children (7 to 10 years) in the hypnosis and distraction conditions were rated as experiencing less pain than youngsters in the standard care condition. However, younger children (3 to 6 years) in the hypnosis condition were rated as experiencing less pain than those in the distraction and control conditions. These findings suggest that older children benefited from both hypnosis and distraction, whereas younger children benefited the most from hypnosis.

Finally, Liossi and Hatira (1999) randomly assigned 30 children between the ages of 5 and 15 undergoing BMAs to hypnosis, cognitive-behavioral, or standard care control conditions. The hypnosis intervention consisted of two 30-minute, live, individual preparation sessions where children were give suggestions for relaxation, visual imagery (a favorite place, activity, or television program), ego-strengthening, and pain reduction. At the end of each session, patients were given a posthypnotic suggestion that the hypnotic experience would be repeated during the BMA. The cognitive-behavioral intervention consisted of two 30-minute preparation sessions and included relaxation training (e.g., progressive muscle relaxation), breathing exercises, and coping self-statements.

The therapist accompanied all children into the treatment room during the BMA. Youngsters in the hypnosis and cognitive behavioral conditions had been instructed to begin using their pain management skills when the therapist stroked them on the cheek. However, the therapist did not provide active intervention (i.e., suggestions) during the procedure. Child self-reports of pain and anxiety during the BMA, as well as observer ratings of distress were significantly lower in the hypnosis and cognitive-behavioral conditions than in the standard care control condition. Moreover, observer ratings of distress and self-reports of anxiety (but not pain) were significantly lower for youngsters receiving hypnosis than those receiving the cognitive-behavioral intervention.

Generally, these studies showed that hypnosis is more effective than standard care in relieving the anxiety experienced by adults (Snow et al., 2012), as well as the pain and anxiety experienced by children (Kuttner et al., 1988; Liossi & Hatira, 1999) undergoing bone marrow aspirations. The latter two studies also demonstrated that hypnosis is at least as effective as distraction and cognitive-behavioral therapy (CBT) in alleviating children's anxiety and pain during this medical procedure.

Lumbar Punctures

In a lumbar puncture (LP), a narrow-gauge needle is inserted between two vertebrae into the spinal column to remove a sample of cerebrospinal fluid or inject medication. Liossi and Hatira (2003) examined the efficacy of two different kinds of hypnotic suggestions for relieving the pain experienced by children undergoing this medical procedure. Participants were 80 youngsters between the ages of 6 and 16 who were randomly assigned to hypnosis with direct suggestions, hypnosis with indirect suggestions, attention control, or standard care control conditions.

The hypnosis interventions involved a 40-minute, live, individual preparation session and both included suggestions for ego-strengthening and comfort. The hypnosis with direct suggestions condition also included suggestions to make the back numb, topical anesthesia (painting numbing medicine on the back), local anesthesia (injecting an anesthetic into the back) and glove anesthesia (transfer numb feelings from the hand to the back). The hypnosis with indirect suggestions condition added suggestions for pleasant, distracting imagery (i.e., the setting sun) or a metaphor for pain reduction (i.e., adjusting to spicy Mexican food). In both hypnosis conditions, the preparation session ended with a posthypnotic suggestion that the experience would be repeated during the LP with the help of the therapist (who provided suggestions live throughout the actual medical procedure).

Children receiving the two hypnosis interventions reported less pain and anxiety, and were rated as exhibiting less behavioral distress than youngsters in the attention control and standard care control conditions during the LP. However, there was no difference between the two hypnosis conditions in reducing pain, anxiety, or distress.

In another study in this series, Liossi et al. (2006) randomized 45 youngsters between the ages of 6 and 16 undergoing LPs to hypnosis, attention control, or standard care control conditions. The hypnosis condition consisted of a 40-minute, live, individual preparation session and included direct suggestions for pain reduction (see direct suggestion condition in Liossi & Hatira, 2003), plus a posthypnotic suggestion that hypnosis would be re-experienced during the actual medical procedure when the therapist stroked the child's cheek. Thus, the therapist did not deliver suggestions live during the LP. Patients in the hypnosis condition reported less pain and anxiety, and were rated as displaying less behavioral distress compared with those in the attention control and standard care control conditions.

The findings of Liossi et al. (2006) and Liossi and Hatira (2003) indicate hypnosis is very effective for helping children and adolescents reduce the pain, anxiety, and distress associated with lumbar punctures. Moreover, the results of the latter study argue that direct suggestions for pain reduction may be no more effective than indirect suggestions in relieving the discomfort associated with this medical procedure.

Venipunctures

A venipuncture involves puncturing a vein with a needle to collect blood or to provide intravenous therapy. Liossi et al. (2009) randomly assigned 45 children between the ages of 7 and 16 undergoing venipunctures to hypnosis, attention control, or standard medical care control conditions. The hypnosis intervention consisted of a 15-minute, live, individual preparation session and included direct suggestions for pain reduction, as well as a posthypnotic suggestion that the hypnosis experience would be repeated during the actual venipuncture when a parent would stroke the child's hand not receiving the venipuncture. During the preparation session, children also received training in self-hypnosis. Suggestions were not delivered live during the medical procedure. Results showed that youngsters assigned to the hypnosis condition reduced pain, anxiety, and distress significantly more than patients in the attention and standard medical care control conditions.

Other Forms of Acute and Procedural Pain

A voiding cystourethrogram (VCUG) is a procedure involving urethral catheterization, insertion of radiologic contrast materials into the bladder, and imaging during urination. Butler et al. (2005) randomly assigned 44 children between the ages of 5 and 15 undergoing VCUG to hypnosis or standard care control conditions. The hypnosis intervention consisted of a 1-hour, live, individual training session and included suggestions to imagine floating in a bath, lake, or hot tub, as well as visualizing an amusement park, friend's house, or playground. Parents and child were instructed to practice the procedure several times a day in preparation for the VCUG. A therapist was present during the procedure to deliver suggestions. Observational ratings of distress during the VCUG were significantly lower in the hypnosis group than in the standard care group. However, there was no difference between the groups in child self-reports of distress.

In a study of the therapeutic benefits of hypnosis for bone fractures, Ginandes and Rosenthal (1999) randomized 12 patients with ankle bone fractures to hypnosis or standard care control conditions. The hypnosis intervention consisted of five live, individual sessions and included suggestions to reduce inflammation and swelling, alleviate pain, and stimulate healing. Patients were given a series of recordings for daily at-home practice to reinforce sessions. Generally, results showed no statistically significant differences between the hypnosis and control conditions in self-reports of pain, although this may have been due to the limited statistical power resulting from the very small number of patients in the study.

Finally, Marc et al. (2007) randomly assigned 29 women undergoing surgical abortions to hypnosis or standard care control conditions. The hypnosis intervention was delivered live beginning 20 minutes before and throughout the abortion, and consisted of suggestions for relaxation, pleasant imagery, numbness in the abdominal area, and reduction of pain. Patients in the hypnosis group used significantly less self-administered nitrous oxide sedation during the procedure than control participants. However, differences between the groups in self-reported pain and anxiety during the procedure were not significant, which the authors attributed to low statistical power.

All in all, the results of these three studies suggest the possibility hypnosis may help to reduce the distress experienced by children undergoing VCUG, but do not provide support for the use of hypnosis to manage the pain associated with bone fractures or surgical abortions. However, it is necessary to qualify this conclusion by noting the small number of participants in these two studies (Ginandes & Rosenthal, 1999; Marc et al., 2007) may have limited the statistical power needed to detect a difference between the hypnosis and control conditions.

Summary of Reviewed Studies

Generally, this review of randomized controlled studies indicates hypnosis is an efficacious method of relieving acute and procedural pain. This includes the pain associated with burn wound care, labor pain, cancer, dental procedures, radiological procedures, biopsies, surgery, bone marrow aspirations, lumbar punctures, and venipunctures. Of 36 studies reviewed, 24 showed hypnosis was significantly more effective than standard care or attention control conditions in reducing pain, behavioral distress, or both.

However, there were three exceptions to this overall pattern of efficacy. First, studies suffering from low statistical power generally failed to produce a significant effect for hypnosis. Had these studies included more participants, it is conceivable they might have demonstrated a statistically significant difference in pain reduction between the hypnosis and control conditions. Unfortunately, it is impossible to foresee the impact of increasing the sample size of a study on the results. Consequently, investigations with low statistical power that failed to show significant differences between the hypnosis and control conditions can best be characterized as inconclusive.

Second, studies in which an audio recording was the only intervention generally failed to show hypnosis was effective in relieving pain. Recordings may have several limitations. A scripted recording cannot take into account the individual preferences of the person being hypnotized. For example, some patients may respond best to direct suggestions for pain reduction and others to suggestions for pleasant, distracting imagery. Furthermore, a recording cannot adapt to the changing needs of patients while they are in pain or undergoing an invasive medical procedure. This review argues hypnosis interventions may be most effective when they are primarily delivered live by a clinician in an individual or group setting. Recordings can be used to reinforce and practice what has been experienced in session with a therapist, but probably should not be the sole or primary mode of delivery.

Finally, this review indicates hypnosis may be more effective when suggestions are delivered immediately before or during the time a patient is experiencing pain or undergoing an invasive medical procedure. Hypnosis appeared to be less effective in studies where there was a large time gap between the delivery of suggestions and the experience of pain, particularly when the intervention lacked a clear mechanism to transfer the experience of hypnosis into the pain situation. It should not be surprising that hypnosis is ineffective when, for example, women in childbirth classes are given suggestions for relaxation and reduced pain, but labor does not take place for days or weeks after the classes end.

Self-hypnosis is one of the most common ways to transfer the experience of hypnosis into a pain situation when a clinician cannot be present. Recently, Eason and Parris (2019) conducted a systematic review and meta-analysis of 22 randomized controlled studies of self-hypnosis as an intervention for a range of symptoms and problems in clinical settings. These investigators defined self-hypnosis as "self-induction into the hypnotic process produced by self-generated suggestions" (p. 262). They concluded self-hypnosis is most likely to be effective when taught as a self-directed skill and when it involves at least three practice sessions before using it in a clinical situation.

The present assessment of the research literature is consistent with the conclusions of Eason and Parris (2019). The current review indicates self-hypnosis is more likely to be beneficial when patients are taught how to deliver suggestions to themselves and given instructions to practice these suggestions on their own multiple times before using them to confront pain. It is less likely to help when patients are simply given a suggestion during a preparation session that they can use self-hypnosis to reduce the pain without being taught how to do this or provided with opportunities for practice.

Overall Impact of Hypnosis on Acute and Procedural Pain

Recently, Milling et al. (2021) reported the results of a comprehensive meta-analysis of all controlled studies of the use of hypnosis for relieving clinical pain. This meta-analysis included controlled studies that utilized both random and nonrandom assignment to condition. The overall mean weighted effect size for 40 trials of hypnosis at the end of active intervention was 0.60. This effect size falls in the medium range according to Cohen's (1988) guideline and suggests the average patient receiving hypnosis reduced pain more than about 73% of control patients. The impact of hypnosis was similar for acute, procedural, and chronic pain. At the end of active intervention, mean weighted effect sizes were 0.63 for 11 trials of acute pain, 0.55 for 17 trials of procedural pain, and 0.64 for 12 trials of chronic pain. These findings confirm that hypnosis is a very beneficial intervention for relieving all forms of pain.

The findings of Milling et al. (2021) indicate the efficacy of hypnosis is similar to that of other popular psychological pain interventions, including distraction, CBT, biofeedback, and mindfulness. Meta-analyses in which each of these interventions were compared with a control condition in alleviating clinical pain typically produce mean weighted effect sizes no larger than 0.60 and confidence intervals that overlap with those reported in Milling et al. This includes effect sizes ranging from 0.44 to 0.62 for distraction (Birnie et al., 2014; Kenney & Milling, 2016), 0.15 to 0.51 for CBT (Haddock et al., 1997; Tatrow & Montgomery, 2006), 0.45 to 0.81 for biofeedback (Nestoriuc & Martin, 2007; Nestoriuc et al., 2008), and 0.23 to 0.45 for mindfulness (Goldberg et al., 2018; Lauche et al., 2013). On average, there does not appear to be a difference in effectiveness between hypnosis and these other popular psychological pain interventions.

However, there is an important qualifier to this conclusion. In their seminal meta-analysis of the effectiveness of hypnotic analgesia, Montgomery et al. (2000) found the impact of hypnosis varied markedly by level of hypnotic suggestibility. For participants scoring in the high suggestibility range, the mean weighted effect size was 1.16, which would be classified as a large effect. For people in the medium suggestibility range, the mean weighted effect size was 0.64, which would be considered a medium effect. Finally, for those in the low suggestibility range, the mean weighted effect size was −0.01, which indicates a negligible effect. This suggests hypnosis may actually be more effective than other popular psychological pain interventions for patients falling in the high suggestibility range and less effective for those in the low range. Therefore, pain patients falling in the high and medium ranges of suggestibility may be especially good candidates for hypnosis.

All in all, the research literature indicates hypnosis is a useful tool for relieving acute and procedural pain. This review suggests the impact of a hypnosis intervention can be maximized if the primary mode of delivery is by having a clinician deliver it live in an individual or group setting rather than via audio recording. Where possible, suggestions designed to reduce pain should be provided immediately before or during the time a patient is in pain or undergoing an invasive medical procedure. Self-hypnosis may be beneficial when patients are explicitly provided with training in self-directed hypnosis skills and given instructions to practice on multiple occasions. Patients falling in the high and medium ranges of hypnotic suggestibility may be especially appropriate candidates for hypnosis, although individuals in the low suggestibility range may possibly derive some benefit from hypnosis interventions as well.

CASE EXAMPLES

This section of the chapter summarizes published case examples of the use of hypnosis for relieving a variety of forms of acute and procedural pain.

Bone Marrow Biopsies

Snow and Warbet (2010) described the application of hypnosis with 64-year-old man who had been diagnosed with acute myelogenous leukemia (AML). Bone marrow aspirations and biopsies are routinely used to monitor the medical status of individuals with AML. The patient indicated he had never been seriously ill prior to the diagnosis of AML. He was hospitalized several times, which ultimately culminated in a bone marrow transplant. The patient had experienced excruciating pain during past bone marrow biopsies and requested hypnosis to relieve the discomfort.

Hypnosis was delivered live during the bone marrow biopsy after lidocaine was injected at the biopsy site. Following a hypnotic induction, the patient was given instructions for progressive muscle relaxation delivered in the context of hypnosis. Thereafter, the patient received suggestions to imagine a quiet beach on a warm sunny day or some other special place. These suggestions emphasized experiencing each of the senses. The patient was also given suggestions that he might experience warmth, coolness, numbness, or slight pressure in his lower back, but no pain. Finally, the patient was given suggestions for dissociation from the pain—as if he could step back from the pain and look at it from a distance.

The patient showed a very positive response to hypnosis. During the first biopsy in which hypnosis was used, the patient became very relaxed. At the next biopsy, the patient grimaced, but remained calm. The patient reported the procedure felt more like pressure than pain. During a subsequent biopsy, the patient remained relaxed and did not grimace. After the biopsy, the patient asked if the procedure had been completed because he did not feel anything at all.

Burn Wound Care

Wallace (1987) illustrated the use of hypnosis with a married woman of unspecified age who had suffered thermal burns resulting from a pan fire. The burns covered 40% of the patient's body, of which 10% were deep full thickness burns on her arms, thighs, and one hand. She complained of unrelenting pain in her hand. The patient recalled that after the accident, she had obtained some relief by placing her hands in cold water offered by her neighbor.

During the hypnosis session, the patient was given suggestions she was placing her hand in a cold bucket of ice water, which caused tingling, cold, numbing sensations. The patient was then told she could transfer the feelings of cool numbness to any part of her body by stroking it with her hand. Thereafter, the patient was given suggestions that while experiencing the sensations of cold, she could float up away from her body into a pleasant, fluffy warm or cool cloud such that she could look down on her body and that nothing would bother her. Additionally, suggestions were offered in which the patient imagined herself relaxing in her favorite armchair at home with her dog curled up beside her. Each time she stroked the dog, she would feel more relaxed and away from it all.

During the session, the patient was encouraged to practice hypnosis on her own as much as possible. She was given a posthypnotic suggestion that she could re-experience these images by focusing on a spot on the ceiling and taking five deep breaths. The patient was given an audio recording of the session, which she used for the remaining 14 days of her hospitalization.

After the hypnosis session, the patient indicated she was deeply relaxed and her hand remained numb and pain-free for 3 hours. During the remainder of her hospital stay, the patient reported great success in using hypnosis to relieve her background levels of pain, and some success in using it to obtain relief during burn dressing changes, physical therapy exercises, and after skin graft surgery.

Hematoma

A hematoma involves the pooling of blood outside of a blood vessel and under the skin. Deltito (1984) demonstrated the use of hypnosis to alleviate the pain caused by a hematoma. The patient was a 21-year-old female college student who presented in the emergency room with a large painful hematoma over the hip after a cycling accident. The hematoma was surgically evacuated during the following week, but the patient returned to the emergency room complaining of a great deal of pain when walking.

The patient indicated she was afraid she would be unable to row for her college crew team, and she did not want to put prescribed analgesics in her body. Under hypnosis, the patient was given the suggestion she had not sustained a permanent injury and that, from now on, it would feel like there was a rubber band wrapped around her hip, which would cause some discomfort but no real pain. After coming out of hypnosis, the patient reported experiencing no pain, told one of the nurses it felt like there was a rubber band around her waist, and walked without a limp. The patient was followed for several weeks and continued to report no pain.

Dental Procedures

Temple and Utting (2014) explained how hypnosis can be utilized to alleviate the discomfort associated with routine dental procedures. The patient was a married woman in her late 30s who was unable to receive dental treatment using local analgesia, intravenous sedation, or general anesthesia because of the risk of precipitating severe nonepileptic seizures.

The initial round of dental treatment was provided over a period of 10 months. The patient was shown how to use glove anesthesia suggestions in which the experience of anesthesia could be induced in her hand and then transferred to the appropriate location in her mouth. Posthypnotic suggestions were given so the patient would experience pain relief for as long as necessary following completion of the dental procedure. The patient underwent several dental restorations and one extraction using hypnosis to effectively control the pain.

Across the next 10 years, the patient continued to receive dental treatment using hypnosis as the method of pain control. However, there was a nearly 4-year gap in the patient's dental care. When she eventually returned to the dentist, she needed a root canal in two teeth. Using glove anesthesia, the patient was able to undergo the root canals without pain. An extraction was also performed on one of these teeth without event.

Hemodialysis

Hemodialysis is a procedure in which a dialysis machine and a dialyzer are used to clean wastes and fluids from the blood when the kidneys are no longer able to do so. During hemodialysis, several needles are placed in the arm, blood is removed from the body, filtered through the dialyzer, and then returned to the body. Dimond (1981) detailed the use of hypnosis to alleviate the pain and anxiety associated with hemodialysis. The patient was a 30-year-old married woman who was referred for intervention because she was very emotional during dialysis, and the technicians were unable to obtain an adequate blood flow. The patient indicated she had a fear of needles and a low tolerance for pain.

The hypnosis intervention was carried out across a series of 12 sessions. Initially, the patient was given suggestions she had a "black box" in her head through which all pain sensations were channeled and that she could control the pain anywhere in her body by removing the appropriate "fuse" or throwing the appropriate "switch" in the box. These suggestions produced immediate relief from pain. The patient was given posthypnotic suggestions in which she was encouraged to practice the pain control imagery on her own.

However, the patient continued to experience difficulties achieving an adequate blood flow during dialysis. The patient was then given suggestions to mentally explore the dialysis equipment at her own pace (as a form of desensitization) and to think of it as a life-sustaining extension of herself. It was suggested to the patient that her growing acceptance of the dialysis equipment might be accompanied by an increase in blood flow. This was followed by an increase in actual blood flow. These improvements in the patient's response to dialysis were maintained for 30 months past the end of hypnosis intervention.

Surgical Pain

Fathi et al. (2019) described the use of hypnosis to control pain during and after surgery. The patient was a 37-year-old man undergoing an anterior cruciate ligament (ACL) surgical reconstruction. This procedure involves creating tunnels in the bones (i.e., tibia, femur) and can be extremely painful. The patient had suffered a left knee trauma 9 months prior to the surgery.

He had experienced pain and instability of the knee despite nonsurgical treatment for more than 6 months. He was referred for hypnosis in response to his requests to relieve severe anxiety.

In the operating room, hypnosis was provided by the anesthesiologist. The surgical procedure was performed without general or neuraxial anesthesia. Hypnosis was induced after prepping and draping the knee. Based on the patient's interests, suggestions were given in which he was asked to imagine walking in a valley between the mountains of his village. The patient was asked to imagine a lake and to focus on the pleasant coolness of the water, with small red fishes nibbling at his knee. This was intended to camouflage when the surgeon touched the patient's knee or made incisions of the skin. The patient was also asked to imagine birds flying around the lake. These suggestions were continued throughout the surgery. During the surgery, and while in hypnosis, the patient was able to talk to the hypnotist and surgeon.

While in the hospital, the patient did not feel the need for any analgesic medications and was discharged the day after the surgery. Six days after the surgery, the patient reported a lack of pain despite not taking any analgesic drugs.

HYPNOSIS PROTOCOL

This section of the chapter presents commonly used hypnotic suggestions for relieving acute and procedural pain. Intervention should begin with a hypnotic induction, which can either be a standardized induction (e.g., Morgan & Hilgard, 1978/1979) or one devised by the practitioner.

Direct Suggestions for Pain Reduction

Perhaps the most frequently employed hypnotic suggestions for acute and procedural pain involve direct suggestions for pain reduction. There are a very wide variety of direct hypnotic pain reduction suggestions and some are as simple as reminding the patient what a numb feeling is and suggesting the affected body part is numb and feels less discomfort. One popular direct hypnotic suggestion for pain reduction is referred to as a *glove anesthesia* or *glove analgesia* suggestion:

"Now, I would like you to pay close attention to your left hand . . . place your left hand flat on the table . . . imagine that your left hand is beginning to feel a little numb . . . you know what a numb feeling is . . . as if your left hand had been placed in a thick, thick glove . . . and you can't feel much of anything through the glove . . . that's right . . .

Your left hand is becoming more and more numb . . . more and more insensitive . . . very numb . . . very dull . . . very insensitive . . . as if it were covered in a thick, thick glove . . . you may not be able to feel anything at all through that glove on your left hand . . . you may not be able to feel anything at all in your left hand . . . completely insensitive . . . completely numb. For a while, you may want to notice how numb and insensitive your hand feels. . . .

And now, touch your left hand to (the affected body part) *and let that numb feeling transfer from your hand to* (the affected body part) *. . ."*

Suggestions for Pleasant or Distracting Imagery

Another kind of hypnotic suggestion that is often used to relieve acute and procedural pain involves making suggestions for pleasant or distracting imagery. Effective suggestions for pleasant or distracting imagery are likely to incorporate the interests of the patient. For example, if a patient indicates he or she enjoys the beach:

"You said you like to go the beach. Imagine you are at the beach right now. Imagine you are standing on a sandy white beach, looking out across the deep blue water of the ocean. It is a beautiful summer day. Some puffy white clouds glide across the pastel blue sky. The beach stretches out before you in the distance as far as you can see. See the waves gently rolling up on the beach. You can smell the salty ocean air . . . and you can occasionally hear sea gulls calling. Feel the wind gently blowing on your skin. It is such a beautiful day at the beach . . .

You begin walking down the beach. As you take each step, you can feel the soft white sand beneath your feet. . . . The breeze gently rustles the leaves of a few palm trees. . . . You notice a weathered beach chair in a peaceful spot and you stop to sit down and relax. . . . Feel the warmth of the sun on your body . . . hear the sound of the waves rolling up on the beach . . . over and over again . . . the rhythmic sound of the waves is so peaceful and relaxing. It's such a relaxing and tranquil day. . . . Just take a few moments to enjoy this beautiful day . . ."

Suggestions for Relaxation

Helping a patient to relax can sometimes be useful in alleviating pain. Most hypnotic inductions include suggestions for relaxation. However, some patients may be able to achieve even greater relaxation by providing instructions for progressive muscle relaxation labeled as hypnotic relaxation and delivered in the context of hypnosis. Consider the following instructions adapted from Goldfried and Davison (1976):

"Hypnotic relaxation involves intentionally tensing and then relaxing various muscle groups. Hypnotic muscle relaxation is a way to relax your whole body a little at a time. People usually find that it is easier to relax little by little than all at once. So, in hypnotic muscle relaxation you will be relaxing all the muscles in your body one group at a time. Hypnotic muscle relaxation involves three steps: (1) turning your attention to the muscles to be relaxed; (2) tensing the muscles, not so that it hurts, but enough so that you can feel the tension; and (3) gradually letting the tension go and feeling the muscles unwind.

Keeping these three steps in mind, please continue to enjoy the experience of hypnosis and listen carefully to the suggestions I am going to make to you. I'm going to make you aware of certain sensations in your body and then show you how you can reduce these sensations. First direct your attention to your left arm, your left hand in particular. . . . Clench your left fist. . . . Clench it tightly and study the tension in the hand and in the forearm. . . . Study those sensations of tension. . . . And now let go. . . . Relax the left hand and let it rest in your lap. . . . And note any difference between the tension and the relaxation. . . . Once again now, clench your left hand into a fist, tightly, noticing any tension in the hand and in the forearm. . . . Study those tensions, and now let go. Let your fingers spread out, now more relaxed, and note any difference once again between muscular tension and muscular relaxation . . ."

(Work your way through each of the muscle groups in the body in a similar fashion, addressing the right hand, biceps, shoulders, face, neck, upper back, lungs, stomach, and legs one muscle group at a time.)

"Now, as you sit there, enjoying the comfort and pleasantness of hypnotic relaxation . . . I'm going to go over the various muscle groups in your body. . . . As I name each group . . . try to notice if there is any tension in those muscles. . . . If there is any . . . try to concentrate on those muscles . . . and send messages to them to relax . . . to loosen. . . . Relax the muscles in your feet, ankles, and calves . . . shins, knees, and thighs . . . buttocks and hips. . . . Loosen the muscles of your lower body. . . . Relax your stomach, waist, lower back . . . upper back, chest, and shoulders. . . . Relax your upper arms, forearms, and hands, right to the tips of your fingers. . . . Let the muscles of your throat and neck loosen. . . . Relax your jaw and facial muscles. . . . Let all the muscles of your body become loose and limp . . . completely comfortable . . . completely relaxed . . ."

Other Types of Suggestions

Other kinds of hypnotic suggestions are sometimes used to relieve acute and procedural pain. For example, *suggestions for dissociation* from the pain may invite the patient to experience the affected body part as if it were no longer part of or connected to the individual. For example, in the case example on burn wound care, the patient was given suggestions that she could float up away from her body into a cloud such that she could look down on her body. In *suggestions for time distortion*, the patient is led to believe the amount of time they experience pain will be short (e.g., an hour may seem like only a minute). *Ego-strengthening suggestions* are designed to enhance a patient's confidence in their ability to cope, including with the pain. These are just some possibilities. The range of hypnotic suggestions that may be helpful in alleviating acute pain is broad and limited only by the creativity of the clinician.

CONCLUSION

The evidence base supporting the efficacy of hypnosis for relieving acute and procedural pain is quite substantial. The research literature suggests the effect of hypnosis is likely to be strengthened if the primary mode of delivery is by having a clinician provide it live immediately before or during the time a patient is in pain. Therefore, clinicians who use hypnosis for analgesia may wish to arrange to be present during or just before the time their patients are experiencing pain. If this is not feasible, clinicians may wish to consider providing patients with explicit training in self-directed hypnosis skills that include instructions to practice on multiple occasions. Patients falling in the high and medium ranges of hypnotic suggestibility may be especially good candidates for hypnosis. Finally, the research literature indicates hypnosis is likely to be beneficial for most, if not all, forms of acute and procedural pain. All in all, hypnosis appears to be a potent and evidence-based tool for relieving acute and procedural pain.

REFERENCES

Apfelbaum, J. L., Chen, C., Mehta, S. S., & Gan, T. J. (2003). Postoperative pain experience: Results from a national survey suggest postoperative pain continues to be undermanaged. *Anesthesia and Analgesia, 97*(2), 534–540. https://doi.org/10.1213/01.ANE.0000068822.10113.9E

Barber, J. (1977). Rapid induction analgesia: A clinical report. *American Journal of Clinical Hypnosis, 19*(3), 138–147. https://doi.org/10.1080/00029157.1977.10403860

Beevi, Z., Low, W. Y., & Hassan, J. (2017). The effectiveness of hypnosis intervention for labor: An experimental study. *American Journal of Clinical Hypnosis, 60*(2), 172–191. https://doi.org/10.1080/00029157.2017.1280659

Birnie, K. A., Noel, M., Parker, J. A., Chambers, C. T., Uman, L. S., Kisely, S. R., & McGrath, P. J. (2014). Systematic review and meta-analysis of distraction and hypnosis for needle-related pain and distress in children and adolescents. *Journal of Pediatric Psychology, 39*(8), 783–808. https://doi.org/10.1093/jpepsy/jsu029

Brennan, F., Carr, D. B., & Cousins, M. (2007). Pain management: A fundamental human right. *Anesthesia & Analgesia, 105*(1), 205–221. https://doi.org/10.1213/01.ane.0000268145.52345.55

Brooks, P. A. (2002). *The use of clinical hypnosis to accelerate the appearance of soft tissue wound resolution and patient recovery in post surgical patients* [Unpublished doctoral dissertation]. The Union Institute, Cincinnati, OH.

Butler, L. D., Symons, B. K., Henderson, S. L., Shortliffe, L. D., & Spiegel, D. (2005). Hypnosis reduces distress and duration of an invasive medical procedure for children. *Pediatrics, 115*(1), e77–e85. https://doi.org/10.1542/peds.2004-0818

Cherry, D. K., Burt, C. W., & Woodwell, D. A. (2003). National ambulatory medical care survey: 2001 summary. *Advance Data, 11*(337), 1–44. https://pubmed.ncbi.nlm.nih.gov/12924075/

Chester, S. J., Tyack, Z., De Young, A., Kipping, B., Griffin, B., Stockton, K., Ware, R. S., Zhang, X., & Kimble, R. M. (2018). Efficacy of hypnosis on pain, wound-healing, anxiety, and stress in children with acute burn injuries: A randomized controlled trial. *Pain, 159*(9), 1790–1801. https://doi.org/10.1097/j.pain.0000000000001276

Cohen, J. (1988). *Statistical power analysis for the behavioral sciences* (2nd ed.). Lawrence Earlbaum Associates.

Deltito, J. A. (1984). Hypnosis in the treatment of acute pain in the emergency department setting. *Postgraduate Medical Journal, 60*(702), 263–266. https://doi.org/10.1136/pgmj.60.702.263

Dimond, R. E. (1981). Hypnotic treatment of a kidney dialysis patient. *American Journal of Clinical Hypnosis, 23*(4), 284–288. https://doi.org/10.1080/00029157.1981.10404038

Eason, A. D., & Parris, B. A. (2019). Clinical applications of self-hypnosis: A systematic review and meta-analysis of randomized controlled trials. *Psychology of Consciousness: Theory, Research, and Practice, 6*(3), 262–278. https://doi.org/10.1037/cns0000173

Eitner, S., Bittner, C., Wichmann, M., Nickenig, H.-J., & Sokol, B. (2010). Comparison of conventional therapies for dentin hypersensitivity versus medical hypnosis. *International Journal of Clinical and Experimental Hypnosis, 58*(4), 457–475. https://doi.org/10.1080/00207144.2010.499350

Enqvist, B., & Fischer, K. (1997). Preoperative hypnotic techniques reduce consumption of analgesics after surgical removal of third mandibular molars: A brief communication. *International Journal of Clinical and Experimental Hypnosis, 45*(2), 102–108. https://doi.org/10.1080/00207149708416112

Fathi, M., Ariamanesh, A. S., Joudi, M., Joudi, M., Sadrossadati, F., & Izanloo, A. (2019). Hypnosis as an approach to control pain and anxiety in anterior cruciate ligament reconstruction and meniscal surgeries: Two case presentations. *Anesthesiology and Pain Medicine, 9*(4), e89277. https://doi.org/10.5812/aapm.89277

Freeman, R. M., Macaulay, A. J., Eve, L., Chamberlain, G. V. P., & Bhat, A. V. (1986). Randomised trial of self hypnosis for analgesia in labour. *British Medical Journal (Clinical Research Ed.), 292*(6521), 657–658. https://doi.org/10.1136/bmj.292.6521.657

Ginandes, C. S., & Rosenthal, D. I. (1999). Using hypnosis to accelerate the healing of bone fractures: A randomized controlled pilot study. *Alternative Therapies in Health and Medicine, 5*(2), 67–75. https://pubmed.ncbi.nlm.nih.gov/10069091/

Goldberg, S. B., Tucker, R. P., Greene, P. A., Davidson, R. J., Wampold, B. E., Kearney, D. J., & Simpson, T. L. (2018). Mindfulness-based interventions for psychiatric disorders: A systematic review and meta-analysis. *Clinical Psychology Review, 59,* 52–60. https://doi.org/10.1016/j.cpr.2017.10.011

Goldfried, M. R., & Davison, G. C. (1976). *Clinical behavior therapy.* Holt, Rinehart & Winston.

Guthrie, K., Taylor, D. J., & Defriend, D. (1984). Maternal hypnosis induced by husbands during childbirth. *Journal of Obstetrics and Gynaecology, 5*(2), 93–95. https://doi.org/10.3109/01443618409109124

Haddock, C. K., Rowan, A. B., Andrasik, F., Wilson, P. G., Talcott, G. W., & Stein, R. J. (1997). Home-based behavioral treatments for chronic benign headache: A meta-analysis of controlled trials. *Cephalalgia, 17*(2), 113–118. https://doi.org/10.1046/j.1468-2982.1997.1702113.x

Harandi, A. A., Esfandani, A., & Shakibaei, F. (2004). The effect of hypnotherapy on procedural pain and state anxiety related to physiotherapy in women hospitalized in a burn unit. *Contemporary Hypnosis, 21*(1), 28–34. https://doi.org/10.1002/ch.285

Harmon, T. M., Hynan, M. T., & Tyre, T. E. (1990). Improved obstetric outcomes using hypnotic analgesia and skill mastery combined with childbirth education. *Journal of Consulting and Clinical Psychology, 58*(5), 525–530. https://doi.org/10.1037/0022-006X.58.5.525

Huet, A., Lucas-Polomeni, M.-M., Robert, J.-C., Sixou, J.-L., & Wodey, E. (2011). Hypnosis and dental anesthesia in children: A prospective controlled study. *International Journal of Clinical and Experimental Hypnosis, 59*(4), 424–440. https://doi.org/10.1080/00207144.2011.594740

Institute of Medicine. (2011). *Relieving pain in America: A blueprint for transforming prevention, care, education, and research.* National Academies Press.

John, M. E., Jr., & Parrino, J. P. (1983). Practical hypnotic suggestion in ophthalmic surgery. *American Journal of Ophthalmology, 96*(4), 540–542. https://doi.org/10.1016/S0002-9394(14)77919-X

Joudi, M., Fathi, M., Izanloo, A., Montazeri, O., & Jangjoo, A. (2016). An evaluation of the effect of hypnosis on postoperative analgesia following laparoscopic cholecystectomy. *International Journal of Clinical and Experimental Hypnosis, 64*(3), 365–372. https://doi.org/10.1080/00207144.2016.1171113

Katz, E. R., Kellerman, J., & Ellenberg, L. (1987). Hypnosis in the reduction of acute pain and distress in children with cancer. *Journal of Pediatric Psychology, 12*(3), 379–394. https://doi.org/10.1093/jpepsy/12.3.379

Kenney, M. P., & Milling, L. S. (2016). The effectiveness of virtual reality distraction for reducing pain: A meta-analysis. *Psychology of Consciousness: Theory, Research, and Practice, 3*(3), 199–210. https://doi.org/10.1037/cns0000084

Kuttner, L., Bowman, M., & Teasdale, M. (1988). Psychological treatment of distress, pain, and anxiety for young children with cancer. *Journal of Developmental and Behavioral Pediatrics, 9*(6), 374–381. https://doi.org/10.1097/00004703-198812000-00010

Lambert, S. A. (1996). The effects of hypnosis/guided imagery on the postoperative course of children. *Journal of Developmental & Behavioral Pediatrics, 17*(5), 307–310. https://doi.org/10.1097/00004703-199610000-00003

Lang, E. V., Benotsch, E. G., Fick, L. J., Lutgendorf, S., Berbaum, M. L., Berbaum, K. S., Logan, H., & Spiegel, D. (2000). Adjunctive non-pharmacological analgesia for invasive medical procedures: A randomised trial. *The Lancet, 355*(9214), 1486–1490. https://doi.org/10.1016/S0140-6736(00)02162-0

Lang, E. V., Berbaum, K. S., Faintuch, S., Hatsiopoulou, O., Halsey, N., Li, X., Berbaum, M. L., Laser, E., & Baum, J. (2006). Adjunctive self-hypnotic relaxation for outpatient medical procedures: A prospective randomized trial with women undergoing large core breast biopsy. *Pain, 126*(1–3), 155–164. https://doi.org/10.1016/j.pain.2006.06.035

Lang, E. V., Berbaum, K. S., Pauker, S. G., Faintuch, S., Salazar, G. M., Lutgendorf, S., Laser, E., Logan, H., & Spiegel, D. (2008). Beneficial effects of hypnosis and adverse effects of empathic attention during percutaneous tumor treatment: When being nice does not suffice. *Journal of Vascular and Interventional Radiology, 19*(6), 897–905. https://doi.org/10.1016/j.jvir.2008.01.027

Lang, E. V., Joyce, J. S., Spiegel, D., Hamilton, D., & Lee, K. K. (1996). Self-hypnotic relaxation during interventional radiological procedures: Effects on pain perception and intravenous drug use. *International Journal of Clinical and Experimental Hypnosis, 44*(2), 106–119. https://doi.org/10.1080/00207149608416074

Lauche, R., Cramer, H., Dobos, G., Langhorst, J., & Schmidt, S. (2013). A systematic review and meta-analysis of mindfulness-based stress reduction for the fibromyalgia syndrome. *Journal of Psychosomatic Research, 75*(6), 500–510. https://doi.org/10.1016/j.jpsychores.2013.10.010

Liossi, C., & Hatira, P. (1999). Clinical hypnosis versus cognitive behavioral training for pain management with pediatric cancer patients undergoing bone marrow aspirations. *International Journal of Clinical and Experimental Hypnosis, 47*(2), 104–116. https://doi.org/10.1080/00207149908410025

Liossi, C., & Hatira, P. (2003). Clinical hypnosis in the alleviation of procedure-related pain in pediatric oncology patients. *International Journal of Clinical and Experimental Hypnosis, 51*(1), 4–28. https://doi.org/10.1076/iceh.51.1.4.14064

Liossi, C., White, P., & Hatira, P. (2006). Randomized clinical trial of local anesthetic versus a combination of local anesthetic with self-hypnosis in the management of pediatric procedure-related pain. *Health Psychology, 25*(3), 307–315. https://doi.org/10.1037/0278-6133.25.3.307

Liossi, C., White, P., & Hatira, P. (2009). A randomized clinical trial of a brief hypnosis intervention to control venepuncture-related pain of paediatric cancer patients. *Pain, 142*(3), 255–263. https://doi.org/10.1016/j.pain.2009.01.017

Mairs, D. A. E. (1995). Hypnosis and pain in childbirth. *Contemporary Hypnosis, 12*(2), 111–118.

Marc, I., Rainville, P., Verreault, R., Vaillancourt, L., Masse, B., & Dodin, S. (2007). The use of hypnosis to improve pain management during voluntary interruption of pregnancy: An open randomized preliminary study. *Contraception, 75*(1), 52–58. https://doi.org/10.1016/j.contraception.2006.07.012

Melzack, R., Kinch, R., Dobkin, P., Lebrun, M., & Taenzer, P. (1984). Severity of labour pain: Influence of physical as well as psychologic variables. *Canadian Medical Association Journal, 130*(5), 579–584. https://pubmed.ncbi.nlm.nih.gov/6697268/

Melzack, R., Taenzer, P., Feldman, P., & Kinch, R. A. (1981). Labour is still painful after prepared childbirth training. *Canadian Medical Association Journal, 125*(4), 357–363. https://pubmed.ncbi.nlm.nih.gov/7272887/

Merskey, H., & Bogduk, N. (1994). *Classification of chronic pain* (2nd ed.). IASP Press.

Milling, L. S., Valentine, K. E., LoStimolo, L. M., Nett, A. M., & McCarley, H. S. (2021). Hypnosis and the alleviation of clinical pain: A comprehensive meta-analysis. *International Journal of Clinical and Experimental Hypnosis, 69*(3), 297–322. https://doi.org/10.1080/00207144.2021.1920330

Montgomery, G. H., Bovbjerg, D. H., Schnur, J. B., David, D., Goldfarb, A., Weltz, C. R., Schechter, C., Graff-Zivin, J., Tatrow, K., Price, D. D., & Silverstein, J. H. (2007). A randomized clinical trial of a brief hypnosis intervention to control side effects in breast surgery patients. *Journal of the National Cancer Institute, 99*(17), 1304–1312. https://doi.org/10.1093/jnci/djm106

Montgomery, G. H., DuHamel, K. N., & Redd, W. H. (2000). A meta-analysis of hypnotically induced analgesia: How effective is hypnosis? *International Journal of Clinical and Experimental Hypnosis, 48*(2), 138–153. https://doi.org/10.1080/00207140008410045

Montgomery, G. H., Weltz, C. R., Seltz, M., & Bovbjerg, D. H. (2002). Brief presurgery hypnosis reduces distress and pain in excisional breast biopsy patients. *International Journal of Clinical and Experimental Hypnosis, 50*(1), 17–32. https://doi.org/10.1080/00207140208410088

Morgan, A. H., & Hilgard, J. R. (1978/1979). The Stanford Hypnotic Clinical Scale for Adults. *American Journal of Clinical Hypnosis, 21*(2–3), 134–147. https://doi.org/10.1080/00029157.1978.10403968

Nahin, R. L. (2015). Estimates of pain prevalence and severity in adults: United States, 2012. *The Journal of Pain, 16*(8), 769–780. https://doi.org/10.1016/j.jpain.2015.05.002

Nestoriuc, Y., & Martin, A. (2007). Efficacy of biofeedback for migraine: A meta-analysis. *Pain, 128*(1–2), 111–127. https://doi.org/10.1016/j.pain.2006.09.007

Nestoriuc, Y., Rief, W., & Martin, A. (2008). Meta-analysis of biofeedback for tension-type headache: Efficacy, specificity, and treatment moderators. *Journal of Consulting and Clinical Psychology, 76*(3), 379–396. https://doi.org/10.1037/0022-006X.76.3.379

Niven, C. A., & Murphy-Black, T. (2000). Memory for labor pain: A review of the literature. *Birth, 27*(4), 244–253. https://doi.org/10.1046/j.1523-536x.2000.00244.x

Ozgunay, S. E., Ozmen, S., Karasu, D., Yilmaz, C., & Taymur, I. (2019). The effect of hypnosis on intraoperative hemorrhage and postoperative pain in rhinoplasty. *International Journal of Clinical and Experimental Hypnosis, 67*(3), 262–277. https://doi.org/10.1080/00207144.2019.1612670

Patterson, D. R., Everett, J. J., Burns, G. L., & Marvin, J. A. (1992). Hypnosis for the treatment of burn pain. *Journal of Consulting and Clinical Psychology, 60*(5), 713–717. https://doi.org/10.1037/0022-006X.60.5.713

Patterson, D. R., & Ptacek, J. T. (1997). Baseline pain as a moderator of hypnotic analgesia for burn injury treatment. *Journal of Consulting and Clinical Psychology, 65*(1), 60–67. https://doi.org/10.1037/0022-006X.65.1.60

Perry, S., Heidrich, G., & Ramos, E. (1981). Assessment of pain in burn patients. *The Journal of Burn Care & Rehabilitation, 2*(6), 322–326. https://doi.org/10.1097/00004630-198111000-00004

Pletcher, M. J., Kertesz, S. G., Kohn, M. A., & Gonzales, R. (2008). Trends in opioid prescribing by race/ethnicity for patients seeking care in US emergency departments. *Journal of the American Medical Association, 299*(1), 70–78. https://doi.org/10.1001/jama.2007.64

Ramírez-Carrasco, A., Butrón-Téllez Girón, C., Sanchez-Armass, O., & Pierdant-Pérez, M. (2017). Effectiveness of hypnosis in combination with conventional techniques of behavior management in anxiety/pain reduction during dental anesthetic infiltration. *Pain Research and Management, 2017.* https://doi.org/10.1155/2017/1434015

Sánchez-Jáuregui, T., Téllez, A., Juárez-García, D., García, C. H., & García, F. E. (2019). Clinical hypnosis and music in breast biopsy: A randomized clinical trial. *American Journal of Clinical Hypnosis, 61*(3), 244–257. https://doi.org/10.1080/00029157.2018.1489776

Sinatra, R. (2010). Causes and consequences of inadequate management of acute pain. *Pain Medicine, 11*(12), 1859–1871. https://doi.org/10.1111/j.1526-4637.2010.00983.x

Snow, A., Dorfman, D., Warbet, R., Cammarata, M., Eisenman, S., Zilberfein, F., Isola, L., & Navada, S. (2012). A randomized trial of hypnosis for relief of pain and anxiety in adult cancer patients undergoing bone marrow procedures. *Journal of Psychosocial Oncology, 30*(3), 281–293. https://doi.org/10.1080/07347332.2012.664261

Snow, A., & Warbet, R. (2010). Hypnosis: Exploring the benefits for the role of the hospital social worker. *Social Work in Health Care, 49*(3), 245–262. https://doi.org/10.1080/00981380903364825

Spiegel, D., & Bloom, J. R. (1983). Group therapy and hypnosis reduce metastatic breast carcinoma pain. *Psychosomatic Medicine, 45*(4), 333–339. https://doi.org/10.1097/00006842-198308000-00007

Syrjala, K. L., Cummings, C., & Donaldson, G. W. (1992). Hypnosis or cognitive behavioral training for the reduction of pain and nausea during cancer treatment: A controlled clinical trial. *Pain, 48*(2), 137–146. https://doi.org/10.1016/0304-3959(92)90049-H

Taenzer, P. (1983). *Self-control of postoperative pain: Effects of hypnosis and waking suggestion* [Unpublished doctoral dissertation]. McGill University, Montreal, Canada.

Tatrow, K., & Montgomery, G. H. (2006). Cognitive behavioral therapy techniques for distress and pain in breast cancer patients: A meta-analysis. *Journal of Behavioral Medicine, 29*(1), 17–27. https://doi.org/10.1007/s10865-005-9036-1

Temple, J., & Utting, S. (2014). The transfer of patient attachment between dental hypnosis practitioners for hypnoanaesthesia: A case report. *Contemporary Hypnosis & Integrative Therapy, 30*(2), 69–75.

Wallace, L. M. (1987). Hypnosis and pain control on an English burns unit. *Intensive Care Nursing, 3*(2), 50–55. https://doi.org/10.1016/0266-612X(87)90024-1

Wright, B. R., & Drummond, P. D. (2000). Rapid induction analgesia for the alleviation of procedural pain during burn care. *Burns, 26*(3), 275–282. https://doi.org/10.1016/S0305-4179(99)00134-5

5 HYPNOSIS AND CHRONIC PAIN

LINDSEY C. McKERNAN AND ERIN L. CONNORS

INTRODUCTION

Chronic pain occurs when pain persists or recurs for 3 months or longer, far beyond the time expected to heal from acute injury and no longer having an adaptive purpose (Clauw et al., 2019; Treede et al., 2019). Chronic pain is recognized as a major public health problem, affecting approximately 20% of U.S. adults and costing the health care system approximately $635 billion annually (Dahlhamer et al., 2018; Gaskin & Richard, 2012). Conditions such as abdominal and low back pain are a primary source of emergency room encounters nationally (Weiss et al., 2014). In addition to substantial societal burden, chronic pain significantly reduces quality of life for affected individuals and is associated with disability, opioid dependence, emotional distress, and the development of co-occurring physical and psychological conditions (Clauw et al., 2019). Recognizing its broad impact and the limited efficacy of pharmacological interventions for pain, leading organizations recommend multidisciplinary management incorporating nonpharmacological strategies to improve a person's quality of life and functioning (Institute of Medicine, 2011).

https://doi.org/10.1037/0000347-005
Evidence-Based Practice in Clinical Hypnosis, L. S. Milling (Editor)

Some of the most common chronic pain conditions include tension-type headache, low back pain, and chronic neck pain. Pain itself can be influenced by one or multiple mechanisms, such as nociceptive, neuropathic, and noci-plastic or "centralized" pain processes. Nociceptive pain includes that associated with actual or threatened tissue damage, such as in arthritis. Neuropathic pain includes that caused by damage or lesion to the somatosensory nervous system. It often involves "burning" or painful "tingling" sensations, present in conditions such as diabetic neuropathy. Nociplastic or centralized pain refers to widespread pain with no observable pathology, with representative conditions including fibromyalgia or irritable bowel syndrome (IBS).

For many, pain conditions may overlap and have multiple mechanisms influencing a person's pain experience. Not surprisingly, having chronic pain can drastically alter a person's willingness to engage in social or physical activity, relating to others, and mood (Clauw et al., 2019). Individuals can become highly attuned to sensations in the body and restrict movement to avoid exacerbating pain. The fear avoidance model of pain (Zale & Ditre, 2015) posits that during acute injury recovery such behavior is adaptive, but in the context of chronic pain becomes counterproductive, triggering additional pain due to physical deconditioning when activity is ultimately initiated. Evidently, more pain reinforces one's fear and hesitancy to move, which in turn increases disability risk. Thus, pain and associated inactivity can lead to a perpetuation of symptoms commonly referred to as the "pain cycle."

Chronic pain conditions are both conceptualized and treated from a biopsychosocial perspective, which accounts for the biological, psychological, and social factors that influence a person's experience of pain (Gatchel et al., 2007). Further, pain is subjective—both a sensory and emotional experience (IASP Task Force on Taxonomy, 2017) informed by sensory, cognitive, and affective factors (Melzack, 2001). With hypnosis, this presents tremendous opportunity to cultivate individualized treatment plans and suggestions unique to each patient's pain experience. In fact, experts in applying hypnosis for pain recommend the application of diverse suggestions that span the many life areas (and brain regions) affected by pain (Jensen & Patterson, 2014). Moreover, treatment goals include both pain reduction and improved overall function. Interestingly, patients can benefit from hypnosis irrespective of pain relief and improve their mood and sleep (Patterson & Jensen, 2003). This again presents an opportunity clinically to attempt hypnosis with even the most complex of cases, as we demonstrate later in this chapter.

This chapter reviews evidence from controlled studies assessing the efficacy of hypnosis for chronic pain, and information regarding patient and treatment-level factors that may influence treatment outcomes. We also provide guidance with case formulation and treatment planning, using a specific case example and step-by-step example treatment plan for reference. It is our hope this information provides a balanced, up-to-date perspective on the topic with practical guidance for practitioners interested in applying hypnosis for chronic pain cases.

REVIEW OF OUTCOME RESEARCH

As was previously mentioned, hypnosis has been applied to a variety of pain conditions including chronic widespread pain, fibromyalgia, cancer, and spinal cord injury, among others. Furthermore, the effectiveness of this intervention to provide pain relief has been shown to vary according to both individual patient characteristics (e.g., degree of hypnotic suggestibility, patient expectations pretreatment) as well as characteristics specific to the delivery of the hypnotic intervention itself (e.g., cognitive-behavioral therapy combined with hypnosis, type of suggestions and visualizations given). Thus, in this section we review controlled studies of the efficacy of hypnosis as an intervention for chronic pain, while highlighting specific variables linked to successful outcomes. These studies are organized where possible according to the International Association for the Study of Pain (IASP) definitions of neuropathic, nociceptive, and nociplastic pain (IASP Task Force on Taxonomy, 2017). Given that many individuals present clinically with overlapping neuropathic, nociceptive, and nociplastic symptoms (Freynhagen et al., 2019), this method of classification is a simplification. Finally, we discuss important takeaways bearing in mind the limitations of current research.

Neuropathic Pain

Despite the fact that controlled studies investigating hypnosis effects on neuropathic pain are limited, the empirical literature does provide preliminary support for the use of hypnosis in the treatment of patients with neuropathic pain conditions such as chronic brachial neuralgia, spinal cord injury, and potentially complex regional pain syndrome. Two different randomized controlled trials (RCTs) have evaluated and compared the efficacy of hypnotherapy with acupressure among patients with chronic brachial neuralgia (Ahmad, 2015; Razak et al., 2019). Overall, both hypnotherapy and acupressure interventions were effective in terms of reducing average pain intensity, but hypnosis evidenced superiority overall. Specifically, acupressure reduced pain intensity faster than hypnotherapy in the first 2 weeks of treatment, but benefits from hypnotherapy were longer-lasting (Razak et al., 2019). Similarly, chronic brachial neuralgia patients reported greater improvements in pain and disability metrics compared with acupressure (Ahmad, 2015), as well as greater improvements in quality of life and mental health 4 months posttreatment (Razak et al., 2019).

Conversely, another trial comparing treatment as usual to hypnosis in 27 burn patients found no meaningful difference between interventions with respect to pain intensity (Wiechman et al., 2019). Along the same lines, Fialka et al. (1996) conducted the only controlled trial to test the benefits of hypnosis in 18 patients with complex regional pain syndrome, finding pain decreased in both hypnosis and treatment-as-usual groups. Furthermore, significant differences were only observed with regard to skin temperature (decreased in hypnosis, increased in control).

Several clinical trials have investigated the effects of hypnosis on spinal cord injury populations. For instance, Jensen et al. (2009) looked at the effects of 10 self-hypnosis sessions compared with EMG-assisted biofeedback relaxation training. Ultimately, both the hypnosis and biofeedback groups reported reductions in pain intensity scores. Nonetheless, participants in the hypnosis condition experienced greater decreases in their daily average pain scores in the pre- to posttreatment phases, which were maintained at 3-month follow-up.

Notably, Jensen and colleagues (2009) characterized spinal cord injury pain into groups of either neuropathic versus nonneuropathic (Jensen et al., 2009) pain types, and neuropathic, nociceptive, or mixed pain types (Jensen et al., 2013, 2014). This is important to mention as hypnosis proved effective for neuropathic pain patients in one study, but those with non-neuropathic chronic pain did not respond to hypnotic analgesia (Jensen et al., 2009). In the other two studies, between group differences were not accounted for, and data for all pain types were reported together.

Many of the previously described studies saw improvements in both the treatment *and* control conditions, with no significant difference between the two. Nonetheless, hypnotic analgesia appears to be associated with substantial reductions in chronic neuropathic pain intensity (Jensen et al., 2009, 2013; Razak et al., 2019). Additionally, the impact of hypnosis extends beyond pain relief. Studies revealed improvements in perceived disability (Ahmad, 2015), ability to regulate skin temperature (Fialka et al., 1996), increased quality of life, and sustained improvements specific to mental health such as limitations in typical activities due to physical and emotional problems, overall social functioning (Razak et al., 2019), and depression (Jensen et al., 2009). Lastly, the benefits of hypnosis were greater for patients with higher presession theta activity (Jensen et al., 2014) as well as for patients with neuropathic pain secondary to spinal cord injury (Jensen et al., 2009).

Nociceptive Pain

Relative to research on neuropathic and nociplastic pain, there are more studies of nociceptive pain (e.g., musculoskeletal and inflammatory conditions). Hypnotic intervention has been found to have superior effect when compared with alternative interventions for some pain-centered outcomes secondary to such nociceptive conditions as temporomandibular disorders, hemophilia, arthritis, Crohn's disease, and low back pain (Abrahamsen et al., 2009; Ferrando et al., 2012; Gay et al., 2002; Lee et al., 2021; Winocur et al., 2002). At the same time, the evidence is inconsistent. Most patients experienced improvements in pain and quality of life outcomes, but this change did not always differ from control conditions.

With regard to temporomandibular disorder-specific pain, one trial compared the effectiveness of "hypnorelaxation" to the use of occlusal appliance or control in the treatment of 40 female patients (Winocur et al., 2002). Both hypnosis and occlusal device treatments were more effective than the minimal treatment condition in diminishing muscle sensitivity, yet only hypnosis resulted in a significant reduction in patient perception of pain (i.e., emotional support and lifestyle recommendations). Likewise, patients in another trial who received hypnosis saw a significant reduction in daily pain at pre- to posttreatment (by 46%), compared with relaxation/visualization controls, whose pain intensity scores increased (by 7%; Abrahamsen et al., 2009). The hypnosis group reported greater overall improvement across measures of sleep quality. Yet, both groups demonstrated declines in pain-driven awakenings, somatization, anxiety, and pain on palpation outcomes. Ferrando et al. (2012) demonstrated that patients in the cognitive-behavioral therapy (CBT) with hypnosis treatment group displayed significant reductions in pain frequency, self-medication frequency, pain intensity, subjective pain index, pain severity, and emotional distress posttreatment as compared with standard treatment controls. Moreover, these differences remained at 9 months follow-up. Nevertheless, no meaningful improvements between groups were observed on measures of pain interference and depression.

Gay et al. (2002) evaluated the effectiveness of Eriksonian hypnosis and Jacobson relaxation compared with no-treatment control for the reduction of osteoarthritis pain. After only 4 weeks, those who received hypnosis reported more than a 50% reduction in pain intensity, whereas the control group reported little change in pain throughout the trial. Similar to neuropathic pain studies described previously, relaxation also evidenced pain relief significant at 8 weeks of treatment, meaning hypnosis produced meaningful changes at an earlier timepoint compared with both relaxation and control interventions. Regarding medication use, both experimental groups produced significant reductions in pain medication at 8 weeks. However, differences between the effects of the hypnosis intervention and the relaxation control on pain reduction were not statistically different overall.

Lee et al. (2021) conducted the first RCT comparing clinical hypnosis to standard care in pediatric patients with Crohn's disease, demonstrating that hypnosis is both a feasible and acceptable intervention associated with improved pain and psychosocial functioning. Compared with waitlist-controls, patients in the hypnosis intervention saw significant decreases in abdominal pain severity, greater improvement in most pain, reduced absences from school (59%), and increased ratings in health-related quality of life. Qualitative data also described improved energy levels, sense of control, school-related stress and anxiety, as well as perceived benefit from other pains (e.g., headaches, arthralgias, and injuries).

In contrast, Bhatt et al. (2017) examined the effect of one 30-minute hypnosis session on peripheral blood flow during thermal pain quantitative sensory testing (QST) in 14 patients with sickle cell disease and 14 healthy controls. Following hypnosis, pain intensity decreased by a moderate amount in patients with sickle cell disease, but this effect was not significant. Interestingly, significant increases in pain threshold and tolerance levels were observed in controls following hypnotic intervention, but no changes were observed in patients with sickle cell disease. From a physiological standpoint, however, patients with sickle cell disease had lower baseline peripheral blood flow and a greater increase in blood flow after hypnosis than controls.

Another study compared pain intensity, pain interference, and sleep quality metrics among 100 veterans with history of chronic low back pain (Tan et al., 2015). All four groups reported improvements in pain intensity, pain interference, and sleep quality due to treatment. Importantly, participants receiving any one of the three hypnosis treatment conditions demonstrated greater reduction in overall pain intensity when compared with surface electromyography (sEMG) biofeedback. Nonetheless, hypnosis was not more effective than biofeedback for improving sleep quality and reducing pain interference.

Another RCT examined the benefits of combining pain education (PE) with clinical hypnosis (CH) in a group setting for patients with chronic nonspecific low back pain (Rizzo et al., 2018). One-hundred patients were randomized to receive either PE alone or PE with CH. No significant difference was detected between the groups in average pain intensity at 2 weeks or 3 months. However, PE with CH was significantly superior on improving worst pain intensity, disability, and catastrophizing, as well as more global perceived benefits at 2 weeks.

Furthermore, data supports the use of hypnosis as an effective intervention to reduce pain interference and promote quality of life in some rare musculoskeletal disorders. For example, Paredes et al. (2019) examined the feasibility, acceptability, and effectiveness of hypnosis for pain management among 20 adults with hemophilia experiencing joint deterioration and associated chronic pain. Compared with treatment as usual (control), the group that received four sessions of hypnosis displayed greater diminished pain interference and greater improvements on health-related quality of life measures (i.e., daily activities, treatment difficulties, physical health, and joints).

Based on the current findings, some studies have found hypnosis to be an effective intervention for nociceptive pain conditions as reflected by significant improvement in daily pain ratings (Abrahamsen et al., 2009) and pain intensity (Gay et al., 2002; Tan et al., 2015) compared with controls. In addition, patients reported reduced muscle sensitivity (Winocur et al., 2002), and improved sleep quality, somatization, anxiety, and pain on palpation (Abrahamsen et al., 2009). At the same time, patients in a few trials saw no significant difference in pain scores (Abrahamsen et al., 2009; Ferrando et al., 2012) and depression (Ferrando et al., 2012) regardless of treatment group. Other trials showed similar improvement in medication usage (Gay et al., 2002) and pain interference (Tan et al., 2015) across experimental conditions.

Nociplastic Pain

Increasing evidence shows the positive impact of hypnosis on nociplastic pain. This form of pain is thought to involve central sensitization, a widely recognized pain-generating mechanism contributing to conditions such as irritable bowel syndrome, fibromyalgia, and chronic widespread pain.

One study analyzed and compared data from 32 children/adolescents with functional abdominal pain (FAP) or irritable bowel syndrome following randomization to two self-administered audio-based interventions: gut-directed hypnotherapy (GDHT), designed to normalize gut function and unspecific hypnotherapy (UHT), designed primarily for relaxation and well-being (Gulewitsch & Schlarb 2017). Findings provided support for the efficacy of both treatment conditions (reduced average days with pain and reduced duration), however UHT was superior for the reduction of pain intensity. Both groups also attained similar improvements across secondary outcomes of pain-related disability, health-related quality of life, and somatic symptoms.

Another study randomized 12 women and four men with chronic widespread pain to either hypnosis or control conditions in a crossover design to evaluate the effect of standardized hypnosis treatment used in general practice (Grøndahl & Rosvold, 2008). Ultimately, individuals who received hypnosis showed significant improvement across measures of pain interference, quality of life, anxiety, fatigue, loneliness, and pessimism, while the control group showed a significant decline in scores. Patients who completed treatment demonstrated maintained improvements when assessed 1 year later.

Derbyshire et al. (2017) delivered hypnotic and nonhypnotic suggestions for low, medium, and high pain to 13 fibromyalgia patients and 15 experimental controls. Both fibromyalgia patients and controls reported significant changes in pain experience after suggestion to increase or decrease pain. However, hypnotic suggestions (following an induction) produced slightly larger changes in pain report. Altogether, formal hypnotic induction strengthened the impact of suggestions and increased sense of control over pain for both groups.

In another RCT with fibromyalgia patients, Castel et al. (2012) compared hypnosis combined with CBT to CBT alone and standard care in a group setting. Compared with individuals in the standard care condition, those who received CBT with hypnosis or CBT alone showed greater improvements in reducing pain intensity, catastrophizing, psychological distress, and sleep disturbances. However, combined therapy was superior to CBT alone in reducing psychological distress at the end of treatment.

Mixed Pain Samples

A number of trials have evaluated the efficacy of hypnosis in the treatment of heterogeneous conditions with diverse pathophysiology. Among these studies, the trend appears to be the same—patients benefit from hypnotherapy, but the findings are mixed as to the extent of superiority to a control and/or standard intervention.

For example, Ardigo et al. (2016) conducted one of the few randomized controlled studies exploring the feasibility and efficacy of hypnosis in pain management for a population of hospitalized elderly patients with varied conditions. Their most important finding was that hypnosis evidenced both feasibility and significant reduction in pain intensity among hospitalized geriatric patients. Additionally, hypnosis demonstrated more sustained analgesic effects compared with massage, and hypnosis improved patient mood, while massage did not. However, hypnosis and massage conditions showed no difference in pain intensity and mood 12 weeks following hospital discharge.

Another prospective study aimed to evaluate the effectiveness of different treatments (i.e., physiotherapy, psychoeducation, physiotherapy with psychoeducation, and self-hypnosis/self-care learning) in reducing disability associated with chronic pain (Vanhaudenhuyse et al., 2015). Each intervention evidenced improved metrics implicated in chronic pain, with the greatest combined changes in emotional functioning. As compared with other groups, the self-hypnosis/self-care group demonstrated a preferential effect on psychological and social factors such as anxiety, depression, pain intensity, pain interference, and quality of life. In fact, decrease in pain intensity was only found in patients assigned to the self-hypnosis/self-care treatment.

Evidence from their earlier study informed Vanhaudenhuyse et al.'s (2018) decision to further investigate differences in self-hypnosis/self-care learning and psychoeducation with physiotherapy with regards to patient attitudes and pain-related beliefs. All treatments occurred in a group format. Both treatment conditions observed significant increases in pain control and decreases in the search for medical "cure" as well as the belief that hurt signifies physical injury. Data also indicated that both self-hypnosis and psychoeducation/physiotherapy were associated with changes in passive to active coping patterns. Nonetheless, improvement of sense of control appeared to be more important for treatment success among patients in the self-hypnosis group compared with controls. Self-hypnosis was found to be superior to psychoeducation/physiotherapy in terms of reduced pain intensity and perceived disability.

Jensen et al. (2020) evaluated the efficacy of four nonpharmacological treatments, including two different hypnotic interventions, cognitive therapy and pain education, in 173 individuals with chronic pain. Improvements in pain intensity, pain interference, and depressive symptoms across all four groups were detected and maintained 12 months posttreatment. In a similar trial, Tonye-Geoffroy et al. (2021) compared pain relief outcomes between transcutaneous electrical nerve stimulation (TENS) with hypnosis and TENS treatment alone among 72 patients with chronic noncancer nociceptive and/or neuropathic pain. While both groups showed a substantial decrease in pain intensity and high treatment compliance at 3 months, they reported no additional effect of combining strategies. Furthermore, no significant difference was observed between the intervention and control groups in quality of life, drug consumption, or compliance.

Patient-Level and Treatment-Level Characteristics

Are there specific differences between individual patients and/or treatment delivery that determine effective response to hypnosis? While still inconclusive, some studies demonstrated that variables such as frequency of self-hypnosis practice, type of hypnotic suggestions (e.g., hyper- vs hypoalgesia), baseline pain levels, emotional comorbidities, mental imagery skills, and hypnotic susceptibility may influence the efficacy of hypnotic treatment and should be considered when tailoring the intervention. Based on secondary outcomes research from studies reviewed in the previous section, we summarize the empirical findings regarding the link between individual and treatment-level factors and response to hypnosis.

Practice

While few studies considered the role of consistent practice in treatment outcomes, the current evidence suggests that practice frequency does not have a significant effect on changes in pain. In one previously described study, Tan et al. (2015) found a weak and nonsignificant association between self-hypnosis home practice frequency and pain reduction. Given that all participants in the hypnosis conditions reported some level of practicing, authors speculated minimal consistent practice may be necessary to have a beneficial impact. Similarly, in discussing their findings that the benefits of hypnosis did not last beyond hospital discharge, Ardigo et al. (2016) inferred this was due to the fact that few individuals continued to practice self-hypnosis after 3 months. Further research needs to be done to confirm this hypothesis but, the evidence suggests the value of postdischarge intervention such as reminders and audio recordings for home practice.

Nonetheless, Gulewitsch and Schlarb (2017) found marginal evidence that treatment adherence (self-hypnosis practice) during the first month predicts treatment outcomes reported by parents at follow-up. Across groups, both parents and children affirmed the usefulness of daily practice with the audio CD. At the same time, roughly 30% of participants dropped out, which could be related to a variety of factors including the demand inherent in practicing daily over a 12-week period. Hence, shorter practice intervals may influence the extent to which patients engage in treatment. Lee et al. (2021) reported a trend toward greater health-related quality of life in patients who practiced self-hypnosis consistently. Researchers in the same study elicited feedback from participants who shared requests for shorter home practice recordings, which may have improved patient compliance.

Brain Activity

Research suggests that certain neural patterns lay the foundation for achieving successful responses to hypnotic analgesia. One study used electroencephalogram (EEG) to compare a single session of four nonpharmacological pain treatments and a control sham transcranial direct current stimulation (tDCS) procedure in 30 individuals with SCI (Jensen et al., 2013). Each nonpharmacological pain treatment produced neural patterns that differed from one another. Specifically, subjects who received hypnosis training showed greater increases in both theta and alpha activity (cortical slowing), and significant decreases in gamma. Using data from their previous study,

Jensen et al. (2014) attempted to predict pain reduction on the basis of measured differences in baseline EEG activity prior to a single session of neurofeedback, meditation, tDCS, and hypnosis. More baseline theta power significantly predicted greater response to hypnotic analgesia. Thus, evidence suggests that different patients respond differently to pain treatments, and variances in treatment responses are dependent upon specific brain states (e.g., higher levels of theta activity).

In a later study, Jensen et al. (2018) tested and found support for these inferences after delivering two interventions (mindfulness meditation or neurofeedback) hypothesized to increase slow-wave activity in individuals with multiple sclerosis. Thus, there are implications for enhancing pain treatment by modifying patient neural activity in preparation for hypnosis and/or matching patients to treatment according to their brain wave patterns. Specifically, evidence for greater slow-wave activation following hypnotic analgesia, signal the importance of inducing a state of relaxation for optimal response (Rainville et al., 1999). Lastly, Abrahamsen et al. (2010) additionally revealed that changes in pain intensity and unpleasantness produced by hypnotically induced hypo- and hyperalgesia are associated with distinctive brain activation patterns that differ significantly from patient to control.

Suggestibility
Attempts to predict outcomes determined by individual differences in hypnotic suggestibility largely found nonsignificant associations, but the evidence still appears mixed. Several trials demonstrated that hypnotizability was not significantly associated with treatment outcome (Abrahamsen et al., 2009; Jensen et al., 2009; Tan et al., 2015). Conversely, Abrahamsen et al. (2010) observed significant correlations between hypnotic susceptibility scores and reduced unpleasantness, implying that the more likely a person is to respond to hypnotic suggestions, the greater reduction in unpleasantness ratings. Similarly, one trial revealed that hypnotizability scores were positively correlated with reduced impact of fibromyalgia on patients' lives and improved affective quality of pain. Another study found that both hypnotic susceptibility and vividness of mental imagery have a moderating effect in hypnosis and relaxation treatments (Gay et al., 2002). Researchers concluded that patients with strong mental imagery and hypnosis abilities will experience more sustainable benefits from hypnosis and relaxation than those with poor imagery or hypnosis skills. Nonetheless, assessing hypnotizability/suggestibility is clinically relevant given that it may help to distinguish between those who respond readily to hypnosis and those who may need additional training or support.

Type of Pain Condition/Baseline Characteristics
Variation across pain conditions and baseline pain-related metrics may be associated with treatment efficacy. As was previously mentioned, Jensen et al. (2009) discovered that patients with neuropathic chronic pain were more likely than patients with nonneuropathic pain to respond to hypnosis, suggesting that hypnosis may be more or less effective for different types of pain problems. What's more, Gulewitsch and Schlarb (2017) found that children/adolescents lost to follow-up in their abdominal pain study reported higher baseline pain severity and more emotional problems, indicating that this group may require more intensive or individualized treatment. Furthermore, another trial in children with IBS/FAP, revealed that being male, shorter duration of symptoms, and having fewer negative beliefs about the abdominal pain predicted treatment success (Rutten et al., 2017). The majority of controlled studies do not include analyses of baseline characteristics, and patients still find benefit from hypnosis despite differences in pain scores at baseline.

Suggestion and Induction
There have been inconsistencies in the field regarding whether or not a formal hypnotic induction is necessary for suggestions to be effective and if variation in type of suggestion impacts results as well. Derbyshire et al. (2017) observed activation patterns in both groups were more marked after a hypnotic induction procedure—which is consistent with other evidence that the induction procedure has a small but possibly significant effect on an individual's responsiveness to suggestion.

With respect to suggestion, Abrahamsen et al. (2010) evidenced that hypnotic suggestions of increased (hyperalgesia) and/or decreased (hypoalgesia) pain intensity alter temporomandibular disorder (TMD) patient's perception of pain and unpleasantness. Similarly, the hypnosis group in another study was given individually tailored pain coping suggestions and only found a statistically relevant effect for the hypnosis condition compared with control condition (relaxation; Abrahamsen et al., 2009). Furthermore, they observed no change among controls, but saw a significant increase in the use of the pain coping strategy "reinterpreting pain sensations" in the hypnosis group during and after treatment. Comparably, Ahmad (2015) tailored inductions with specific analgesia suggestions based upon patient's needs. Patients in the hypnotherapy group reported significant improvement in pain interference, implying that customized suggestions to patient need are associated with treatment efficacy.

Lastly, Gulewitsch and Schlarb (2017) concluded that hypnotherapeutic metaphors focused on the gut region in children/adolescents with IBS/FAP are probably not necessary for effective pain relief and might even contribute to maintenance of the symptoms in a home-based setting. Unlike the gut-directed group, the unspecific hypnosis condition received suggestions for relaxation and ego-strengthening, which evidenced superiority in terms of pain intensity reduction. Another trial compared the relative effects of analgesic suggestions and relaxation suggestions on fibromyalgia pain, finding that suggestions of analgesia have a greater effect on the intensity of pain (sensory component) and the unpleasantness (affective component) of pain than hypnosis followed by suggestions of relaxation (Castel et al., 2007). Conversely, Castel et al. (2009) concluded that hypnosis with analgesic suggestions (i.e., imagining a cool blue treatment soothing body parts) appeared more effective on the affective (unpleasantness) dimension of pain than on the sensory (intensity) dimension, implying that different suggestions benefit different aspects of pain.

Used in Combination
How can hypnosis best be combined with other therapies? Hypnosis used in combination with other forms of psychological intervention has been understudied in clinical trials of chronic pain. One controlled trial demonstrated that patients with fibromyalgia who received CBT plus hypnosis showed slightly more benefit to pain intensity than the CBT-alone condition, however between-group differences were not significant (Castel et al., 2009). Ferrando et al. (2012) reported similar results, in that CBT plus hypnosis significantly improved pain and emotional distress outcomes in TMD patients when compared with standard treatment alone (splint use education, jaw exercises, and pharmacological support).

Delivery Format (Number, Duration, Frequency, Setting)
Several controlled trials provided evidence that the success of hypnosis is not limited to the traditional treatment format of hypnosis guided by a therapist in an individual treatment setting. For example, the results from one study suggested that effective hypnotic interventions can be delivered without provider contact (i.e., remotely), increasing accessibility to chronic pain treatment for hard-to-reach populations (Gulewitsch & Schlarb, 2017). Similarly, Grøndahl and Rosvold (2008) demonstrated the efficacy and feasibility of delivering hypnosis in general practice settings for patients with chronic widespread pain, while Ardigo et al. (2016) found significant reduction in pain intensity when delivered during hospitalization. What's more, hypnosis for chronic pain has been delivered in trials with observed benefit in group formats as well as in relatively brief time periods. In fact, results from one study provided support to the efficacy of hypnotic analgesia as a brief (effects in as

few as two sessions) nonpharmacological treatment in the management of chronic low back pain (Tan et al., 2015). Similarly, meaningful changes were observed following brief hypnosis interventions of only four sessions in another study (Abrahamsen et al., 2009). Both Castel et al. (2009) and Rizzo et al. (2018) found support for the superiority of hypnosis as an intervention offered in group settings.

Additional Factors

Few controlled trials assessed whether or not treatment expectations and pain coping strategies influenced the efficacy of hypnosis treatment. Nonetheless, Jensen et al. (2009) reported that expectations of treatment were not associated with outcome in treatment of neuropathic pain. Furthermore, another trial found that treatment expectations were similar across groups at all assessment points, concluding that the expectation of improvement does not have a biased effect on the findings (Gulewitsch & Schlarb, 2017). With regard to pain coping, Vanhaudenhuyse et al. (2018) revealed that a better sense of control over pain was more important in predicting treatment outcomes for patients included in the self-hypnosis/self-care group than the control group. Hence, mobilizing patient resources to physically move and reinforcing sense of self-worth might be important aspects of suggestion for patients with chronic pain.

Several limitations of the above-reviewed controlled studies are important to consider, including (a) numbers of patients in the majority of described trials are low (limiting power to detect statistical differences), (b) hypnotic interventions varied widely between studies, (c) baseline characteristics differed between control and experimental groups in several studies, (d) control conditions may have used components of hypnosis, (e) many studies used cross-sectional designs or were exploratory, and (f) a few studies were controlled but did not randomize comparator groups. In general, the number of controlled studies are limited, and this highlights the need for more research.

In the following section, we further explore how to modify specific components of hypnosis (e.g., inductions, suggestions) from the outset through a case example of an individual with a common chronic pain condition.

CASE EXAMPLE

This is a case of a 35-year-old woman referred for chronic low back and leg pain secondary to arachnoiditis after subarachnoid hemorrhage (SAH). At intake, the client reported long-standing history of depression and IBS, both of which improved on and off during periods of low job stress. Up to this point, she had tried various interventions for symptom relief, including medications, stem cell transplant, and physical therapy, without significant positive results. Having undergone several procedures and assessments from different specialists, she noted feeling a sense of hopelessness about her prognosis. Shortly after referral and initiating additional services at our clinic, including individual psychotherapy, she declared bankruptcy from medical debt, making it especially difficult to engage in an integrative treatment plan. Arguably as a last resort, the client was recommended to work with a nonbilling provider to learn self-hypnosis for pain management. Hence, the client began working with the second author of this chapter, a postdoctoral fellow in psychology, to complete eight sessions of a self-hypnosis for chronic pain protocol (Jensen, 2011).

During the first session, she described chronic and persistent pain, numbness, debilitating spasms/muscle cramps, and a characteristic burning pain in both her lower back and legs. As a result of these symptoms, the client experienced significant interference with work, relationships (especially with her husband), and quality of life. Furthermore, she described herself as a passionate musician, making a career for herself as director of a local music program. While she previously found immense joy in this work, daily physical pain restricted her ability to teach full-time and caused her to feel "burned out." Thus, her primary goal was to improve symptoms that impaired daily functioning, and ultimately to balance her health care needs with larger work and life-related goals.

Biopsychosocial Approach to Treatment

Consistent with the biopsychosocial approach described previously, we assessed the biological, psychological, and social–environmental factors pertinent to this client's presentation to tailor treatment goals and target suggestions. This assessment is summarized in Figure 5.1 and outlined in detail thereafter.

Format of Sessions

Each session was similar in that it lasted 60 minutes, including 20 to 30 minutes of formal hypnosis that was audio-recorded and provided to the client to encourage daily practice between each appointment. However, hypnotic inductions and suggestions varied session to session to address the different components of her pain experience and its effects, which could change day-to-day. After an initial biopsychosocial evaluation of symptoms and goals, the client was introduced to the process of hypnosis, followed by identifying pleasant and unpleasant sensations, as well as exploring the qualities of a

FIGURE 5.1. Summary of Biopsychosocial Assessment

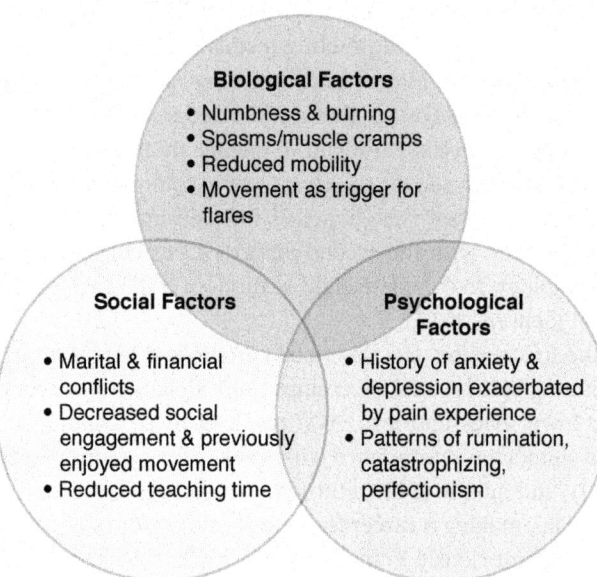

"favorite place" that she would be invited to visit in subsequent sessions for deepening. Next the therapist guided the client through an induction that typically involved progressive muscle relaxation (e.g., envisioning tension relief from the top of head to the bottom of feet) with subsequent suggestions tailored to the individual. Additional sessions began with reviewing and exploring home practice and collaboratively addressing thoughts, concerns, and/or questions that the client had. The therapist used motivational interviewing techniques to reinforce her efforts to practice, as well as her insight to utilize the hypnosis skills to focus her attention in different ways. These techniques are informed by principles and protocols outlined by Patterson (2010) and Jensen (2011) for the use of hypnosis with chronic pain.

Biological

In evaluating biological components of pain, we considered the primary underlying pathophysiological mechanisms responsible for her condition, useful pharmacological treatments, physical symptoms she found most bothersome, and outlined what sensations felt pleasant or unpleasant. She noted muscle tension and guarding in response to pain. Given that her pain was driven by both neuropathic and musculoskeletal factors equally, suggestions were incorporated to modify pain control and lifestyle changes related to these mechanisms. Specifically, suggestions were designed to facilitate increased comfort and acceptance of all sensations. For example, using the metaphor of a radio dial to turn down pain volume noting that *"as your comfort grows . . . any feelings or sensations of discomfort just seem to be drifting farther and farther away and becoming smaller and smaller."* In one session, the client was excited to share that while practicing over the last week, she effectively turned down the volume on painful sensations from callouses she frequently acquired from playing her instrument. While not specific to leg or back pain, it demonstrated her ability to apply these suggestions in various areas of her life. Lastly, although we did not measure her baseline hypnotizability level, administering a scale of hypnotizability might be useful to some clinicians as a means of informing tailored treatment strategies to varying mind styles. One potential would be the Elkins Hypnotizability Scale, which has been developed for clinical settings and can be conducted in approximately 20 minutes (Elkins, 2013).

Psychological
With respect to psychological functioning, we identified both adaptive and maladaptive thought patterns and coping strategies and later targeted these for increased or decreased use similar to the approach for painful sensations. Suggestions encouraged a shift from maladaptive beliefs (*"I can't do anything because of pain"*), coping and cognitive processes (e.g., catastrophizing, perfectionism), to more helpful and reassuring ones. Some of the sessions were split to provide psychoeducation and discuss the relationship between her pain and mood, as well as how pain impacted cognition and beliefs. Specifically, we spent one session identifying automatic negative thinking patterns, which included a daily thought record for homework. In a subsequent session, we reviewed the thoughts she had tracked, all of which related to teaching music. Positive thoughts included *"I am a clever problem-solver"* and negative thoughts included *"I am an ineffective teacher."* As a result of completing this exercise, the client noted gaining insight into how experiences before pain influenced her presently, stating, *"my mom catastrophizes everything."* We then identified thoughts she wanted to have that were realistic, reassuring, and helpful and incorporated them into suggestions to increase frequency and automaticity. Hence, one particular session concluded by conducting hypnosis with suggestions to bring to her awareness thoughts about her body, sensations, and coping. Moreover, our final session used a time progress suggestion to increase adaptive pain-related thought content.

The client's emotional history (anxiety and depression) and reactivity was also targeted in treatment. Given her increasing stress as well as features of obsessive–compulsive disorder, including time and focus spent on dietary modifications and rumination over her financial situation, we first focused on learning to relax and calm the regulatory system, and then on learning to change the relationship she had with anxiety. Similar to biological processes, we incorporated suggestions around decreasing anxiety-related bodily distress—dialing down anxiety and experiencing how her physiological body could shift. We used visual imagery to soften tension in the body (preference for warm vs. cold), such as feeling the sun's rays, and as the rays touched each tense body part, feeling the release of tension. Lastly, we developed a "favorite place" to build and establish a space she could take with her that brings a sense of comfort and calm. Posthypnotic cues of taking a deep breath and/or noticing ruminating behavior were used to help her come back to the safe place outside of sessions. While visualizing this place in one session, the client became noticeably tearful and after alerting, she folded forward with her hands in her lap to cry. While processing later she stated, "that was really intense for me" and explained the experience had reminded her of what it was like to be genuinely happy and made her sad to think about how long pain had dictated her life.

Social–Environmental

When they are perceived as supportive, social relationships and the patient's environment have the potential to enhance patient coping and quality of life or be detrimental. Social–environmental factors played an important role in this client's pain experience, as she was prone to withdraw from relationships, activities, and physical movement that used to feel meaningful due to pain. We began by focusing on her core values—how would her current lifestyle be different if her pain could be managed more effectively? The client reported that she would be able to engage more with her music work and have stronger relationships. Then we targeted suggestions to focus on participation in meaningful activities. For instance, this client reported that she hadn't felt able to sit through church service in some time, engage in yoga without flaring her symptoms, or go hiking with her husband without conflict. Therefore, having her visualize how she wanted to be and how she wanted to respond to pain, anxiety, and depression during trance was an important component of treatment. Recalibrating and connecting again to her values through suggestions for ego-strengthening and self-confidence were also employed. For example, reflecting that, *"every day you will develop much more confidence in yourself. . . . More confidence in your ability to do what you need to do or want to do to achieve your most valued goals."*

Results

Overall, this case took a layered biopsychosocial approach to suggestions that in brief included pain reduction, enhanced coping, and core values.

After the first session, she reported developing new awareness of just how tense she was throughout the day, especially while driving. Additionally, she reported a better sense of control over pain and improvement in her marital relationship as a result. Nearly one year later, she wrote to this provider stating, *"I am happy to say I am doing well. I haven't been diligent about practicing regularly, but I do practice sporadically, and I think my awareness of my bracing and tension is still heightened from our sessions. Also, my yoga practices have been totally different and better since working together."*

HYPNOSIS PROTOCOL

The following hypnosis protocol includes a script for a general induction and hypnotic suggestions that can be applied to a wide variety of chronic pain problems.

Induction

"Okay . . . just settling back . . . and allowing the eyes to close if that feels comfortable or focusing a soft gaze on a spot on the floor . . . that's right . . .

I'm going to talk to you for a while . . . all you have to do is listen to what I'm saying and consider allowing yourself to feel more comfortable and relaxed than you might expect in this moment . . . beginning by adjusting yourself to whatever position feels most comfortable for you . . . maybe sitting feels best, . . . or maybe lying down . . . knowing that throughout the time you're listening to my voice, you can adjust yourself to a different position to help yourself be comfortable, and this will not interrupt your concentration or ability to maintain a deep state of comfortable relaxation.

So, you've come here this afternoon, and you're making yourself comfortable now . . . that's right . . . listening to the sound of my voice, and already beginning to get a sense of how deeply you can relax here today . . .

Maybe you can notice how much more comfortable you can feel by taking a big, deep, satisfying breath. Go ahead . . . draw a deep, satisfying breath into your belly . . . gently hold the breath for as long as it feels comfortable . . . and let it go.

Repeat that process again, inhaling deeply into your belly . . . holding it for a moment . . . and letting it go.

Allowing the whole body to relax. . . . Allowing all the muscles to go limp. . . . Maybe noticing that where there was once tension in your body, your muscles have become a little softer . . . as you exhale, you might notice more space between your shoulders and ears . . . notice how comfortable your eyes can feel when they close . . . and when they close, just let them rest closed . . . that's right, just noticing . . . beginning to sink in a little more . . . and perhaps as you sit there, listening to me, you might begin to notice a pleasant feeling of drowsiness.

Maybe beginning to notice the top of your head is feeling more relaxed and comfortable . . .

Letting that relaxation and comfort spread down through your fore-head, over your eyelids, into your jaw, down the neck, deep, relaxing, and comfortably . . . letting this sensation of comfort spread down through your shoulders, deep, warm, and heavy . . . moving gently down your entire body . . .

You already know how to relax, don't you? . . . And because you already know how to relax, you can relax even deeper here today as you listen to the sound of my voice . . . breathing in and out, listening to my voice . . . ."

Deepening

"In a moment I am going to count from one to ten. With each number I count, you will find yourself becoming deeper and deeper relaxed. The larger the number . . . the more comfortable you can feel. . . . The number 10 being a signal to your brain to become profoundly comfortable, deeply relaxed . . . breathing in and out, listening to my voice . . . let's begin now.

One . . . starting to focus more on your comfort . . . you might already be noticing a sense of warmth or heaviness, a sense of the muscles letting go even more.

Two . . . one level into deeper comfort . . . breathing in and out, listening to my voice . . .

Three . . . deeper into yourself . . . focusing more and more on the sound of my voice without even trying . . .

Four . . . perhaps noticing places in your body beginning to relax more and more. . . . You might even notice a restful heaviness in your forehead beginning to spread and flow . . . down, across your eyes, your face, down into your mouth and jaw, moving into your neck, deep, restful, heavy . . .

Five . . . halfway there now . . .

Six . . . allowing that sense of comfort to move down the muscles of the left arm, into the left hand, left fingertips . . . then the right arm, the right hand, the right fingertips . . . that's right, gently relaxing the muscles of the arms . . .

Seven . . . maybe starting to notice that all the sounds that once were distracting or pulling you away from this experience . . . are now becoming a part of your experience of comfort and relaxation . . . gently *fading into the background . . . anything you can notice becomes a part of your experience of comfort and relaxation . . .*

Eight . . . that's right . . . how easy and effortless it is to relax more and more, more and more . . . so much so that the relaxation spreads down your spine, wrapping around your abdomen . . . warm, pleasant sensation . . .

Nine . . . allowing yourself to relax more and more . . . comfort moving across your hips, down, heavy down, into the left leg, left foot . . . right leg, right foot. . . . Noticing your whole body, from head to toe, comfort washing over you as you move into a deeply relaxed state at your own pace. Almost there . . .

Ten . . . deeply and profoundly relaxed now . . . taking a moment to notice what it feels like to be here . . . not a care in the world . . . breathing in and out . . . listening to the sound of my voice."

Safe Place

"Now there may have been a time and a place in your life where you've felt perfectly relaxed, and perfectly at ease. And I wonder if you're able to get a sense of that right now? (pause for several seconds to allow them to call to mind this place)

If nothing comes to you right away, that's perfectly alright. Call to mind a place that you know you could feel comfortable and at ease . . . settling into this place now . . .

Notice what you are able to see in front of you, really notice what you can see . . . (pause about 5 seconds) *the colors . . . the view. . . . Now notice what you are able to hear . . .* (pause about 5 seconds) *. . . perhaps the sounds that are closer to you, and then picking up on the ones further in the distance.*

Notice what you can smell and taste (pause about 5 seconds)

What do you feel in this place? (pause about 5 seconds) *perhaps the temperature is just right . . . maybe you notice a softness in your body . . . the absence of tension . . .*

As you become more and more absorbed into your state of comfort . . . looking around again, taking in the small details around you. Noticing any new sensations, smells, sounds . . .

Taking a another big, deep, breath now . . . then letting it all the way out, and as you do, just let yourself sink even deeper, into an even more profound level of relaxation. And as you are deeply comfortable in this place, taking several additional deep breaths. Notice how calm you feel,

how peaceful this is, and enjoying the pleasurable experience . . . breathing
in and out, listening to my voice . . ."

Suggestions

"Now we're going to talk to that powerful resource, that part of your brain
that allows your heart to beat without you having to think about it; it
allows you to breathe, easy and comfortably, naturally and automatically,
without asking it to do so; it even allows the hair to grow on your body
without you having to will it to do so . . . and I wonder in what ways
this resource will serve you today? I wonder in what ways your mind can
help you to feel more comfortable, more at ease? Breathing in and out,
listening to my voice . . .

Maybe it's a nice cool soothing liquid . . . a treatment of some kind
starting at the top of your spine working its way down your lower back and
spreading throughout your body, acting on the places that feel uncomfort-
able, painful . . . it might even feel like your pain disappears altogether . . .
or perhaps you just find that you aren't thinking about your comfort level
any longer. Breathing in and out, listening to my voice . . .

Or maybe you can imagine that in your mind there's a dimmer switch
of some kind, and you can turn down the feeling of pain in your body
like turning down the dial on a radio . . . you can turn it up or down. . . .
I wonder what it feels like to imagine that now . . . those unpleasant sensa-
tions changing . . . (pause for a few seconds) *. . . I don't know what's going*
to happen or how your mind is going to serve you today, but I do know
you'll feel surprisingly more comfortable . . . more at ease. . . . It may be
that you simply forget about the pain; that the amount of time you have
experienced discomfort dramatically shifts, and you look back in time and
have difficulty remembering exactly when it bothered you . . .

Breathing in and out, listening to my voice . . .

Yes, your mind can serve you in a number of unusual ways. . . . It may be
that you find yourself placing your discomfort in a box and locking it with
a key. Then picking that box of discomfort up and placing it in another
box . . . then locking that one. Then continuing to do this until the dis-
comfort is soooo muffled . . . so muffled in fact that you barely notice it.
Just notice what that feels like in your body . . . then I wonder what happens if
you send this series of boxes out to sea or to space miles and miles away . . .
watching the discomfort disappear into the distance . . .

I wonder how pleasant that feels . . . noticing how the pleasant and
comfortable sensations just wash over everything. Such a pleasure to be
able to experience . . . to bring about such comfort.

Breathing in and out, listening to my voice . . .

These areas of your body are feeling more and more comfortable as the feelings of comfort spread. And I wonder what lessons this resource in your mind will give you today . . . your body knows . . . and you might find that somewhere inside of you, you will find the motivation, the confidence to start doing the things that make you feel better . . . that allow you to take care of your body. . . . I don't know what you will do, and part of you may not know either. Yet, your body knows, and won't it be interesting to see how you start taking better care of yourself? And won't it also be nice to notice that you are far less bothered by things?

Breathing in and out, listening to my voice . . .

And I want to remind you that any comfortable sensations that you are experiencing right now . . . those sensations . . . and this experience of comfort . . . can remain with you, for minutes, hours, days . . . and years . . . you can call upon that automatic resource we all have in our brains at any time. . . . Long after you listen to these ideas. . . . And your eyes are open and you start thinking about something else, the feelings of comfort can remain with you . . . always there . . . longer and longer, stronger and stronger, automatically and easily. Just drifting comfortably, your eyes remain closed . . ."

Posthypnotic Suggestions

"And now we have reached the time to extend what has been most useful to you in this session into the rest of your day, and your daily life . . .

And now, while you are still here absorbing the experience, before we make our way back together. . . . Notice how your body feels. So deeply comfortable. Remembering that you can return to this feeling at any time, and how easy it will be to do so. All you will need to do is listen to the recording or even close your eyes, take a big deep satisfying breath, and you will be right back here . . . safe, comfortable, relaxed . . . your mind will be able to use these skills, automatically, so that you can create comfort and relaxation, and an inner strength, whenever you need it.

And as we begin to return to the room and a state of alertness . . . I want you to remember that the process does not stop at the point you find your eyes opening.

Now . . . getting ready to return. You are looking at the number 10 in front of you. And in a moment, I am going to start counting with you as we move back up into a state of alertness, from 10 to 1. With each number I count you will feel more alert, awake, and refreshed.

Breathing in and out, listening to my voice . . .

Let's begin now." (beginning to speak in a more alert tone)

Alerting

"Ten. Perhaps you can see the number, right in front of you.

Nine, slowly going upward, becoming more and more awake, more and more refreshed.

Eight, even more awake . . . noticing your body, perhaps gently moving your fingers and toes.

Seven . . . and six.

And now, picturing the room around you . . . what it looks like . . . the colors in the walls and ceiling, the textures in the carpet and chairs.

Five, more and more awake, more and more refreshed.

Four, that's right, more and more alert. Feeling profoundly relaxed, but also alert and refreshed, and perhaps energized.

Three . . . two . . . and, when we reach the final number, your eyes will stay closed for a bit longer, and you will find them open only when you are ready to become alert and complete with your experience . . . and now . . .

One."

CONCLUSION

It should be noted that current evidence is both promising and methodologically limited. No single trial definitively supports the use of hypnosis for *all* patients with chronic pain, and the heterogeneity of current studies remains a challenge to identifying specific characteristics of either the hypnotic intervention or the patients themselves that lead to optimal benefit. The existing evidence does suggest that hypnosis may be an effective intervention to improve the distress, intensity, disability, and interference associated with chronic pain. Although nociceptive and nociplastic pain conditions seem to receive more attention in empirical trials, the literature suggests that hypnosis may have a greater impact on neuropathic pain than nociceptive and nociplastic conditions (Jensen et al., 2009). Having said that, there is research support for the positive role of hypnosis to treat nociceptive pain conditions (e.g., temporomandibular disorders, Crohn's disease, chronic low back pain, and hemophilia) and nociplastic pain disorders (e.g., fibromyalgia, irritable bowel syndrome, and chronic widespread pain).

There are also benefits to patients that extend beyond pain relief, including improved sleep and well-being following hypnosis. The findings of controlled studies reviewed in this chapter are echoed by previous reviews including controlled and uncontrolled studies (e.g., Dillworth & Jensen, 2010; Hammond, 2010; Jensen & Patterson, 2006). Consistent across most systematic reviews is the observation that we still do not know for whom hypnotic intervention works best and which of the many possible hypnotic protocols produce the most benefit.

Additionally, there is some evidence to suggest that a combination of suggestions (pain-specific and otherwise) may best suit chronic pain populations (Dillworth & Jensen, 2010), and varying suggestions to meet the complex needs of pain presentations is recommended (Jensen & Patterson, 2014).

At the same time, results across studies varied, and thus the specific needs and individual characteristics important to treatment outcome are likely unique to each person. Therefore, in working with chronic pain cases, a biopsychosocial assessment is ideal when possible to inform treatment (Patterson, 2010). This will help to facilitate a treatment plan and generate suggestions unique to the individual and their circumstances.

REFERENCES

Abrahamsen, R., Dietz, M., Lodahl, S., Roepstorff, A., Zachariae, R., Østergaard, L., & Svensson, P. (2010). Effect of hypnotic pain modulation on brain activity in patients with temporomandibular disorder pain. *Pain, 151*(3), 825–833. https://doi.org/10.1016/j.pain.2010.09.020

Abrahamsen, R., Zachariae, R., & Svensson, P. (2009). Effect of hypnosis on oral function and psychological factors in temporomandibular disorders patients. *Journal of Oral Rehabilitation, 36*(8), 556–570. https://doi.org/10.1111/j.1365-2842.2009.01974.x

Ahmad, T. S. (2015). Hypnotherapy and accupressure for brachial neuralgia. *BMC Proceedings, 9*(S3), A82. https://doi.org/10.1186/1753-6561-9-S3-A82

Ardigo, S., Herrmann, F. R., Moret, V., Déramé, L., Giannelli, S., Gold, G., & Pautex, S. (2016). Hypnosis can reduce pain in hospitalized older patients: A randomized controlled study. *BMC Geriatrics, 16*(1), 14. https://doi.org/10.1186/s12877-016-0180-y

Bhatt, R. R., Martin, S. R., Evans, S., Lung, K., Coates, T. D., Zeltzer, L. K., & Tsao, J. C. (2017). The effect of hypnosis on pain and peripheral blood flow in sickle-cell disease: A pilot study. *Journal of Pain Research, 10*, 1635–1644. https://doi.org/10.2147/JPR.S131859

Castel, A., Cascón, R., Padrol, A., Sala, J., & Rull, M. (2012). Multicomponent cognitive-behavioral group therapy with hypnosis for the treatment of fibromyalgia: Long-term outcome. *The Journal of Pain, 13*(3), 255–265. https://doi.org/10.1016/j.jpain.2011.11.005

Castel, A., Pérez, M., Sala, J., Padrol, A., & Rull, M. (2007). Effect of hypnotic suggestion on fibromyalgic pain: Comparison between hypnosis and relaxation. *European Journal of Pain, 11*(4), 463–468. https://doi.org/10.1016/j.ejpain.2006.06.006

Castel, A., Salvat, M., Sala, J., & Rull, M. (2009). Cognitive-behavioural group treatment with hypnosis: A randomized pilot trail in fibromyalgia. *Contemporary Hypnosis, 26*(1), 48–59. https://doi.org/10.1002/ch.372

Clauw, D. J., Essex, M. N., Pitman, V., & Jones, K. D. (2019). Reframing chronic pain as a disease, not a symptom: Rationale and implications for pain management. *Postgraduate Medicine, 131*(3), 185–198. https://doi.org/10.1080/00325481.2019.1574403

Dahlhamer, J., Lucas, J., Zelaya, C., Nahin, R., Mackey, S., DeBar, L., Kerns, R., Von Korff, M., Porter, L., & Helmick, C. (2018). Prevalence of chronic pain and high-impact chronic pain among adults–United States, 2016. *MMWR Morbidity and Mortality Weekly Report, 67*(36), 1001–1006. https://doi.org/10.15585/mmwr.mm6736a2

Derbyshire, S. W., Whalley, M. G., Seah, S. T., & Oakley, D. A. (2017). Suggestions to reduce clinical fibromyalgia pain and experimentally induced pain produce parallel effects on perceived pain but divergent functional MRI-based brain activity. *Psychosomatic Medicine, 79*(2), 189–200. https://doi.org/10.1097/PSY.0000000000000370

Dillworth, T., & Jensen, M. P. (2010). The role of suggestions in hypnosis for chronic pain: A review of the literature. *The Open Pain Journal, 3*(1), 39–51. https://doi.org/10.2174/1876386301003010039

Elkins, G. (2013). *Hypnotic relaxation therapy: Principles and applications.* Springer.

Ferrando, M., Galdón, M. J., Durá, E., Andreu, Y., Jiménez, Y., & Poveda, R. (2012). Enhancing the efficacy of treatment for temporomandibular patients with muscular diagnosis through cognitive-behavioral intervention, including hypnosis: A randomized study. *Oral Surgery, Oral Medicine, Oral Pathology and Oral Radiology, 113*(1), 81–89. https://doi.org/10.1016/j.tripleo.2011.08.020

Fialka, V., Korpan, M., Saradeth, T., Paternostro-Slugo, T., Hexel, O., Frischenschlager, O., & Ernst, E. (1996). Autogenic training for reflex sympathetic dystrophy: A pilot study. *Complementary Therapies in Medicine, 4*(2), 103–105. https://doi.org/10.1016/S0965-2299(96)80026-4

Freynhagen, R., Parada, H. A., Calderon-Ospina, C. A., Chen, J., Rakhmawati Emril, D., Fernández-Villacorta, F. J., Franco, H., Ho, K. Y., Lara-Solares, A., Li, C. C.-F., Mimenza Alvarado, A., Nimmaanrat, S., Dolma Santos, M., & Ciampi de Andrade, D. (2019). Current understanding of the mixed pain concept: A brief narrative review. *Current Medical Research and Opinion, 35*(6), 1011–1018. https://doi.org/10.1080/03007995.2018.1552042

Gaskin, D. J., & Richard, P. (2012). The economic costs of pain in the United States. *The Journal of Pain, 13*(8), 715–724. https://doi.org/10.1016/j.jpain.2012.03.009

Gatchel, R. J., Peng, Y. B., Peters, M. L., Fuchs, P. N., & Turk, D. C. (2007). The biopsychosocial approach to chronic pain: Scientific advances and future directions. *Psychological Bulletin, 133*(4), 581–624. https://doi.org/10.1037/0033-2909.133.4.581

Gay, M.-C., Philippot, P., & Luminet, O. (2002). Differential effectiveness of psychological interventions for reducing osteoarthritis pain: A comparison of Erickson hypnosis and Jacobson relaxation. *European Journal of Pain, 6*(1), 1–16. https://doi.org/10.1053/eujp.2001.0263

Grøndahl, J. R., & Rosvold, E. O. (2008). Hypnosis as a treatment of chronic wide-spread pain in general practice: A randomized controlled pilot trial. *BMC Musculo-skeletal Disorders, 9*(1), 124. https://doi.org/10.1186/1471-2474-9-124

Gulewitsch, M. D., & Schlarb, A. A. (2017). Comparison of gut-directed hypnotherapy and unspecific hypnotherapy as self-help format in children and adolescents with functional abdominal pain or irritable bowel syndrome: A randomized pilot study. *European Journal of Gastroenterology & Hepatology, 29*(12), 1351–1360. https://doi.org/10.1097/MEG.0000000000000984

Hammond, D. C. (2010). Hypnosis in the treatment of anxiety- and stress-related disorders. *Expert Review of Neurotherapeutics, 10*(2), 263–273. https://doi.org/10.1586/ern.09.140

IASP Task Force on Taxonomy. (2017, December 14). *IASP terminology*. International Association for the Study of Pain. https://www.iasp-pain.org/Education/Content.aspx?ItemNumber=1698#Pain

Institute of Medicine. (2011). *Relieving pain in America: A blueprint for transforming prevention, care, education, and research*. National Academies Press. https://doi.org/10.17226/13172

Jensen, M. P. (2011). *Hypnosis for chronic pain management: Therapist guide*. Oxford University Press.

Jensen, M. P., Barber, J., Romano, J. M., Hanley, M. A., Raichle, K. A., Molton, I. R., Engel, J. M., Osborne, T. L., Stoelb, B. L., Cardenas, D. D., & Patterson, D. R. (2009). Effects of self-hypnosis training and EMG biofeedback relaxation training on chronic pain in persons with spinal-cord injury. *International Journal of Clinical and Experimental Hypnosis, 57*(3), 239–268. https://doi.org/10.1080/00207140902881007

Jensen, M. P., Battalio, S. L., Chan, J. F., Edwards, K. A., Day, M. A., Sherlin, L. H., & Ehde, D. M. (2018). Use of neurofeedback and mindfulness to enhance response to hypnosis treatment in individuals with multiple sclerosis: Results from a pilot ran-domized clinical trial. *International Journal of Clinical and Experimental Hypnosis, 66*(3), 231–264. https://doi.org/10.1080/00207144.2018.1460546

Jensen, M. P., Mendoza, M. E., Ehde, D. M., Patterson, D. R., Molton, I. R., Dillworth, T. M., Gertz, K. J., Chan, J., Hakimian, S., Battalio, S. L., & Ciol, M. A. (2020). Effects of hypnosis, cognitive therapy, hypnotic cognitive therapy, and pain education in adults with chronic pain: A randomized clinical trial. *Pain, 161*(10), 2284–2298. https://doi.org/10.1097/j.pain.0000000000001943

Jensen, M. P., & Patterson, D. R. (2006). Hypnotic treatment of chronic pain. *Journal of Behavioral Medicine, 29*(1), 95–124. https://doi.org/10.1007/s10865-005-9031-6

Jensen, M. P., & Patterson, D. R. (2014). Hypnotic approaches for chronic pain man-agement: Clinical implications of recent research findings. *American Psychologist, 69*(2), 167–177. https://doi.org/10.1037/a0035644

Jensen, M. P., Sherlin, L. H., Askew, R. L., Fregni, F., Witkop, G., Gianas, A., Howe, J. D., & Hakimian, S. (2013). Effects of non-pharmacological pain treatments on brain states. *Clinical Neurophysiology, 124*(10), 2016–2024. https://doi.org/10.1016/j.clinph.2013.04.009

Jensen, M. P., Sherlin, L. H., Fregni, F., Gianas, A., Howe, J. D., & Hakimian, S. (2014). Baseline brain activity predicts response to neuromodulatory pain treatment. *Pain Medicine, 15*(12), 2055–2063. https://doi.org/10.1111/pme.12546

Lee, A., Moulton, D., McKernan, L., Russell, A., Slaughter, J. C., Acra, S., & Walker, L. (2021). Clinical hypnosis in pediatric Crohn's disease: A randomized controlled pilot study. *Journal of Pediatric Gastroenterology and Nutrition, 72*(3), e63–e70. https://doi.org/10.1097/MPG.0000000000002980

Melzack, R. (2001). Pain and the neuromatrix in the brain. *Journal of Dental Education, 65*(12), 1378–1382. https://doi.org/10.1002/j.0022-0337.2001.65.12.tb03497.x

Paredes, A. C., Costa, P., Fernandes, S., Lopes, M., Carvalho, M., Almeida, A., & Pinto, P. R. (2019). Effectiveness of hypnosis for pain management and promotion of health-related quality-of-life among people with haemophilia: A randomised controlled pilot trial. *Scientific Reports, 9*(1), 13399. https://doi.org/10.1038/s41598-019-49827-1

Patterson, D. R. (2010). *Clinical hypnosis for pain control.* American Psychological Association. https://doi.org/10.1037/12128-000

Patterson, D. R., & Jensen, M. P. (2003). Hypnosis and clinical pain. *Psychological Bulletin, 129*(4), 495–521. https://doi.org/10.1037/0033-2909.129.4.495

Rainville, P., Hofbauer, R. K., Paus, T., Duncan, G. H., Bushnell, M. C., & Price, D. D. (1999). Cerebral mechanisms of hypnotic induction and suggestion. *Journal of Cognitive Neuroscience, 11*(1), 110–125. https://doi.org/10.1162/089892999563175

Razak, I., Chung, T. Y., & Ahmad, T. S. (2019). A comparative study of two modalities in pain management of patients presenting with chronic brachial neuralgia. *Journal of Alternative and Complementary Medicine, 25*(8), 861–867. https://doi.org/10.1089/acm.2019.0052

Rizzo, R. R. N., Medeiros, F. C., Pires, L. G., Pimenta, R. M., McAuley, J. H., Jensen, M. P., & Costa, L. O. P. (2018). Hypnosis enhances the effects of pain education in patients with chronic nonspecific low back pain: A randomized controlled trial. *The Journal of Pain, 19*(10), 1103.e1–1103.e9. https://doi.org/10.1016/j.jpain.2018.03.013

Rutten, J. M. T. M., Vlieger, A. M., Frankenhuis, C., George, E. K., Groeneweg, M., Norbruis, O. F., Tjon a Ten, W., van Wering, H. M., Dijkgraaf, M. G. W., Merkus, M. P., & Benninga, M. A. (2017). Home-based hypnotherapy self-exercises vs individual hypnotherapy with a therapist for treatment of pediatric irritable bowel syndrome, functional abdominal pain, or functional abdominal pain syndrome: A randomized clinical trial. *JAMA Pediatrics, 171*(5), 470–477. https://doi.org/10.1001/jamapediatrics.2017.0091

Tan, G., Rintala, D. H., Jensen, M. P., Fukui, T., Smith, D., & Williams, W. (2015). A randomized controlled trial of hypnosis compared with biofeedback for adults with chronic low back pain. *European Journal of Pain, 19*(2), 271–280. https://doi.org/10.1002/ejp.545

Tonye-Geoffroy, L., Mauboussin Carlos, S., Tuffet, S., Fromentin, H., Berard, L., Leblanc, J., & Laroche, F. (2021). Efficacy of a combination of hypnosis and transcutaneous electrical nerve stimulation for chronic non-cancer pain: A randomized controlled trial. *Journal of Advanced Nursing, 77*(6), 2875–2886. https://doi.org/10.1111/jan.14833

Treede, R.-D., Rief, W., Barke, A., Aziz, Q., Bennett, M. I., Benoliel, R., Cohen, M., Evers, S., Finnerup, N. B., First, M. B., Giamberardino, M. A., Kaasa, S., Korwisi, B., Kosek, E., Lavand'homme, P., Nicholas, M., Perrot, S., Scholz, J., Schug, S., . . . Wang, S. J. (2019). Chronic pain as a symptom or a disease: The IASP classification of chronic pain for the International Classification of Diseases (ICD-11). *Pain, 160*(1), 19–27. https://doi.org/10.1097/j.pain.0000000000001384

Vanhaudenhuyse, A., Gillet, A., Malaise, N., Salamun, I., Barsics, C., Grosdent, S., Maquet, D., Nyssen, A. S., & Faymonville, M. E. (2015). Efficacy and cost-effectiveness:

A study of different treatment approaches in a tertiary pain centre. *European Journal of Pain, 19*(10), 1437–1446. https://doi.org/10.1002/ejp.674

Vanhaudenhuyse, A., Gillet, A., Malaise, N., Salamun, I., Grosdent, S., Maquet, D., Nyssen, A. S., & Faymonville, M. E. (2018). Psychological interventions influence patients' attitudes and beliefs about their chronic pain. *Journal of Traditional and Complementary Medicine, 8*(2), 296–302. https://doi.org/10.1016/j.jtcme.2016.09.001

Weiss, A. J., Wier, L. M., Stocks, C., & Blanchard, J. (2014, June). Overview of emergency department visits in the United States, 2011 (Statistical Brief #174). In *HCUP statistical briefs: Healthcare cost and utilization project*, Agency for Healthcare Research and Quality (U.S.). https://www.ncbi.nlm.nih.gov/books/NBK235856/

Wiechman, S., McMullen, K., Carrougher, G., Baker, C., & Gibran, N. (2019). A randomized controlled trial of hypnosis for pain and itch following burn injury. Conference Abstract. *Journal of Burn Care & Research, 40*(Suppl. 1), S100. https://doi.org/10.1093/jbcr/irz013.166

Winocur, E., Gavish, A., Emodi-Perlman, A., Halachmi, M., & Eli, I. (2002). Hypnorelaxation as treatment for myofascial pain disorder: A comparative study. *Oral Surgery, Oral Medicine, Oral Pathology, Oral Radiology, 93*(4), 429–434. https://doi.org/10.1067/moe.2002.122587

Zale, E. L., & Ditre, J. W. (2015). Pain-related fear, disability, and the fear-avoidance model of chronic pain. *Current Opinion in Psychology, 5*, 24–30. https://doi.org/10.1016/j.copsyc.2015.03.014

6
APPLICATIONS OF HYPNOSIS IN BEHAVIORAL MEDICINE

GARY R. ELKINS AND MORGAN SNYDER

INTRODUCTION

Behavioral medicine is a "multidisciplinary field concerned with the development and integration of biomedical and behavioral knowledge relevant to health and disease, and the application of this knowledge to prevention, health promotion, diagnosis, treatment, rehabilitation, and care" (Dekker et al., 2017, p. 4). It has been increasingly recognized that behavioral interventions, such as hypnosis (Elkins et al., 2015), are an important aspect of treatment for many medical conditions, symptoms, and disorders.

Hypnosis has numerous applications in behavioral medicine in the treatment of medical and psychophysiological disorders. Research has demonstrated that hypnosis interventions are of benefit to individuals suffering from hypertension, cancer-related symptoms, menopause and hot flashes, irritable bowel syndrome (IBS), and sleep. The use of hypnosis in behavioral medicine may be as a stand-alone intervention or adjunctive, for these conditions. This chapter discusses research examining hypnosis interventions for aspects of behavioral medicine and the important characteristics of these hypnosis interventions.

https://doi.org/10.1037/0000347-006
Evidence-Based Practice in Clinical Hypnosis, L. S. Milling (Editor)

REVIEW OF OUTCOME RESEARCH

This section of the chapter reviews studies of five promising applications of clinical hypnosis in behavioral medicine.

Hypertension

It is estimated that approximately 45% of adults in the United States have hypertension (Centers for Disease Control and Prevention [CDC], 2020). Hypertension, or high blood pressure, occurs in two stages with Stage 1 being defined as systolic blood pressure at 130 to 139 mm Hg or diastolic blood pressure at 80 to 89 mm Hg and Stage 2 being defined as systolic blood pressure greater than or equal to 140 mm Hg or diastolic blood pressure greater than or equal to 90 mm Hg (Whelton et al., 2018). Hypertension increases risk for heart disease and stroke (CDC, 2020), and nearly half a million deaths in the United States were attributable to hypertension in 2018 (CDC, 2020). Hypertension costs the United States about $131 billion each year (Kirkland et al., 2018). It is estimated that only 24% of adults who are diagnosed with hypertension have it under control (CDC, 2020); therefore, interventions to address hypertension are important.

Research has examined the use of hypnosis for lowering blood pressure and targeting risk factors of hypertension such as anxiety and stress. One randomized controlled trial examined the efficacy of hypnosis for reducing mild hypertension and also whether the effect is influenced by hypnotizability and imagery skills. In this study, 30 participants were randomized to either a hypnosis or wait-list control condition. Hypnosis treatment consisted of eight weekly sessions that were 30 minutes long. A standardized relaxation induction was used and indirect suggestions of blood pressure regulation were given, but never referred directly to hypertension. Participants were encouraged to practice self-hypnosis and suggestions for self-hypnosis practice were given at the end of each session.

Participants in the hypnosis condition had lowered diastolic blood pressure after 8 weeks of treatment, at a 6-month follow up, and at a 12-month follow up compared with the control condition, which had stable or slightly increased diastolic blood pressure levels (Gay, 2007). Additionally, participants in the hypnosis condition had lower systolic blood pressure levels at each time point when compared to controls (Gay, 2007). There was no significant relationship between self-hypnosis practice and blood pressure levels, and participants who practiced fewer than four times a week had blood pressure levels similar to those who practiced four or more times per week at end-point and follow-up. No significant relationships were found between hypnotizability or imagery ability and blood pressure levels. Authors suggest that the lack of effect of hypnotizability may be due to the small sample size in this study. The decreased blood pressure shown in this study seemed to occur independently of anxiety, although hypnosis was shown to be effective in reducing anxiety. Overall, this study supports the use of hypnosis to treat hypertension.

Additionally, a small pilot study examined the use of hypnosis in combination with cognitive restructuring for lowering blood pressure among patients with hypertension. Participants were randomly assigned to receive cognitive experiential therapy (which is a combination of hypnosis and cognitive restructuring), hypnosis, cognitive restructuring, or attention placebo. Each of the groups met weekly for 8 weeks with sessions lasting approximately 75 minutes. Results demonstrated that participants who received cognitive restructuring and hypnosis showed greater improvement on diastolic blood pressure than all other treatments (Tosi et al., 1992). Interestingly, participants who received hypnosis showed greater improvement in systolic blood pressure compared to all other treatments. Results of this small randomized controlled trial indicated that hypnosis, either alone or in combination with cognitive restructuring, has a beneficial effect on blood pressure and could be beneficial for treating hypertension.

Self-hypnosis may also be beneficial for lowering blood pressure among individuals with hypertension. A study conducted by Raskin et al. (1999) taught participants self-hypnosis during four 30-minute sessions, and then participants were instructed to practice twice per day at home. This study showed that participants who were taught self-hypnosis had lower diastolic blood pressure compared to controls (Raskin et al., 1999). In addition, participants in the self-hypnosis condition did not require increased medication doses during the course of the study, while 32% of controls did. Instructing individuals in self-hypnosis could be beneficial for reducing blood pressure, and this only required four sessions of instruction, making it a short and easy to administer intervention. This mode of delivery could be beneficial for making hypnosis treatment more accessible to individuals with hypertension.

Hypnosis may also reduce anxiety (Golden, 2012) and stress, which are risk factors of hypertension. One randomized controlled trial examined the efficacy of audio-recorded hypnosis for reducing stress and showed that hypnosis was effective in relieving stress (Cardeña et al., 2013). Given that stress and anxiety are risk factors for hypertension, the reduction of stress and anxiety with hypnosis could prevent hypertension or could be a mechanism in which hypnosis contributes to lowered blood pressure.

The mechanisms underlying the efficacy of hypnosis for lowering blood pressure are not known. One potential mechanism that has been explored is that hypnosis lowers sympathetic nervous system activity. Sympathetic nervous system activity is implicated in hypertension, and research has shown that hypnosis lowers sympathetic nervous system activity compared with control conditions matched on relaxation, such as listening to music (Kekecs et al., 2016). Another proposed mechanism is that hypnosis lowers anxiety and stress, which are strongly related to high blood pressure. One study discussed previously (Gay, 2007) found that hypnosis reduced blood pressure independent of anxiety. However, other studies have shown hypnosis to be effective for reducing stress (Cardeña et al., 2013). Therefore, stress and anxiety reduction is a mechanism that future studies should explore further.

The use of hypnosis to lower blood pressure among individuals with hypertension has been demonstrated in a few small randomized studies. However, large randomized controlled trials are needed to establish efficacy and to be able to recommend hypnosis as a treatment option for individuals with hypertension. Future research should include larger randomized controlled trials and should further explore the mechanisms of hypnosis for lowering blood pressure and treating hypertension.

Cancer-Related Symptoms

Cancer is the second leading cause of death in the United States, and 1,701,315 new cases of cancer were reported in 2017 (U.S. Cancer Statistics Working Group, 2020). There are many different types of cancer and varying levels of severity; nevertheless, a cancer diagnosis is anxiety provoking and often associated with negative consequences resulting from cancer itself as well as the treatments. There are several aspects of cancer that can benefit from the use of hypnosis, and a few of these will be discussed in this section. Specifically, research has shown that hypnosis is beneficial for reducing nausea and vomiting associated with chemotherapy, hot flashes in breast cancer survivors, managing distress, and improving immune function.

One of the most distressing side effects that can result from cancer treatment is chemotherapy-induced nausea and vomiting (CINV; de Boer-Dennert et al., 1997). Chemotherapy-induced nausea and vomiting is common, and it is estimated that up to 40% of patients suffer from CINV. Hypnosis has been studied as a treatment for relieving CINV. Though there are just a few clinical trials, conducted mainly in children, preliminary evidence supports the efficacy of hypnosis for reducing chemotherapy-induced nausea and vomiting.

Hypnosis may be especially beneficial for reducing CINV when it is used in addition to standard antiemetic medications. For example, one small randomized controlled trial assigned women with cancer to receive standard treatment or self-hypnosis training in addition to standard antiemetic medications.

The intervention included two 1-hour sessions where participants received training in self-hypnosis techniques, and these sessions occurred prior to the first dose of chemotherapy. Results showed that women who practiced self-hypnosis in addition to taking the antiemetic medications experienced less nausea than patients only taking the medications (Hurley et al., 2012). This was a small controlled trial; however, the results demonstrate that self-hypnosis in addition to standard pharmacological treatment may be beneficial for reducing nausea related to chemotherapy.

Overall, research demonstrates that hypnosis is helpful for reducing CINV, as one systematic review and meta-analysis on the topic showed a large effect size when compared with standard treatment and a small effect size when compared to cognitive-behavioral therapy (Richardson et al., 2007). This meta-analysis included six studies total, and five out of the six of the studies included in this review were conducted with children. Therefore, a large portion of the research in the area has been done with children, and further research on this topic, specifically in adult cancer patients, is warranted as evidence points to hypnosis being beneficial for CINV.

In addition, hypnosis has been shown to reduce anticipatory nausea and vomiting (ANV) among cancer patients in many case studies and other small nonrandomized studies, but the field is lacking large randomized controlled studies on this topic. Anticipatory nausea and vomiting occurs prior to any administration of chemotherapy; factors that may contribute to ANV include classical conditioning, demographic factors, treatment-related factors, and anxiety or negative experiences (Kamen et al., 2014). Approximately 20% of patients experience ANV prior to chemotherapy treatment (Morrow, 1982), therefore, effective treatments for ANV are necessary. Anticipatory nausea and vomiting are difficult to control with pharmacological treatments, but behavioral treatments do seem to be effective for treating ANV. One small randomized controlled trial showed that children who received hypnosis treatment experienced less anticipatory nausea than controls (Jacknow et al., 1994). In this study, children were randomized to hypnosis or standard treatment control conditions. In the hypnosis condition, children were taught self-hypnosis during the first course of chemotherapy. There were approximately two sessions and these included an explanation of hypnosis, as well as a discussion of the child's interests to aid in creating personalized imagery. Suggestions were given for feeling safe and well and being able to experience a pleasant place they had enjoyed during the session on their own. If nausea or vomiting occurred during chemotherapy, the subsequent sessions would use more direct suggestions to address that problem, for example, turning off the "vomiting-control center." Children were asked to practice self-hypnosis twice a day and were provided with an audio recording after their second

144 • *Elkins and Snyder*

session to aid in that practice. The children who were taught self-hypnosis reported less anticipatory nausea than controls at 1 to 2 months post-diagnosis. However, there were no significant differences between groups at the 4- to 6-month follow-up; the authors reasoned that this may have been the result of self-hypnosis practice decreasing over the course of treatment. The authors suggested that booster sessions with a therapist may be necessary in order to encourage the children to maintain self-hypnosis practice during the course of chemotherapy (Jacknow et al., 1994).

Another study conducted in children demonstrated that hypnosis was effective for reducing ANV (Hawkins et al., 1995). In this study, children who were about to begin chemotherapy treatment were randomized to hypnosis training, a therapist contact control group, or a treatment as usual control group. The hypnosis intervention included one outpatient training session conducted before inpatient admission for chemotherapy. This training session included an explanation of hypnosis and its benefits for reducing nausea and vomiting, a relaxation induction and visual imagery, as well as suggestions for feeling calm, confident, and relaxed about chemotherapy. Indirect suggestions were also given using metaphors associated with decreases in ANV, for example, envisioning a calming lake after a storm and a young pirate who was seasick and then felt relief from that when the water calmed. At the end of the session, the children were given posthypnotic suggestions for pleasant experiences to be repeated on the days that they would receive chemotherapy. The children in the hypnosis condition had a 33% reduction in vomiting episodes, a 40% reduction in anticipatory nausea after the intervention, and had significantly less anticipatory nausea and vomiting compared with both the therapist contact control and treatment as usual control conditions (Hawkins et al., 1995).

In another small study, hypnosis was shown to control anticipatory nausea and vomiting among adult cancer patients undergoing treatment. In this study, six patients received hypnosis including deep muscle relaxation and suggestions for relaxing imagery with pleasant scenes such as sitting on a swing rocking back and forth, watching the waves of the ocean go in and out, and becoming more and more relaxed while stepping down a staircase. Suggestions for absence of nausea and comfort were also given. The hypnosis intervention was utilized during each of the patient's chemotherapy sessions. Results showed that hypnosis controlled anticipatory nausea and vomiting, and when hypnosis was not used, anticipatory nausea and vomiting came back (Redd et al., 1982).

Taken together, the studies discussed above demonstrate that hypnosis is beneficial for reducing anticipatory nausea and vomiting. However, most of the randomized controlled studies have been small and conducted with children, therefore, the evidence is stronger in children than adults. Future research should include larger randomized trials and should examine the efficacy of hypnosis for reducing anticipatory nausea and vomiting in adults.

Another distressing consequence of cancer, namely, breast cancer and prostate cancer, is experiencing hot flashes. Research has demonstrated that hypnosis is beneficial for reducing hot flashes among breast cancer survivors (Elkins et al., 2008); more information about this topic will be discussed in the section on menopause and hot flashes. It is important to note in this section that hot flashes can be an extremely distressing aspect of cancer, and that research supports the use of hypnosis to reduce hot flashes in breast cancer survivors. Very little research has been conducted with individuals with prostate cancer and could be an important focus for future research.

Research also suggests that hypnosis may positively affect the immune system and improve immune function. Researchers within the field of psychoneuroimmunology have conducted several studies examining the effects of behavioral interventions on immune system functioning and support has been found for the positive influence behavioral interventions have on improving immune system function. For example, research has demonstrated that hypnosis could lower interleukin-6 (IL-6) levels (Schoen & Nowack, 2013). High levels of IL-6 are implicated in cancer, and IL-6 is found in high levels near tumors in the body. This cytokine plays a role in promoting tumorigenesis, which is the transformation of normal cells into cancer cells (Kumari et al., 2016). Hypnosis as an intervention to reduce IL-6 levels could be especially important for individuals with cancer, and future research should examine the efficacy of hypnosis to reduce IL-6 levels for cancer patients.

In addition, hypnosis has been shown to have the potential to increase the number of natural killer (NK) cells in women with breast cancer (Bakke et al., 2002). This is important because increased numbers of NK cells are associated with decreased tumor size (Whiteside & Herberman, 1995). In this study, women with breast cancer received hypnotic-guided imagery and were encouraged to develop imagery of their own immune system being effective. The imagery that each patient developed was unique, and examples include imagining cancer cells being destroyed by an NK cell and warriors representing NK cells protecting an area. The sessions focused on making these images as vivid and effective as possible, and the sessions were recorded so that participants were able to practice between sessions. This study demonstrates the important influence that imagery can have on the immune system for individuals with cancer.

Furthermore, one randomized study examined the effects of hypnosis on the immune system by measuring immunoglobulin A, an indicator of stress and immune system response, from saliva. Participants were randomized to one of four conditions, three of which included hypnosis: (a) light trance induction using progressive muscle relaxation, (b) guided imagery, (c) deep trance with suggestions targeting the immune system response, or (d) control. Hypnotizability was not correlated with changes in immunoglobulin A levels. Individuals randomized to the deep trance hypnosis intervention showed significant changes in immunoglobulin A levels from pre- to postintervention, however, the light trance induction using progressive muscle relaxation group and the guided imagery group did not show significant changes in levels of immunoglobulin A levels (Barling & Raine, 2005). Results of the study showed that the hypnotic-guided imagery intervention increased the number of NK cells (Bakke et al., 2002). This demonstrates that hypnosis utilizing deep trance technique can be beneficial for improving immune system functioning.

More recently, a study examined the effects of hypnosis on cytokines among women with breast cancer (Téllez et al., 2020). This study included 40 women with breast cancer who were nonrandomly assigned to a hypnosis condition or a standard treatment control condition. The hypnosis intervention included suggestions to strengthen the immune system and reduce stress, anxiety, and depression, and improve optimism and self-esteem. Hypnosis was delivered in groups and included 24 sessions that lasted approximately 1 hour each. At the end of chemotherapy, the control condition showed increased levels of granulocyte colony stimulating factor (G-CSF) and tumor necrosis factor (TNF-α), while these levels remained stable in the hypnosis condition. This is meaningful because G-CSF and TNF-α may promote tumor growth (Ham et al., 2016; Kowanetz et al., 2010); therefore, stability of these levels in the hypnosis condition could be a positive outcome. Though not statistically significant, this study also showed improved granulocyte macrophage colony-stimulating factor (GM-CSF) and vascular endothelial growth factor (VEGF) levels in the hypnosis condition compared to the control condition. High levels of VEGF are associated with worse cancer outcomes, such as relapse and lower survival rate for women with breast cancer (Gasparini, 2000). Tumors secrete GM-CSF, and GM-CSF and VEGF together may have a harmful and immunosuppressive effect on the immune system (Kusmartsev & Gabrilovich, 2002). These results show that hypnosis can influence important cytokines that are related to cancer outcomes for women with breast cancer. Taken together, the studies discussed in this section demonstrate that hypnosis may be a beneficial intervention for improving the immune function of cancer patients.

To conclude, research has demonstrated that hypnosis is beneficial for multiple aspects of a cancer diagnosis and treatment. Hypnosis has been shown to reduce chemotherapy-induced nausea and vomiting, especially in children, aid in stress management, and improve immune system functioning.

Future research should continue to examine the potential of hypnosis to improve the lives of individuals with cancer.

Menopause and Hot Flashes

Menopause is marked by hormonal changes and the cessation of the menstrual cycle in women. It is projected that 1.2 billion women will be menopausal or postmenopausal by the year 2030 (Hill, 1996). Problematic symptoms are common during menopause and include hot flashes, night sweats, insomnia, vaginal dryness, mood disorders, and weight gain (Sussman et al., 2015). Symptoms of menopause are distressing and pharmacological treatment options are often associated with side effects. For example, hormone replacement therapy (HRT) is effective for treating hot flashes, however, its use is often accompanied by a variety of side effects including nausea, headache, breast tenderness, and increased risk of certain cancers (Writing Group for the Women's Health Initiative Investigators, 2002). Therefore, nonpharmacological treatment options for hot flashes and other symptoms of menopause are necessary. Hypnosis is a safe and effective treatment that is recommended by the North American Menopause Society (NAMS; 2015) for the treatment of menopausal symptoms.

Vasomotor symptoms, namely, hot flashes and night sweats, are the most common symptoms of menopause (Sussman et al., 2015). Research has demonstrated the effectiveness of hypnosis for reducing hot flashes among postmenopausal women. In one randomized clinical trial, postmenopausal women were assigned to receive clinical hypnosis or structured-attention control. Hot flashes were reduced approximately 80% on average in the hypnosis condition, corresponding to an average reduction of about 18 hot flashes per week, which is highly clinically significant (Elkins, Fisher, et al., 2013). The hypnosis intervention was also effective for reducing the interference of hot flashes on multiple aspects of daily life including work and social activities (Elkins, Fisher, et al., 2013).

The hypnosis intervention that was utilized in the randomized clinical trial discussed above included five weekly sessions that were approximately 45 minutes each. The intervention consisted of hypnotic inductions and suggestions for mental imagery for coolness, relaxation, and safe place imagery. The specific suggestions were individualized, based on patient preferences. Preferred imagery most often included images of coolness, including cool mountains, water, air or wind, snow, trees, leaves, or forests (Elkins et al., 2010). None of the participants preferred imagery that was associated with warmth. In addition to the sessions, an audio recording of a hypnotic induction was provided and participants were asked to practice daily at home. Participants were also trained in the practice of self-hypnosis.

This randomized clinical trial also assessed the role of hypnotizability, and results showed that hypnotizability was a significant moderator of the effect of group assignment (clinical hypnosis or structured-attention control) on hot flash frequency. In fact, participants who scored higher in hypnotizability reported fewer hot flashes than individuals who scored lower in hypnotizability (Sliwinski & Elkins, 2017). Hypnotizability may play a role in the effectiveness of hypnosis interventions for reducing hot flashes, and it is important to assess hypnotizability in future studies.

Additionally, a recent pilot randomized clinical trial demonstrated that hypnosis was as effective as venlafaxine, an antidepressant medication commonly used for the treatment of hot flashes, with both treatments reducing hot flashes by about 50% (Barton et al., 2017). Given that antidepressants such as venlafaxine could be associated with negative and unwanted side effects, hypnosis may represent an alternative treatment option for women experiencing hot flashes.

Self-hypnosis may also be a treatment option for hot flashes that could be very convenient and accessible. In one pilot randomized controlled study, self-hypnosis was shown to reduce hot flashes in postmenopausal women and was nearly as effective as therapist-delivered hypnotherapy in previous studies, with hot flashes decreasing by approximately 72% (Elkins, Johnson, et al., 2013). In this study, women received five sessions of guided self-hypnosis and were provided an audio recording. At each session, participants were instructed on home practice with the recording and at the third session were taught brief self-hypnosis without an audio recording. The audio recording included suggestions for mental imagery involving coolness, symptom reduction, and hypnotic relaxation. Results of this study demonstrate that self-hypnosis may be an effective intervention for reducing hot flashes.

In addition, research has demonstrated that hypnosis can be beneficial for improving other symptoms of menopause, such as sleep quality and sexual function. Sexual dysfunction is common during menopause, with postmenopausal women being 2.3 times more likely to experience sexual dysfunction compared to women who are premenopausal (Gracia et al., 2007). One randomized clinical trial found that hypnosis is beneficial for improving sexual pleasure and discomfort in postmenopausal women (Johnson et al., 2016) and demonstrated that hypnosis could be a beneficial intervention to improve sexual functioning for this population who frequently experience sexual dysfunction. In addition, hypnosis has been shown to improve sleep in postmenopausal women. Poor sleep is a commonly reported symptom during menopause (Sussman et al., 2015). In randomized controlled trials where sleep was examined as a secondary outcome, hypnosis was shown to improve sleep among breast cancer survivors (Elkins et al., 2008) and postmenopausal women (Elkins, Johnson, et al., 2013).

In summary, hypnosis is beneficial for postmenopausal women who are experiencing hot flashes and associated symptoms such as sexual dysfunction and sleep disturbances. Hypnosis has been shown to reduce hot flashes in several randomized controlled trials and has been recommended as an effective treatment by NAMS. Hypnosis should be offered as a treatment option for postmenopausal women, and future studies should aim to examine ways in which hypnosis for hot flashes could be made more widely available for postmenopausal women.

Irritable Bowel Syndrome

Irritable bowel syndrome (IBS) is a common, chronic condition with approximately 4% to 5% of individuals in the United States affected, based on the Rome IV criteria (Palsson et al., 2020). Symptoms characteristic of IBS include diarrhea, frequent stools, constipation, bloating, and abdominal pain or cramping. Given the distressing nature of the characteristic symptoms, there are many negative ramifications associated with IBS including decreased quality of life and daily functional impairment (Ballou & Keefer, 2017).

Common treatments for IBS include dietary modifications, over-the-counter and prescription medications, and psychological treatments. Cognitive-behavioral therapy (CBT) is a commonly used treatment for IBS, and efficacy of CBT for IBS has been demonstrated in numerous randomized clinical trials (Li et al., 2014). Hypnosis is another psychological treatment that has been shown to be highly effective for treating symptoms of IBS (Palsson, 2015). Randomized controlled studies provide the best evidence of efficacy of hypnosis for relieving symptoms of IBS and several randomized controlled trials have demonstrated beneficial effects of hypnosis for IBS.

The first randomized controlled trial that investigated the efficacy of hypnosis for IBS was conducted by Whorwell et al. (1984). In this study, 30 participants received either hypnotherapy or placebo and supportive psychotherapy. The hypnotherapy group showed significantly greater improvement in symptoms of IBS when compared with the placebo and supportive psychotherapy group, and this trial was the first to demonstrate the efficacy of hypnosis for treating symptoms of IBS. Since this first randomized controlled trial, several other studies have investigated the use of hypnosis for relieving IBS symptoms.

Several studies have compared hypnosis to other treatments of IBS. One study that compared brief hypnosis with biofeedback found that both groups showed similar improvement in symptoms (Dobbin et al., 2013). Another study compared hypnosis with diet modification, specifically the low FODMAP diet, and found that both hypnosis and the low FODMAP diet showed improvement with no significant difference between groups; however, individuals who received hypnosis showed greater improvement in psychological factors such as symptoms of anxiety and depression (Peters et al., 2016). It could be argued that hypnosis is a less burdensome and a more pleasurable treatment option for IBS patients when compared to diet modification.

The characteristics of hypnosis interventions studied in randomized controlled trials vary widely in number of sessions, length of sessions, and length of treatment period. Number of sessions ranged from approximately three (Dobbin et al., 2013) to seven (Lowén et al., 2013), and length of sessions generally ranged from 30 minutes (Roberts et al., 2006) to 1 hour (Lowén et al., 2013). The length of the treatment periods ranged from approximately 5 weeks to 12 weeks. Although there are many variations in session timing, the hypnosis interventions generally had the same goals and used similar suggestions. The interventions generally included an induction, deepening strategies, and suggestion for relaxation and gut-directed imagery. Several studies described using suggestions for imagery of altered flow of a river to target constipation or diarrhea (Forbes et al., 2000; Roberts et al., 2006). In addition, suggestions for clearing a blocked river were also used for treating certain symptoms of IBS (Lindfors et al., 2012). There are two scripted hypnosis protocols for IBS: the Manchester Protocol (Gonsalkorale, 2006) and the North Carolina Protocol (Palsson, 2006). Some of the studies mentioned using these; however, other studies did not mention use of either scripted protocol. Nearly all of the hypnosis interventions included utilization of an audiotape for participants to listen to daily in between sessions.

The mechanisms explaining the effectiveness of hypnosis for IBS are unknown but have been explored in several studies. Proposed physiological mechanisms include relaxing the smooth muscle of the intestine, reducing arousal, and lessening pain sensitivity (Palsson et al., 2002). Potential psychological mechanisms involve reducing anxiety and somatization (Palsson et al., 2002). One study found that somatization and psychological distress were improved by hypnosis treatment (Palsson et al., 2002). Another study found that hypnosis may influence brain responses to visceral stimuli, which has been shown to be altered in individuals with IBS (Lowén et al., 2013). IBS patients treated with hypnosis showed brain responses similar to those of individuals who did not have IBS during rectal distensions. This suggests hypnosis may have influenced the abnormal visceral stimuli processing often observed in patients with IBS.

There is substantial evidence from randomized controlled studies that hypnosis is effective for treating IBS. Hypnosis is a safe and pleasant intervention that should be considered when looking at treatment options.

Sleep

Sleep is important for overall health and well-being. In fact, short sleep duration is associated with increased risk of diabetes, hypertension, obesity, and cardiovascular disease (Itani et al., 2017). Approximately 40% of the U.S. population reports difficulty falling asleep and staying asleep, and average sleep duration in this population is decreasing (Hisler et al., 2019). Thus, interventions to improve sleep are important. Interventions for improving sleep include both pharmacological and nonpharmacological options. Sedative-hypnotic medications are a common pharmacological option but are associated with negative side effects (Kripke, 2000). Cognitive-behavioral therapy for insomnia (CBT-I) is an effective and commonly used nonpharmacological treatment option (van Straten et al., 2018).

Hypnosis has also been proposed as an intervention for improving sleep. Several randomized controlled trials have examined the efficacy of hypnosis for sleep with sleep as a primary or secondary outcome. One randomized controlled trial examined the efficacy of hypnosis for treating insomnia. In this study, the use of disease-specific suggestions was compared to generic suggestions. Disease-specific suggestions included use of the counter-hyperarousal hypnotic exercise and visualization techniques for managing insomnia-related anxieties. Generic suggestions included suggestions for self-care and self-confidence. Each group received four weekly 1-hour sessions with a therapist. Results showed that hypnosis utilizing both disease-specific and generic suggestions was effective for improving sleep efficiency, sleep onset latency, wake after sleep onset, and total sleep time (Lam et al., 2018). These results suggest that hypnosis may be a beneficial intervention for improving sleep outcomes among individuals with insomnia.

In addition, hypnosis has been shown to increase slow wave sleep (SWS), which is a critical stage for restorative sleep that is associated with improved immune function and memory (Besedovsky et al., 2012; Diekelmann, 2014). One study investigated the use of hypnosis to increase the amount of SWS and showed that suggestions given to sleep deeper did increase the amount of SWS during the nap that followed (Cordi et al., 2014). In this study, participants listened to an audio recording of hypnosis or a control tape as they were lying in a bed preparing to sleep. Suggestions for sleeping deeper included a metaphor of a fish swimming deeper into the water. In another randomized controlled study, listening to a hypnosis audio recording before nighttime sleep also increased the amount of SWS in highly hypnotizable individuals (Cordi et al., 2020). It is important to note that hypnotizability was associated with the outcome in these studies, and individuals who benefitted from the hypnosis interventions were highly hypnotizable. Therefore, hypnotizability may play an important role in hypnosis interventions for improving sleep outcomes. In another randomized controlled study, listening to a hypnosis audio recording before nighttime sleep also increased the amount of SWS in highly hypnotizable individuals (Cordi et al., 2020).

The efficacy of hypnosis for improving sleep has also been demonstrated in systematic reviews and meta-analyses. A recent systematic review found that 58.3% of included studies showed that hypnosis was beneficial for sleep outcomes (Chamine et al., 2018), and suggested that future research with large sample sizes and rigorous methodology continue to investigate this topic. This systematic review also summarized the hypnosis intervention procedures and mentioned that the hypnosis interventions varied widely between studies. For instance, the lengths of the interventions varied from 13-minute audio recordings to eight sessions lasting 1 hour each. Home practice was encouraged in a majority of the studies. Suggestions utilizing a metaphor of drifting down deeper and deeper as a fish might drift down to the ocean floor were used for deeper sleep. In addition, the studies reported that suggestions were given for good sleep, relaxation and relaxing imagery, as well as suggestions for self-confidence.

Summary of Outcome Research

There is strong evidence demonstrated in several randomized controlled studies that hypnosis is beneficial for treating symptoms of IBS, as well as menopause and hot flashes. Additionally, there is preliminary evidence that hypnosis is beneficial for treating hypertension and improving sleep, and moderate evidence of hypnosis for relieving cancer-related symptoms; however, more research in these areas is needed. In addition, hypnotizability appears to be associated with outcomes particularly for hot flashes and sleep. Future research should continue to investigate the role of hypnotizability. Overall, studies to date have consistently demonstrated beneficial effects of hypnosis in behavioral medicine outcomes. Larger randomized controlled trials with these outcomes are needed to strengthen the evidence of efficacy.

CASE EXAMPLE

This case study involves a 52-year-old female breast cancer survivor who sought hypnosis intervention due to stress, hot flashes, and sleep disturbances. Rebecca (pseudonym) is married and employed as an elementary school teacher. Her husband is employed as an accountant, and they have two adult children aged 24 and 22. Rebecca reported being diagnosed with Stage I breast cancer at age 50. She stated that she initially "noticed a lump" in her breast and consulted her gynecologist. She underwent a biopsy, and the diagnosis was confirmed. She then underwent surgery, 3 months of chemotherapy, and radiation. She describes this as a stressful time, as she was very concerned about her health, had to take a leave of absence from work, and had to travel about 150 miles to a major cancer center for treatment. She reports the treatment was successful, and her oncologist started her on Tamoxifen to prevent recurrence of breast cancer in the future. She states that she will need to take Tamoxifen for at least 5 years and that she is having significant side effects from the medication including severe hot flashes and disturbed sleep.

Rebecca was referred by her physician for hypnosis to assist with management of her symptoms. At the time of the initial screening, the patient had been experiencing hot flashes for approximately 2 years. She reported that she had previously taken 75 mg of Effexor for hot flashes but had discontinued this medication due to side effects, and that she found it to be of limited benefit in her case. She had discontinued all pharmacological treatments for hot flashes for 2 months before beginning hypnotherapy. At baseline, she completed a hot flash daily diary that revealed she was having approximately nine hot flashes per day including night sweats occurring two to three times per night, which greatly interfered with her sleep. She estimated getting 5 or fewer hours of sleep per night. As a result, she felt fatigued and irritable during the day. She stated that she had returned to work, but the hot flashes were sometimes so severe that she experienced intense sweating, which was embarrassing and caused significant discomfort and anxiety. She was receptive to the referral for hypnosis stating that she was "so miserable and ready for anything that would work." The goals of intervention were to reduce hot flashes and night sweats, improve sleep, and reduce stress and anxiety.

HYPNOSIS PROTOCOL

The following hypnosis protocol describes the treatment of the patient in the case example. The patient was instructed that her treatment would consist of clinical hypnosis as a behavioral medicine intervention that involves focused attention, relaxation, mental imagery and suggestion. The patient was asked to record the frequency of hot flashes using a "hot flash daily diary" throughout the first 5 weeks of intervention. The initial five sessions were directed toward reduction of hot flashes and night sweats. This involved goal-directed hypnotic inductions utilizing suggestions for deep relaxation and mental imagery associated with coolness and comfort. The sessions were audio recorded and the patient was asked to practice "self-administered" hypnosis using the audio recordings on a daily basis.

During the patient's first hypnosis session, a hypnotic induction was completed. The patient was asked to sit in a recliner and focus her attention on a spot on the wall. Suggestions were given that she could become more relaxed and that she could imagine a *"wave of relaxation"* spreading from the top of her head down to her feet. She was instructed to let her eyelids close as she became aware of feelings of relaxation and *"letting go"* of tension. It was then suggested that she could deepen relaxation and hypnosis by walking down a path in a forest *"and with each step noticing the coolness and as you do, going deeper relaxed."*

At the end of the first week the patient's hot flashes had decreased to an average of seven per day (ranging from six to eight per day). She reported decreases in severity of hot flashes as well. At the third session of clinical hypnosis, it became apparent that the patient's preferred imagery was of a snow-covered mountain scene with suggestion for coolness and comfort. Suggestions were given for reduction of the frequency and severity of hot flashes. For example, *"As you enter a deeper level of hypnosis, you will soon experience coolness. The coolness of snow as you experience being in the mountains on a beautiful day. It is cool here and there is a light snow, and you can feel the soft cool snow on your face. There is a cool breeze and there is snow on the trees. As you walk down a mountain path, feel the snow and the coolness, relaxing deeper and deeper, and any hot flashes become less and less; less and less frequent. . . ."* She continued to keep a record of her hot flashes, noting the frequency and severity of hot flashes each day utilizing the hot flash daily dairy (Loprinzi et al., 1994).

In addition, Rebecca was provided with instructions in self-hypnosis (i.e., focus attention, relax, image coolness) and was encouraged to practice self-hypnosis without the audio recordings. She reported good compliance with practice of self-hypnosis. The patient was seen for an additional two sessions of hypnotherapy. At the end of her fifth visit, her hot flashes had decreased to three hot flashes for the entire week, all reported as mild severity. The reduction in hot flashes is shown in Figure 6.1.

As Rebecca's hot flashes decreased she also experienced improvement in sleep. She reported decreased night sweats and more restful sleep. An additional session included a 15-minute hypnotic induction with suggestions for

FIGURE 6.1. Hot Flash Frequency Reduction for Weeks 1–5 of Hypnosis Intervention

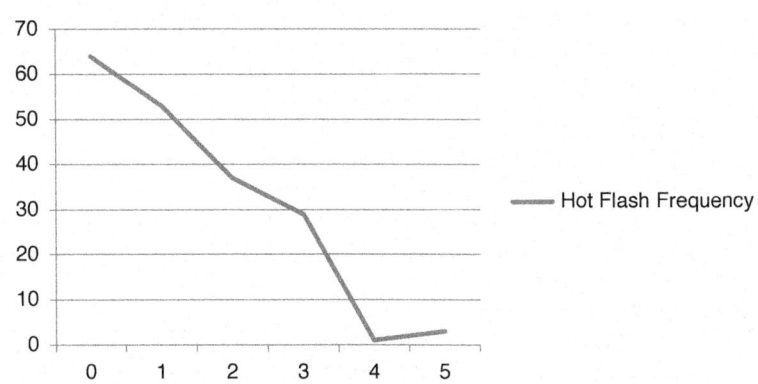

improved sleep. The session was recorded and included suggestions that, *"As you experience the mental imagery of walking down the mountain path, with snow all around, becoming more and more relaxed. Up ahead you can see a cabin in the mountains. It is a safe and secure place. As you go toward this cabin feeling safe and secure . . . soon you are inside the cabin and there is a comfortable place to lie down. You can see the snow coming down. Imagine a single snow flake high in the clouds . . . it drifts down and as you can imagine it drifting down, so you can begin to drift into deep relaxed sleep . . . good deep sleep . . . as the snow flake drifts down, down past the tops of the trees, and drifts down to rest."*

Rebecca indicated she practiced with the audio recordings at night before going to sleep. She found this to be very helpful and over the next 4 weeks her sleep continued to improve until she reported sleeping 7 or more hours per night with few interruptions. She was seen for a total of 10 sessions, and in addition to reducing hot flashes and improving sleep, Rebecca stated she felt less stressed and less anxious. She reported feeling more confident at work and more able to deal with stresses without becoming overly anxious. She was very satisfied with the hypnosis intervention and was encouraged to continue to practice self-hypnosis and use the audio recordings as needed in the future.

CONCLUSION

To conclude, research has shown hypnosis is beneficial in behavioral medicine applications for improving multiple outcomes, including hypertension, cancer-related symptoms, IBS, hot flashes, and sleep. Hypnosis is a safe, nonpharmacological option that can be utilized as a stand-alone intervention or as an adjunct to cognitive-behavioral therapy. The current case example illustrates how hypnosis interventions can provide an effective and time efficient behavioral medicine intervention. Future research can help to identify additional applications and ways to optimize hypnosis interventions in behavioral medicine.

REFERENCES

Bakke, A. C., Purtzer, M. Z., & Newton, P. (2002). The effect of hypnotic-guided imagery on psychological well-being and immune function in patients with prior breast cancer. *Journal of Psychosomatic Research*, *53*(6), 1131–1137. https://doi.org/10.1016/S0022-3999(02)00409-9

Ballou, S., & Keefer, L. (2017). The impact of irritable bowel syndrome on daily functioning: Characterizing and understanding daily consequences of IBS. *Neurogastroenterology and Motility*, *29*(4), e12982. https://doi.org/10.1111/nmo.12982

Barling, N. R., & Raine, S. J. (2005). Some effects of hypnosis on negative affect and immune system response. *Australian Journal of Clinical & Experimental Hypnosis*, *33*(2), 160–177.

Barton, D. L., Schroeder, K. C. F., Banerjee, T., Wolf, S., Keith, T. Z., & Elkins, G. (2017). Efficacy of a biobehavioral intervention for hot flashes: A randomized controlled pilot study. *Menopause*, *24*(7), 774–782. https://doi.org/10.1097/GME.0000000000000837

Besedovsky, L., Lange, T., & Born, J. (2012). Sleep and immune function. *Pflügers Archiv—European Journal of Physiology*, *463*(1), 121–137. https://doi.org/10.1007/s00424-011-1044-0

Cardeña, E., Svensson, C., & Hejdström, F. (2013). Hypnotic tape intervention ameliorates stress: A randomized, control study. *International Journal of Clinical and Experimental Hypnosis*, *61*(2), 125–145. https://doi.org/10.1080/00207144.2013.753820

Centers for Disease Control and Prevention. (2020, September 8). *Facts about hypertension*. https://www.cdc.gov/bloodpressure/facts.htm

Chamine, I., Atchley, R., & Oken, B. S. (2018). Hypnosis intervention effects on sleep outcomes: A systematic review. *Journal of Clinical Sleep Medicine*, *14*(2), 271–283. https://doi.org/10.5664/jcsm.6952

Cordi, M. J., Rossier, L., & Rasch, B. (2020). Hypnotic suggestions given before nighttime sleep extend slow-wave sleep as compared to a control text in highly hypnotizable subjects. *International Journal of Clinical and Experimental Hypnosis*, *68*(1), 105–129. https://doi.org/10.1080/00207144.2020.1687260

Cordi, M. J., Schlarb, A. A., & Rasch, B. (2014). Deepening sleep by hypnotic suggestion. *Sleep*, *37*(6), 1143–1152. https://doi.org/10.5665/sleep.3778

de Boer-Dennert, M., de Wit, R., Schmitz, P. I. M., Djontono, J., van Beurden, V., Stoter, G., & Verweij, J. (1997). Patient perceptions of the side-effects of chemotherapy: The influence of 5HT3 antagonists. *British Journal of Cancer*, *76*(8), 1055–1061. https://doi.org/10.1038/bjc.1997.507

Dekker, J., Stauder, A., & Penedo, F. J. (2017). Proposal for an update of the definition and scope of behavioral medicine. *International Journal of Behavioral Medicine*, *24*(1), 1–4. https://doi.org/10.1007/s12529-016-9610-7

Diekelmann, S. (2014). Sleep for cognitive enhancement. *Frontiers in Systems Neuroscience, 8,* Article 46, 1–12. https://doi.org/10.3389/fnsys.2014.00046

Dobbin, A., Dobbin, J., Ross, S. C., Graham, C., & Ford, M. J. (2013). Randomised controlled trial of brief intervention with biofeedback and hypnotherapy in patients with refractory irritable bowel syndrome. *Journal of the Royal College of Physicians of Edinburgh, 43*(1), 15–23. https://doi.org/10.4997/JRCPE.2013.104

Elkins, G., Johnson, A., Fisher, W., Sliwinski, J., & Keith, T. (2013). A pilot investigation of guided self-hypnosis in the treatment of hot flashes among postmenopausal women. *International Journal of Clinical and Experimental Hypnosis, 61*(3), 342–350. https://doi.org/10.1080/00207144.2013.784112

Elkins, G., Marcus, J., Bunn, J., Perfect, M., Palamara, L., Stearns, V., & Dove, J. (2010). Preferences for hypnotic imagery for hot-flash reduction: A brief communication. *International Journal of Clinical and Experimental Hypnosis, 58*(3), 345–349. https://doi.org/10.1080/00207141003761239

Elkins, G., Marcus, J., Stearns, V., Perfect, M., Rajab, M. H., Ruud, C., Palamara, L., & Keith, T. (2008). Randomized trial of a hypnosis intervention for treatment of hot flashes among breast cancer survivors. *Journal of Clinical Oncology, 26*(31), 5022–5026. https://doi.org/10.1200/JCO.2008.16.6389

Elkins, G. R., Barabasz, A. F., Council, J. R., & Spiegel, D. (2015). Advancing research and practice: The revised APA Division 30 definition of hypnosis. *The American Journal of Clinical Hypnosis, 57*(4), 378–385. https://doi.org/10.1080/00029157.2015.1011465

Elkins, G. R., Fisher, W. I., Johnson, A. K., Carpenter, J. S., & Keith, T. Z. (2013). Clinical hypnosis in the treatment of postmenopausal hot flashes: A randomized controlled trial. *Menopause, 20*(3), 291–298. https://doi.org/10.1097/gme.0b013e31826ce3ed

Forbes, A., MacAuley, S., & Chiotakakou-Faliakou, E. (2000). Hypnotherapy and therapeutic audiotape: Effective in previously unsuccessfully treated irritable bowel syndrome? *International Journal of Colorectal Disease, 15*(5–6), 328–334. https://doi.org/10.1007/s003840000248

Gasparini, G. (2000). Prognostic value of vascular endothelial growth factor in breast cancer. *The Oncologist, 5*(S1), 37–44. https://doi.org/10.1634/theoncologist.5-suppl_1-37

Gay, M.-C. (2007). Effectiveness of hypnosis in reducing mild essential hypertension: A one-year follow-up. *International Journal of Clinical and Experimental Hypnosis, 55*(1), 67–83. https://doi.org/10.1080/00207140600995893

Golden, W. L. (2012). Cognitive hypnotherapy for anxiety disorders. *American Journal of Clinical Hypnosis, 54*(4), 263–274. https://doi.org/10.1080/00029157.2011.650333

Gonsalkorale, W. M. (2006). Gut-directed hypnotherapy: The Manchester approach for treatment of irritable bowel syndrome. *International Journal of Clinical and Experimental Hypnosis, 54*(1), 27–50. https://doi.org/10.1080/00207140500323030

Gracia, C. R., Freeman, E. W., Sammel, M. D., Lin, H., & Mogul, M. (2007). Hormones and sexuality during transition to menopause. *Obstetrics and Gynecology, 109*(4), 831–840. https://doi.org/10.1097/01.AOG.0000258781.15142.0d

Ham, B., Fernandez, M. C., D'Costa, Z., & Brodt, P. (2016). The diverse roles of the TNF axis in cancer progression and metastasis. *Trends in Cancer Research, 11*(1), 1–27. https://pubmed.ncbi.nlm.nih.gov/27928197/

Hawkins, P. J., Liossi, C., Ewart, B. W., Hatira, P., Kosmidis, V. H., & Varvutsi, M. (1995). Hypnotherapy for control of anticipatory nausea and vomiting in children with cancer: Preliminary findings. *Psycho-Oncology, 4*(2), 101–106. https://doi.org/10.1002/pon.2960040203

Hill, K. (1996). The demography of menopause. *Maturitas, 23*(2), 113–127. https://doi.org/10.1016/0378-5122(95)00968-X

Hisler, G. C., Muranovic, D., & Krizan, Z. (2019). Changes in sleep difficulties among the U.S. population from 2013 to 2017: Results from the National Health Interview Survey. *Sleep Health, 5*(6), 615–620. https://doi.org/10.1016/j.sleh.2019.08.008

Hurley, R., Trezona, P., Peczalska, E., Jirik, C., Anderson, E., & Heinrich, R. (2012). A randomized trial of self-hypnosis to control nausea in women receiving moderately emetogenic chemotherapy. *Journal of Clinical Oncology, 23*(16), 8182. https://doi.org/10.1200/jco.2005.23.16_suppl.8182

Itani, O., Jike, M., Watanabe, N., & Kaneita, Y. (2017). Short sleep duration and health outcomes: A systematic review, meta-analysis, and meta-regression. *Sleep Medicine, 32*, 246–256. https://doi.org/10.1016/j.sleep.2016.08.006

Jacknow, D. S., Tschann, J. M., Link, M. P., & Boyce, W. T. (1994). Hypnosis in the prevention of chemotherapy-related nausea and vomiting in children: A prospective study. *Journal of Developmental and Behavioral Pediatrics, 15*(4), 258–264. https://doi.org/10.1097/00004703-199408000-00007

Johnson, A. K., Johnson, A. J., Barton, D., & Elkins, G. (2016). Hypnotic relaxation therapy and sexual function in postmenopausal women: Results of a randomized clinical trial. *International Journal of Clinical and Experimental Hypnosis, 64*(2), 213–224. https://doi.org/10.1080/00207144.2016.1131590

Kamen, C., Tejani, M. A., Chandwani, K., Janelsins, M., Peoples, A. R., Roscoe, J. A., & Morrow, G. R. (2014). Anticipatory nausea and vomiting due to chemotherapy. *European Journal of Pharmacology, 722*, 172–179. https://doi.org/10.1016/j.ejphar.2013.09.071

Kekecs, Z., Szekely, A., & Varga, K. (2016). Alterations in electrodermal activity and cardiac parasympathetic tone during hypnosis. *Psychophysiology, 53*(2), 268–277. https://doi.org/10.1111/psyp.12570

Kirkland, E. B., Heincelman, M., Bishu, K. G., Schumann, S. O., Schreiner, A., Axon, R. N., Mauldin, P. D., & Moran, W. P. (2018). Trends in healthcare expenditures among US adults with hypertension: National estimates, 2003–2014. *Journal of the American Heart Association, 7*(11), e008731. https://doi.org/10.1161/JAHA.118.008731

Kowanetz, M., Wu, X., Lee, J., Tan, M., Hagenbeek, T., Qu, X., Yu, L., Ross, J., Korsisaari, N., Cao, T., Bou-Reslan, H., Kallop, D., Weimer, R., Ludlam, M. J. C., Kaminker, J. S., Modrusan, Z., van Bruggen, N., Peale, F. V., Carano, R., . . . Ferrara, N. (2010). Granulocyte-colony stimulating factor promotes lung metastasis through mobilization of Ly6G+Ly6C+ granulocytes. *Proceedings of the National Academy of Sciences, 107*(50), 21248–21255. https://doi.org/10.1073/pnas.1015855107

Kripke, D. F. (2000). Chronic hypnotic use: Deadly risks, doubtful benefit: Review article. *Sleep Medicine Reviews, 4*(1), 5–20. https://doi.org/10.1053/smrv.1999.0076

Kumari, N., Dwarakanath, B. S., Das, A., & Bhatt, A. N. (2016). Role of interleukin-6 in cancer progression and therapeutic resistance. *Tumor Biology, 37*(9), 11553–11572. https://doi.org/10.1007/s13277-016-5098-7

Kusmartsev, S., & Gabrilovich, D. I. (2002). Immature myeloid cells and cancer-associated immune suppression. *Cancer Immunology, Immunotherapy, 51*(6), 293–298. https://doi.org/10.1007/s00262-002-0280-8

Lam, T. H., Chung, K. F., Lee, C. T., Yeung, W. F., & Yu, B. Y. (2018). Hypnotherapy for insomnia: A randomized controlled trial comparing generic and disease-specific suggestions. *Complementary Therapies in Medicine, 41*, 231–239. https://doi.org/10.1016/j.ctim.2018.10.008

Li, L., Xiong, L., Zhang, S., Yu, Q., & Chen, M. (2014). Cognitive-behavioral therapy for irritable bowel syndrome: A meta-analysis. *Journal of Psychosomatic Research, 77*(1), 1–12. https://doi.org/10.1016/j.jpsychores.2014.03.006

Lindfors, P., Unge, P., Arvidsson, P., Nyhlin, H., Björnsson, E., Abrahamsson, H., & Simrén, M. (2012). Effects of gut-directed hypnotherapy on IBS in different clinical settings—Results from two randomized, controlled trials. *American Journal of Gastroenterology, 107*(2), 276–285. https://doi.org/10.1038/ajg.2011.340

Loprinzi, C. L., Goldberg, R. M., O'Fallon, J. R., Quella, S. K., Miser, A. W., Mynderse, L. A., Brown, L. D., Tschetter, L. K., Wilwerding, M. B., Dose, M., & Oesterling, J. E. (1994). Transdermal clonidine for ameliorating post-orchiectomy hot flashes. *Journal of Urology, 151*(3), 634–636. https://doi.org/10.1016/S0022-5347(17)35034-6

Lowén, M. B. O., Mayer, E. A., Sjöberg, M., Tillisch, K., Naliboff, B., Labus, J., Lundberg, P., Ström, M., Engström, M., & Walter, S. A. (2013). Effect of hypnotherapy and educational intervention on brain response to visceral stimulus in the irritable bowel syndrome. *Alimentary Pharmacology & Therapeutics, 37*(12), 1184–1197. https://doi.org/10.1111/apt.12319

Morrow, G. R. (1982). Prevalence and correlates of anticipatory nausea and vomiting in chemotherapy patients. *Journal of the National Cancer Institute, 68*(4), 585–588. https://doi.org/10.1093/jnci/68.4.585

The North American Menopause Society. (2015). Nonhormonal management of menopause-associated vasomotor symptoms: 2015 Position statement of The North American Menopause Society. *Menopause, 22*(11), 1155–1174. https://doi.org/10.1097/GME.0000000000000546

Palsson, O. S. (2006). Standardized hypnosis treatment for irritable bowel syndrome: The North Carolina protocol. *International Journal of Clinical and Experimental Hypnosis, 54*(1), 51–64. https://doi.org/10.1080/00207140500322933

Palsson, O. S. (2015). Hypnosis treatment of gastrointestinal disorders: A comprehensive review of empirical evidence. *American Journal of Clinical Hypnosis, 58*(2), 134–158. https://doi.org/10.1080/00029157.2015.1039114

Palsson, O. S., Turner, M. J., Johnson, D. A., Burnett, C. K., & Whitehead, W. E. (2002). Hypnosis treatment for severe irritable bowel syndrome: Investigation of mechanism and effects on symptoms. *Digestive Diseases and Sciences, 47*(11), 2605–2614. https://doi.org/10.1023/A:1020545017390

Palsson, O. S., Whitehead, W., Törnblom, H., Sperber, A. D., & Simren, M. (2020). Prevalence of Rome IV functional bowel disorders among adults in the United States, Canada, and the United Kingdom. *Gastroenterology, 158*(5), 1262–1273.e3. https://doi.org/10.1053/j.gastro.2019.12.021

Peters, S. L., Yao, C. K., Philpott, H., Yelland, G. W., Muir, J. G., & Gibson, P. R. (2016). Randomised clinical trial: The efficacy of gut-directed hypnotherapy is similar to that of the low FODMAP diet for the treatment of irritable bowel syndrome. *Alimentary Pharmacology & Therapeutics, 44*(5), 447–459. https://doi.org/10.1111/apt.13706

Raskin, R., Raps, C., Luskin, F., Carlson, R., & Cristal, R. (1999). Pilot study of the effect of self-hypnosis on the medical management of essential hypertension. *Stress*

Medicine, 15(4), 243–247. https://doi.org/10.1002/(SICI)1099-1700(199910)15: 4<243::AID-SMI820>3.0.CO;2-O

Redd, W. H., Andresen, G. V., & Minagawa, R. Y. (1982). Hypnotic control of anticipatory emesis in patients receiving cancer chemotherapy. *Journal of Consulting and Clinical Psychology, 50*(1), 14–19. https://doi.org/10.1037/0022-006X.50.1.14

Richardson, J., Smith, J. E., McCall, G., Richardson, A., Pilkington, K., & Kirsch, I. (2007). Hypnosis for nausea and vomiting in cancer chemotherapy: A systematic review of the research evidence. *European Journal of Cancer Care, 16*(5), 402–412. https://doi.org/10.1111/j.1365-2354.2006.00736.x

Roberts, L., Wilson, S., Singh, S., Roalfe, A., & Greenfield, S. (2006). Gut-directed hypnotherapy for irritable bowel syndrome: Piloting a primary care-based randomised controlled trial. *British Journal of General Practice, 56*(523), 115–121. https://www.ncbi.nlm.nih.gov/pmc/articles/PMC1828217/

Schoen, M., & Nowack, K. (2013). Reconditioning the stress response with hypnosis CD reduces the inflammatory cytokine IL-6 and influences resilience: A pilot study. *Complementary Therapies in Clinical Practice, 19*(2), 83–88. https://doi.org/10.1016/j.ctcp.2012.12.004

Sliwinski, J. R., & Elkins, G. R. (2017). Hypnotherapy to reduce hot flashes: Examination of response expectancies as a mediator of outcomes. *Journal of Evidence-Based Complementary & Alternative Medicine, 22*(4), 652–659. https://doi.org/10.1177/2156587217708523

Sussman, M., Trocio, J., Best, C., Mirkin, S., Bushmakin, A. G., Yood, R., Friedman, M., Menzin, J., & Louie, M. (2015). Prevalence of menopausal symptoms among midlife women: Findings from electronic medical records. *BMC Women's Health, 15,* Article 58. https://doi.org/10.1186/s12905-015-0217-y

Téllez, A., Rodríguez-Padilla, C., Juárez-García, D. M., Jaime-Bernal, L., Sanchez-Jáuregui, T., Almaraz-Castruita, D., & Vielma-Ramírez, H. (2020). Hypnosis in women with breast cancer: Its effects on cytokines. *American Journal of Clinical Hypnosis, 62*(3), 298–310. https://doi.org/10.1080/00029157.2019.1611536

Tosi, D. J., Rudy, D. R., Lewis, J., & Murphy, M. A. (1992). The psychobiological effects of cognitive experiential therapy, hypnosis, cognitive restructuring, and attention placebo control in the treatment of essential hypertension. *Psychotherapy: Theory, Research, & Practice, 29*(2), 274–284. https://doi.org/10.1037/0033-3204.29.2.274

U.S. Cancer Statistics Working Group. (2020). *United States cancer statistics: Data visualizations.* U.S. Department of Health and Human Services, Centers for Disease Control and Prevention, and National Cancer Institute. https://gis.cdc.gov/Cancer/USCS/DataViz.html

van Straten, A., van der Zweerde, T., Kleiboer, A., Cuijpers, P., Morin, C. M., & Lancee, J. (2018). Cognitive and behavioral therapies in the treatment of insomnia: A meta-analysis. *Sleep Medicine Reviews, 38,* 3–16. https://doi.org/10.1016/j.smrv.2017.02.001

Whelton, P. K., Carey, R. M., Aronow, W. S., Casey, D. E., Jr., Collins, K. J., Dennison Himmelfarb, C., DePalma, S. M., Gidding, S., Jamerson, K. A., Jones, D. W., MacLaughlin, E. J., Muntner, P., Ovbiagele, B., Smith, S. C., Jr., Spencer, C. C., Stafford, R. S., Taler, S. J., Thomas, R. J., Williams, K. A., Sr., . . . Wright, J. T., Jr. (2018). 2017 ACC/AHA/AAPA/ABC/ACPM/AGS/APhA/ASH/ASPC/NMA/PCNA Guideline for the prevention, detection, evaluation, and management of high blood pressure in adults: Executive summary: A report of the American College of

Cardiology/American Heart Association Task Force on Clinical Practice Guidelines. *Hypertension, 71*(6), 1269–1324. https://doi.org/10.1161/HYP.0000000000000066

Whiteside, T. L., & Herberman, R. B. (1995). The role of natural killer cells in immune surveillance of cancer. *Current Opinion in Immunology, 7*(5), 704–710. https://doi.org/10.1016/0952-7915(95)80080-8

Whorwell, P. J., Prior, A., & Faragher, E. B. (1984). Controlled trial of hypnotherapy in the treatment of severe refractory irritable-bowel syndrome. *Lancet, 324*(8414), 1232–1234. https://doi.org/10.1016/S0140-6736(84)92793-4

Writing Group for the Women's Health Initiative Investigators. (2002). Risks and benefits of estrogen plus progesterone in healthy postmenopausal women: Principal results From the Women's Health Initiative randomized controlled trial. *Journal of the American Medical Association, 288*(3), 321–333. https://doi.org/10.1001/jama.288.3.321

7 HYPNOSIS FOR THE TREATMENT OF SMOKING

JOSEPH P. GREEN AND STEVEN JAY LYNN

INTRODUCTION

In this chapter, we will discuss the health dangers associated with smoking and the ability of the body to heal following smoking cessation. We will review research supporting the use of nicotine replacement therapy, medications, and behavioral counseling for stopping smoking. However, our main focus will be on the use of hypnosis as a promising cost-effective intervention that can be combined to advantage with empirically supported smoking cessation methods. Through a case illustration, we will showcase how hypnosis can be integrated successfully into a broad-spectrum cognitive-behavioral approach for smoking cessation.

Cigarette smoking causes cancer in almost every organ of the body and is a leading cause of premature death (Hartmann-Boyce et al., 2021; U.S. Department of Health and Human Services, 2014). Smoking accounts for nearly 90% of all lung cancer mortalities and more than 80% of deaths associated with chronic obstructive pulmonary disease (COPD) and complications associated with bronchitis and emphysema (U.S. Department of Health and Human

https://doi.org/10.1037/0000347-007
Evidence-Based Practice in Clinical Hypnosis, L. S. Milling (Editor)

Services, 2014). The risk of developing coronary heart disease or suffering a stroke is two to four times greater among smokers than nonsmokers (U.S. Department of Health and Human Services, 2014). Smoking is also linked with high blood pressure, diabetes, arthritis, tuberculosis, cataracts, and tooth and gum disease (U.S. Department of Health and Human Services, 2010). In addition, smoking delays and impairs wound healing (Kokkinidis et al., 2020; McDaniel & Browning, 2014) and can contribute to sleep impairment and bruxism (Kwiatkowski et al., 1996; Lavigne et al., 1997). Smoking is linked with the dysregulation of pain signals and is associated with increased frequency and severity of lower back pain complaints (Postol et al., 2020). Analyzing data from over 3,700 women who participated in the Kentucky Women's Health registry, Schmelzer et al. (2016) found that smokers were 1.5 times more likely to suffer from persistent back pain relative to nonsmokers even after controlling for body mass, age, education, and other socioeconomic status variables. Bakhshaie et al. (2016) linked more chronic and severe pain with stronger tobacco dependence suggesting that individuals may smoke to cope with pain. The authors suggest that treating underlying pain symptoms could aid tobacco cessation interventions within chronic pain populations.

Smoking can negatively affect fertility and sexual performance in men and women (Bhattacharyya et al., 2020; Choi et al., 2015). Based on 5,000 infertile men, De Brucker et al. (2020) found lower sperm concentration in male smokers compared to men who did not smoke. Smoking is also associated with increased risk of morphological defects within sperm (Bundhun et al., 2019) and is an independent risk factor for erectile dysfunction (Kovac et al., 2015). Women who smoke face increased risks of miscarriages and birth defects (U.S. Department of Health and Human Services, 2010, 2014). Primary female infertility is linked to smoking as well as exposure to secondhand smoke (Hyland et al., 2016). Choi et al. (2015) found a dose-effect relation between smoking and sexual dysfunction among premenopausal women. Ju et al. (2021) found higher rates of sexual arousal disorders, orgasmic disorders, and decreased sexual satisfaction among female smokers in China. Whereas active smoking posed the strongest risk, passive smoking (i.e., exposure to secondhand smoke) also increased risk of female sexual dysfunction. Bhattacharyya et al. (2020) concluded that "nicotine dependence is directly related to sexual dysfunction, and it affects various states of the sexual response cycle" (p. 295).

Although smoking rates in the United States have declined since the 1964 Surgeon General's warning that smoking causes cancer, estimates indicate over 36 million U.S. citizens continue to smoke, more than 16 million Americans battle smoking-related disease, and nearly half a million people die each year from a smoking-related illness (U.S. Department of Health and Human

Services, 2014). The average lifespan of a smoker is about 10 years less than that of a nonsmoker (Jha et al., 2013).

Smoking rates in the European Union (EU) are higher than in the United States. The European Commission Special Eurobarometer (2017) estimated that 28% of EU citizens smoke, resulting in around 700,000 premature deaths annually, and that the lives of smokers are shortened by 14 years, on average, relative to nonsmokers. Fortunately, smoking rates in the EU are declining, by about 6% between 2006 and 2017. The EU Directorate General of Health & Human Safety concluded, "Tobacco consumption is the single largest avoidable health risk in the European Union" (European Commission Special Eurobarometer, 2017).

Globally, smoking rates have declined slightly. The World Health Organization (2017) estimated that 21% of the adult population smoked in 2015, down from 24% in 2007. Most individuals who smoke report wanting to stop (Hartmann-Boyce et al., 2021). Surveys in the United States suggest that upwards of 70% wish that they could stop smoking and more than half have tried to stop within the past year (U.S. Department of Health and Human Services, 2014). Similarly, more than half of the smokers responding to the Eurobarometer reported that they tried quitting in the past, yet a relatively small percentage (around 25%) sought professional assistance to stop smoking. Stopping smoking is difficult, and statistically unlikely without assistance. For example, less than 10% of smokers stop on their own during initial quit attempts (Brose et al., 2011).

Given sustained efforts from health officials to educate the public about the dangers of smoking and the benefits of stopping smoking, it is both surprising and concerning that the downward trend in smoking rates may have stalled (U.S. Department of Health and Human Services, 2010). It may be that those who continue to smoke belong to a cohort that is more "hard core" than previous generations of smokers. This presents a challenge for treatment, as prospective participants may smoke more on average, have a longer history of smoking, and be more resistant to change.

The good news is that stopping smoking can restore health and reverse many smoking-related risks (Hartmann-Boyce et al., 2021). For example, lung cancer risk can be cut nearly in half after a decade smoking abstinence (U.S. Department of Health and Human Services, 2010). Smoking cessation reduces cardiovascular risks too. For example, the risk of stroke is similar among previous smokers who have stopped for at least 5 years and those who have never smoked (U.S. Department of Health and Human Services, 2010). Stopping smoking before the age of 40 reduces the risk of dying from a smoking-related disease by nearly 90% (Jha et al., 2013). The U.S. Department of Health and Human Services (2010) estimates that smoking cessation would eliminate upwards of one-third of cancer-related deaths. Jha et al. (2013) estimated that the likelihood of a lifelong smoker living to the age of 79 is about half that of a nonsmoker, and the age at which a person stops smoking is directly related to longevity. Stopping smoking between the ages of 25 and 34 resulted in an average increase in longevity of 10 years; stopping between the ages of 35 and 44 resulted in a gain of 9 years; and stopping between the ages of 45 and 54 was associated with a 6-year increase in longevity (Jha et al., 2013).

REVIEW OF OUTCOME RESEARCH

This section of the chapter reviews empirical studies of the efficacy of popular interventions for smoking cessation, including hypnosis.

Medications, Nicotine Replacement Therapies, and Counseling Approaches

Both Chantix (varenicline tartrate) and Zyban (bupropion hydrochloride) are U.S. FDA-approved, effective medications for smoking cessation (Stead et al., 2012; Tønnesen, 2009). Gonzales et al. (2006) examined the effectiveness of varenicline, bupropion, and placebo in a randomized controlled trial with over 1,000 patients. They reported 1-year continuous abstinence rates of 21.9%, 16.1%, and 8.4%, respectively. According to Wilkes (2008), as many as 20% of smokers stopped smoking for 1 year after taking bupropion. In addition to medications, nicotine replacement therapy is routinely prescribed for smoking cessation. Tønnesen (2009) reported a 1-year success rate of 26.5% associated with the nicotine patch, 36.5% from a combined nicotine replacement therapy approach (the patch and gum), and 33.2% from medication (varenicline). In a large study contrasting medication and nicotine replacement therapy, Baker et al. (2016) randomized over 1,000 smokers to either the patch, a combination of the patch and nicotine lozenges, or varenicline and found no differences in success rates. Upward of 27% of participants stopped at 6 months and around 20% were successful at 12 months.

A recent Cochrane review found that behavioral interventions and counseling increased stopping smoking rates at 6 months and beyond (Hartmann-Boyce et al., 2021). Hartmann-Boyce et al. (2021) cited evidence that financial incentives for stopping smoking positively impacted success rates. Stand-alone behavioral interventions tend to be successful with 20% to 25% of participants (Glasgow & Lichtenstein, 1987). For example, Cinciripini et al. (1996) reported that 22% of participants were successful after 9 weeks of cognitive-behavioral therapy targeting smoking cessation. Wittchen et al.

(2011) randomly assigned smokers to cognitive-behavioral therapy, medication, nicotine replacement therapy, or a minimal intervention featuring brief advice on how to stop smoking. The first three options included four to five counseling sessions over 9 to 12 weeks focusing on maintaining motivation, discussing situations and reasons why participants smoked, planning to implement alternative behaviors to smoking, coping with withdrawal symptoms (or medication side effects), and preventing relapse. No significant differences in success rates among the groups were observed, with 26% of participants reporting that they had stopped smoking at the 1-year follow-up.

Drug treatment trials and nicotine replacement therapy efficacy studies often include counseling or social support along with the medication (see Gold et al., 2002). Combining counseling with pharmacotherapy improves success rates, perhaps as much as doubling it (e.g., Agency for Health Care Policy and Research, 2008; Baker et al., 2016; Stead et al., 2012). Importantly, more intensive treatment approaches secure better outcomes (Agency for Health Care Policy and Research, 2008). Current U.S. clinical practice guidelines recommend the use of pharmacotherapy (e.g., nicotine replacement therapy or medication) combined with behavioral counseling for smoking cessation (Agency for Health Care Policy and Research, 2008; Hughes, 1995).

Hypnosis as a Tool for Smoking Cessation

Hypnosis can potentiate treatment gains across a number of psychological and medical conditions (e.g., Green et al., 2014; Kirsch et al., 1995; Lynn et al., 2010; Nash et al., 2009). Hypnosis is a popular approach for smoking cessation and holds promise as a cost-effective intervention (Green & Lynn, 2017, 2019; Green, Lynn, & Montgomery, 2006, 2008; Lynn et al., 2010, 2019). Case studies, anecdotal reports, and narrative reviews suggest that hypnosis is helpful as an adjunctive approach to smoking cessation interventions (e.g., Green & Lynn, 2000, 2017; Law & Tang, 1995). Meta-analytic reviews further support the use of hypnosis for smoking cessation (e.g., Green, Lynn, & Montgomery, 2006, 2008; Tahiri et al., 2012; Viswesvaran & Schmidt, 1992) with success rates in the 25% to 35% range (Green & Lynn, 2000). Viswesvaran and Schmidt (1992) concluded from their review of over 600 studies involving more than 71,000 patients that hypnosis was highly effective, reaching an average success rate of 36%.

Public surveys suggest that people commonly view hypnosis as a viable treatment for smoking (e.g., Sood et al., 2006). Still, public opinion is no substitute for empirical evidence. Results from studies of hypnosis for smoking are mixed and marked by a number of limitations. Many of the studies included in earlier reviews do not qualify as randomized controlled trial, leading some to conclude that hypnosis has not been shown to be superior to placebo or alternative treatments (e.g., Abbot et al., 2000; Barnes et al., 2019; Carmody, 2011; Green & Lynn, 2000). Many, perhaps most, hypnosis-based approaches include elements of cognitive-behavioral therapy, mindfulness and acceptance-based approaches, or weave general counseling and supportive strategies into treatment, rendering it difficult to identify effects specific to hypnosis. Studies with dismantling designs could help identify the extent to which hypnosis contributes to change when it is embedded within multicomponent treatment approaches. Rigorous comparison studies investigating the potential benefit of adding hypnosis to established treatments for smoking cessation are limited in number. Lack of randomization, nonstandardized treatments, variability in types of hypnotic suggestions offered, inadequate follow-up periods, reliance on self-report when determining abstinence from smoking, and nonclassification of drop outs as failures are a few of the criticisms of existing studies precluding more definitive conclusions about the effectiveness of hypnosis for smoking cessation (Carmody, 2011; Green & Lynn, 2000, 2017, 2019; Lynn et al., 2010).

If only randomized controlled trials are considered, optimism for the usefulness of hypnosis for smoking cessation fades. For example, in a recent Cochrane review, Barnes et al. (2019) reviewed 14 randomized controlled trials involving hypnosis for smoking cessation compared with other interventions or no treatment. To be included, studies had to randomize participants to conditions and provide follow-up data for at least 6 months posttreatment. If determinable, participants who dropped out of treatment or were otherwise unavailable for follow-up testing were considered treatment failures. Each included study was evaluated for biases. Many studies were judged to be at possible risk of *selection bias* due to insufficient details about how participants were randomized, precluding determination of whether a random sequence generator was used. Multiple studies failed to verify self-reported claims about smoking with biochemical tests, raising questions about *detection bias.* Moreover, studies that did not report the number of participants lost at follow-up were judged to be at risk of *attrition bias.* The authors reported that the studies were diverse in nature and could not be combined in a meta-analysis. Their overall conclusion was that there was "insufficient evidence to determine whether hypnotherapy is more effective for smoking cessation than other forms of behavioural support or unassisted quitting. If a benefit is present, current evidence suggests the benefit is small at most" (p. 2).

The authors acknowledged that a handful of studies found support for adding hypnosis to existing behavioral treatments; however, they judged the totality of the evidence as inconclusive due to too few studies, small sample sizes, and heterogeneous findings. The authors concluded that there was no reason to believe that hypnosis-based interventions produce harmful effects; however, there was little evidence on the topic of iatrogenesis. They called for larger and more rigorous investigations into the efficacy of hypnosis for smoking cessation.

Of the studies included in the Barnes et al. (2019) review, only one was judged to be of low risk of bias across multiple domains. More specifically, Carmody et al. (2008) examined the efficacy of an earlier version of our two-session hypnosis-based cognitive-behavioral therapy program for smoking cessation. The approach featured audiotaped suggestions for smoking cessation, guided imagery and visualization exercises, urge resistance and behavioral substitution strategies, mood management, and general health promotion (Gorassini & Spanos, 1986; Green, 1996, 1999, 2010; Lynn et al., 1993). The authors randomized 286 smokers at the San Francisco VA Medical Center to receive either the hypnosis-based intervention or standard counseling for smoking cessation. Both groups of participants received nicotine replacement therapy as well. At 6 months, 26% of participants in the hypnosis group and 18% of those in the counseling group reported being abstinent for the past 7 days. Self-reported abstinence was confirmed by biochemical verification or by proxy confirmation (e.g., spouse). At 12 months, the rates were 20% versus 14%, respectively. Of interest, the authors reported that the number of dropouts was lower among participants assigned to hypnosis. Whereas none of the group comparisons reached statistical significance, the results showed that people can benefit from hypnosis-based interventions and that hypnosis is appealing to a range of people trying to stop smoking. It is possible that success rates would increase among self-selected (vs. randomized) individuals specifically interested in using hypnosis. Indeed, part of the impact of hypnosis likely stems from its overall appeal, its perception as a powerful mental tool, and the excitement it generates among people interested in trying it (Green & Lynn, 2017).

While not meeting the threshold for inclusion in the latest Cochrane Review (Barnes et al., 2019), we present two additional studies with promising findings. Hasan et al. (2014) contrasted three active treatment approaches with a self-help condition. Participants were 164 hospitalized patients suffering from cardiac or pulmonary illnesses. Treatment consisted of a 90-minute hypnosis session, nicotine replacement therapy, or a combination of both. Patients interested in hypnosis or nicotine replacement therapy were randomized to one of the conditions. Those uninterested in using hypnosis or nicotine replacement therapy were assigned to a self-help condition. All groups received reading materials on quitting smoking and counseling. Those in the active treatment conditions received additional supportive contacts after discharge from the hospital. At 6 months, 36.6% of those receiving hypnosis versus 18% of those receiving nicotine replacement therapy reported that they successfully stopped smoking. Adding nicotine replacement therapy to hypnosis did not improve the success rate of hypnosis alone. Impressively, the (nonrandomized) self-help group achieved a 27% success rate. Whereas none of the group differences reached statistical significance, the results suggested, once again, that hypnosis can be an effective complement to counseling for smoking cessation.

Elkins et al. (2006) randomly assigned 20 participants to either 8 weeks of hypnosis and supportive counseling or to a wait-list control condition. At 6 months follow-up, 40% of the treated smokers reported being abstinent from smoking over the past 7 days compared with 0% of those in the control condition. Importantly, these results were confirmed through expired carbon monoxide testing. Furthermore, 30% of those treated reported continuous abstinence since treatment (compared with 0% in the control group). The authors concluded,

> This rate of smoking cessation is comparable to or higher than that achieved through pharmacological or nonhypnotic behavioral interventions. In this small sample, the hypnosis intervention was well accepted, and the overall results of the present study support the efficacy of an intensive approach to hypnotherapy for adult smokers. (p. 309)

In short, while hypnosis is both popular and at times a seemingly beneficial complement to behavioral and counseling approaches to smoking cessation, we lack sufficiently large and methodologically rigorous investigations to support the claim that hypnosis is an empirically supported treatment for smoking. Nevertheless, it is important to distinguish between approaches that feature hypnosis as an *exclusive* or *primary* intervention from those that incorporate hypnosis into more comprehensive approaches based on established smoking cessation treatments (e.g., cognitive-behavioral therapy, behavioral counseling, and nicotine replacement therapy). Our enthusiasm for hypnosis rests within this latter framework (Green & Lynn, 2000, 2017, 2019). Indeed, we have argued that hypnosis may be beneficial in a number of domains associated with successful treatment. These include the potential to boost motivation, enhance self-efficacy, promote self-acceptance, provide a vehicle to mentally practice alternative behaviors to smoking, and to visualize successfully coping with urges to smoke and contend with discomfort and withdrawal symptoms. We encourage participants to use hypnosis to review and mentally practice key elements of cognitive behavioral strategies for stopping smoking that are embedded within our protocol (Green & Lynn, 2019). We now turn to an illustration of our approach.

CASE EXAMPLE

The following case illustrates our smoking cessation program from assessment through follow-up. Complete details of our approach, including our hypnosis scripts and an assortment of treatment materials, are provided in our treatment manual (Green & Lynn, 2019). The case that follows features a female client who completed our program, achieved smoking abstinence, and provided follow-up data up to 2 years posttreatment. Certain details of the case (e.g., name, biographical information, personal history) were added, modified, or created to conceal her identity. The sequence of our group-based treatment and follow-up contacts included: an initial assessment and program overview meeting followed by two treatment sessions (each lasting approximately 2 hours); a brief phone-based support call 5 to 10 days after the second treatment session; two 45 to 60 minute support sessions held 2 and 4 weeks after treatment; an in-person, individually scheduled 3-month follow session (15–20 minutes); and short follow-up assessments at 6, 12, and 24 months conducted via mail. The targeted "quit date" was identified as the end of the second treatment session.

Background Information

Susan (pseudonym) had just turned 59 years of age when she enrolled in our program. She identified as White, was taller than average, and was the mother of two adult children. She was athletic and played soccer in high school. She completed 2 years of college and earned good grades. She dropped out of school at the start of her junior year after learning she was pregnant. A few months later, she married Richard (pseudonym), an engineering student and father of her child. Three years after their first child was born, they had a second. The youngest child had some significant food allergies and digestive issues that required a special diet and regular doctor visits. They moved four different times during the first decade of their marriage, as Richard pursued better positions at different engineering firms. When the children were young, Susan worked as a stay-at-home mom and reported that it was a struggle to keep up with monthly bills, doctors' visits, and managing the household but added that she "loved every minute of it." When the youngest child started elementary school, she took a part-time job as a sales assistant within a large retail store. By the time her children were in high school, she had been promoted to manager and was working full time.

Susan's husband worked long hours and traveled throughout the year. About 5 years ago, her husband announced that he was moving out, was no longer in love with her, and wanted a divorce. Susan reported she was "shocked and emotionally devastated" but steadfastly added that she "regained control over her life" after about a week of learning the news. She attributed her resilience to her athletic background: "In sports, you learn that when the odds are against you, you toughen up, work hard, and persevere." She stated that she and her husband are amicable now and that he is highly involved in their children's lives. She proudly reported that both of her children graduated from college and matured into "great, responsible people."

Susan started smoking when she was 19 years of age. She said that her roommate smoked and had been pressuring her to smoke as well. "I hated it at first," she said. "But then, after a while, it sort of grew on me, and I started smoking after a stressful test or whenever something was bothering me. And, sometimes I would smoke just to fit in or chill with my friends. It seemed like no big deal because so many of my friends at that time were also smoking," she added. During her pregnancies, she paused from smoking but resumed the habit soon after giving birth, "I'd smoke a few each day—maybe 5, maybe 10, maybe a few more sometimes." Her husband smoked more heavily, upwards of a pack a day. Susan reported wanting to stop smoking, knowing that it was bad for her health and financially expensive. She successfully stopped for a couple of months "three or four times over the years but something would upset me, or I'd get bored, and then I'd go back to my old routine." She never received counseling or outside support during her past quit attempts. She had not tried nicotine replacement therapy or medications to aid her quitting. She stated that gaining weight was a "very big concern" and that fear of gaining weight had been a major stumbling block.

Around the same time that her divorce was finalized, Susan entered menopause. She reported suffering from a lack of energy and decreased endurance. She said that she had sloughed off exercising and had gained "a considerable amount of weight" over the past several years. She weighed 228 pounds when she began our program. She acknowledged that she was sad during her divorce but denied lingering effects or clinical depression. She had no psychiatric history. She appeared motivated, confident, and eager to begin the program: "I know I can stop smoking if I make doing so a priority and stop making excuses."

Session 1: Overview, Orientation, and Assessment

We advertised our 7-week, group format, smoking cessation program by posting notices in doctors' offices and publicizing the class through a newsletter and online forums operated by an area hospital. The first author (JPG) and a respiratory therapist cofacilitated the program. A total of 10 participants enrolled in the class. The initial session involved introductions, completing a few assessment forms, and discussing goals, fears, and concerns. With the aid of a PowerPoint slide presentation, we reviewed details regarding the content of the program, format, and timeline.

Susan scored within normal limits on a depression screen and within the average range on a measure of self-perceived ability, determination, and resolve to achieve long-term goals. She reported smoking an average of 10 cigarettes per day, which was confirmed by our initial expired carbon monoxide breath test. Susan reported high levels of motivation to stop smoking, belief in her ability to stop, and determination to completely abstain from cigarettes. She did not anticipate difficulty going a couple of hours without smoking. In fact, she reported that the *urge to smoke* after 2 hours of not smoking would only be "3" on a 0 (*not very strong*) to 10 (*very strong*) scale. However, she reported that her *urge to smoke* would skyrocket to a "10" over an entire day of not smoking. We applauded her honesty and acknowledged that stopping smoking is difficult but doable. We also reinforced her high level of motivation, determination to achieve her goal, and confidence in her ability to stop smoking.

In a group format, we invited participants to discuss their reasons to stop smoking. Susan announced that her health was the primary reason. She was scared by a recent illness and increasingly worried about her lung functioning. About 6 months previous, she suffered debilitating influenza and was hospitalized for 2 days. Tests revealed that her lungs had been compromised from smoking. About 2 weeks after leaving the hospital, she returned to work but suffered from a lingering cough. Her coughing was a distraction at work and throughout the day, but was especially problematic when trying to sleep. During a follow-up appointment with her physician, she was told that she was in the early stages of chronic obstructive pulmonary disease. Her doctor also warned that her smoking and weight were high risk factors for cardiovascular disease and other health consequences. To the physician's credit, and with Susan's consent, a staff person within the doctor's office called to enroll her in our program.

Highlights of Our Program: Treating Susan for Smoking

Whereas health concerns are the primary reason for participants to enroll in our smoking cessation program, other reasons surface as well, including the financial cost of smoking, insurance incentives, and increased pressure to comply with company-mandated no smoking policies. We talked about the risks of secondhand smoke and tied concerns about the health of children, grandchildren, and even pets to our conversation about reasons to stop smoking. We promoted the benefits of not smoking and living a healthier life such as feeling stronger, having more stamina, fresher breath, healthier teeth, hair and clothes that smell better, and living consistent with values. In addition to reasons not to smoke, we asked participants to disclose fears, anxieties, and anticipated problems or obstacles associated with stopping smoking. It is not unusual for some participants to become emotional while disclosing their need to stop smoking alongside their fear that they will not be able to stop. Some project that stopping smoking is akin to "losing a friend" because they've associated smoking with positive short-term benefits (e.g., relieving stress, mental stimulation). We challenged the logic of this view (e.g., *"Is smoking really a friend?"*; *"Would a true friend be so damaging your health/life?"*). We acknowledged that there may be short term benefits that people have come to associate with smoking (e.g., relaxation, stress relief, enhanced attention), and we highlighted that our program teaches how participants can substitute other behaviors that are more healthy and less costly to achieve these ends. We reframed *giving up* smoking as *gaining* health, *gaining* money, and *gaining* control.

We utilized basic group counseling skills to address anxieties and fears associated with past failures, guilt, or embarrassment stemming from not being able to stop or feelings of shame for continued smoking. As treatment facilitators, we strive to remain upbeat, supportive, and encouraging. We invited members to participate in discussions. We emphasized that the program provides step-by-step guidance for achieving their goal of not smoking. Participants identified a "treatment buddy" they could call or speak to when feeling stressed, overwhelmed, and when tempted to smoke. As the group dynamic coalesced around a common goal, participants seemed reassured that they were not alone and gained confidence that the program could be helpful. We encouraged participants to inform loved ones, friends, and coworkers about their plan to stop smoking and talked about the pros and cons of making such a public announcement. Support and encouragement can be gained from others knowing what you are trying to achieve, while participants may also risk embarrassment or disappointment from others if they go back to smoking or fail to achieve their goal. We also noted that some friends and colleagues who smoke might actually *want you to fail.* We stated, "They might use your failure as justification for their own lack of motivation to stop smoking and then use your failure to belittle programs such as ours so that they don't have to think about signing up!" We stressed that most people—especially true friends and loved ones—will be encouraging and supportive. We challenged participants to make the most out of this opportunity and to steel their resolve to achieve what is arguably "the most important thing for your health." Susan reported that her best friend— also a smoker—was very supportive, praising Susan for enrolling in our class. However, her friend was unwilling to join Susan because she "wasn't quite ready to stop." Susan's children were other social support agents who would regularly call to discuss progress.

Towards the end of the first meeting, we discussed how hypnosis can be an effective tool for smoking cessation. We used Wilson and Barber's (1983) Creative Imagination Scale (CIS) as an introduction to how imagery and mental absorption can lead to altered subjective experiences and how mental preparation can increase the chances of success by anticipating obstacles in difficult situations and implementing prepared responses or action plans. Because most of our clients have no previous experience with hypnosis, we have found that a "nonhypnotic" imagination-based exercise can be disarming. Following the Creative Imagination Scale, we shared experiences and discussed reactions. We stressed that is it not unusual for people who initially score low or otherwise report little subjective involvement during the exercise, to later become "good at hypnosis" with practice.

We suggested that people can learn to use their cognitive abilities to focus, enhance motivation, and practice successfully resisting the urge to smoke. We invited participants to return for the first official *treatment* session, scheduled for the following week, where we go through the nuts and bolts of our treatment. We informed participants that they will be invited to engage in a facilitator-guided hypnosis session towards the end of the next session. As a homework assignment, we instructed participants to monitor smoking on a daily basis, recording the time, activity, emotional state, and physical location. We also asked participants to read a number of handouts and supplemental materials that we provided in their take-home booklet.

Susan scored at the low end of the medium range on the Creative Imagination Scale. She reported that she enjoyed the exercise and that her experience of a couple of the suggested events "seemed pretty real." She acknowledged that she was a bit hesitant to let herself go because she wasn't sure what to expect. She was optimistic that she would be open to suggestion-related ideas at our next session, saying, "I'm really looking forward to next week."

First Treatment Session

We began the first treatment session with a review and discussion of the self-monitoring forms compiled over the previous week. We discussed past quit attempts and how the process of self-monitoring increases awareness of cues and triggers associated with smoking. We inquired about stressors and social support. We talked about how negative affect, stress, or boredom can contribute to relapse. We stressed that withdrawal symptoms are strongest over the first few days to a week following cessation and noted that they then typically diminish over a few weeks. We focused on past successes, even if only for a brief period, rather than conceptualizing past attempts as *failures*. That is, we reinforced previous quit attempts as evidence that participants have the willpower and strength to stop, and that perhaps with the assistance of our comprehensive program, they can stop the destructive habit for good.

The centerpiece of our first treatment session features the various strategies embedded within our cognitive-behavioral approach to smoking cessation. To guide program facilitators, we have provided a detailed script, downloadable slides and video clips, and other ancillary materials (Green & Lynn, 2019). The educational presentation is organized via topics or *suites* of information. The slide presentation is designed to be part of an interactive forum lasting about 60 minutes. Participants complete handouts and worksheets, and we allot time for discussion. To keep on pace, participants begin many of the handouts during the presentation and then complete them at home.

The presentation provides a brief history of the development of the program, dubbed The Winning Edge. We use this catchphrase to refer to the collective tools, knowledge, and strategies embedded within the program. We provide a brief overview of cognitive-behavioral therapy, noting that it is the gold standard for behavioral change. The program emphasizes self-empowerment and stresses individual responsibility for choices and actions. It includes mindfulness-based strategies to become aware of emotions (e.g., irritability, frustration), smoking urges (e.g., "I'd really like to smoke right now"), and smoking-related behaviors (e.g., fiddling with an unlit cigarette) without moral judgement. We distinguished thoughts, feelings, and behaviors. In other words, it is "normal" and participants should expect to have urges, cravings, and desires to smoke. The goal is to not engage in smoking *behavior.* We encouraged change by concentrating on participants' motivation to live a healthier life and challenged hesitancy or uncertainty to fully commit to the program by reiterating the importance of stopping smoking, using participants' own words whenever possible. For example, Susan stated that stopping smoking was an "absolute necessity" and that she "had to complete the program to still be alive in 10 to 15 years." Later, however, she seemed to equivocate, saying, "I'm not sure I'm ready to do this." We simply reminded her of her initial proclamation and encouraged her to give it her all. We argued that the presence of each participant in the group signified that *they* have concluded that the benefits of not smoking outweigh any perceived value of continued smoking.

We framed smoking as a learned behavior. With effort and practice, we stressed that participants can unlearn their smoking behavior and establish new, healthier patterns. During the presentation, Susan, along with the other participants, estimated the number of times she raised a cigarette to her lips. With the aid of a worksheet, she multiplied the average number of cigarettes that she smoked daily by the number 10 (representing an average number of puffs per cigarette), then by 365 (number of days within a year), and finally, by the number of years that she smoked. Susan reported smoking an average of around 10 cigarettes per day for approximately 40 years. Using these numbers, Susan estimated that she raised a cigarette to her lips *1,460,000 times!* She was shocked by this number and needed to recalculate it to confirm its accuracy. We asked all participants to consider *their number* as an indication of how often they have reinforced their smoking habit. We acknowledged that stopping smoking is difficult, but stressed that it is doable, as people successfully stop smoking every day. We noted that participants should anticipate temporary setbacks and difficulties along the way to total abstinence. And, just as they didn't count or think about each time they raised a cigarette to their lips, we argued that a new behavioral pattern will be established and strengthened following each moment where they resist the urge to smoke and after each time that they substitute a healthier behavior for smoking. Individual moments of success accumulate, eventually leading to longer term, more firmly established and automatized decisions and behaviors.

The presentation featured a video message from a health care professional detailing many of the health risks associated with smoking as well as the benefits of stopping smoking. We provided worksheets for participants to list individualized reasons for stopping smoking. We encouraged participants to include specific details. For example, we coaxed Susan to change her generic goal of being "alive and healthy for my children and future grandkids" to "being alive and healthy for (name of oldest child) and (name of youngest child) and future grandkids." Participants transferred their top reasons onto wallet-sized cards that slip inside the cellophane cover of a cigarette box (or taped onto it) as a reminder of their goal not to smoke. We encouraged them to place other "reminder cards" throughout their home (e.g., on the refrigerator, desk, computer stand, next to their TV chair) and at various sites where they work (e.g., desk area, on locker door), if appropriate and allowed. Participants completed other handouts focusing on "triggers"—situations, persons, or environments associated with smoking. Following a discussion of triggers and proposing different ways to avoid or minimize them, participants completed a handout detailing their plan to cope with triggers by substituting alternative behaviors to smoking.

A key component of our program is enhancing motivation and addressing ambivalence (Green & Lynn, 2017). Susan reported that while she wanted to stop smoking for health reasons, she often enjoyed smoking and found it relaxing. We encouraged participants to do a cost–benefit analysis contrasting the long-term benefits of not smoking against the short-term benefits they associate with smoking. Among the various strategies that we employ, we ask who in the group would stop smoking for $1,000,000. Invariably, everyone laughs and raises their hand in response to this question. We then invite participants to think about whether their life and health is worth any amount of money. We also stress social support as another important ingredient for success. Participants list the names of friends, family members, coworkers, and perhaps other group members that will support them. Participants are encouraged to both inform everyone on their list of their goal of not smoking and to ask them to regularly check in and provide support. Participants also complete a behavioral contract not to smoke as a symbol of their commitment. As a homework assignment, they are instructed to have witnesses cosign their contract and display it publicly within their home (e.g., on their refrigerator). Participants also generate short and long-term rewards contingent on remaining smoke free over extended periods of time.

We challenged several common counterproductive beliefs. For example, we distinguished between facts and emotional reasoning: "Just because you may *feel* hopeless or *feel* like a failure doesn't mean that you *are* a failure . . . or that you *can't* stop smoking." We also discouraged magnification (e.g., "it would be *terrible* to have an urge to smoke"). We provided a short handout examining faulty thinking, counterproductive beliefs, and misconceptions related to smoking and smoking cessation. We presented smoking cessation as part of an overall lifestyle of making healthy choices. Our program encourages a healthy diet, proper amounts of sleep, and regular exercise. We advise participants to consult their physician before initiating any dramatic change to their diet or exercise routine.

A major concern among participants is fear of (or actually) gaining weight. We discuss the possibility of weight gain post cessation. For example, Tian et al. (2015) reported an average weight increase of 2.6 kg (5.7 lbs.) among quitters relative to continued smokers over the course of 5 years. We stressed, however, that this is an *average,* and not everyone gains significant amounts of weight. Our program attempts to minimize weight gain by including strategies and suggestions to eat slowly while savoring food, eat in moderation, drink plenty of water, and maintain a manageable exercise regimen. We argued that the benefits of stopping smoking typically far outweigh any mild increase in weight, especially if the gain is short term (see Clair et al., 2013). We suggest that once smoking cessation is achieved, participants could apply many of the program tools and strategies to assist with weight management, fitness, or other goals. Susan was particularly concerned about gaining weight. She enlisted a friend to walk with her in the evenings, and she decided to more meticulously monitor her eating. She liked our suggestion to park her car further away from the entrance of her workplace or grocery store to increase the daily steps she completed.

We strive to bolster self-efficacy by inviting participants to identify with being a nonsmoker. We asked group members to close their eyes and repeat to themselves in a convincing manner, *"I am a nonsmoker."* We encouraged them to develop and reinforce this newfound identity by saying, *"I am a nonsmoker"* whenever they feel good, happy, enjoy the company of others, experience the awe of nature, or when something positive happens during their day. Following this exercise, Susan reported that the phrase rang hollow because she still was smoking, noting it "felt weird" to say that she was a nonsmoker at this time. We discussed how even though she smokes on occasion throughout the day, she does not smoke *all the time*. We asked her to consider that she doesn't smoke while asleep—often upwards of a third of the hours of each day. Furthermore, she previously stated that she would often go for stretches of 2 to 4 hours at work without smoking. So, in truth, we argued, she was never a "full-time" smoker. Instead, we stated that it would be more accurate to label her as a "part-time" smoker and one who was now on her way to becoming a "previous smoker." We challenged group members to change their self-imposed label of "smoker" to "part-time smoker" and to begin to embrace the fact that they do not smoke during a majority of moments throughout the day. With time and work, their imagined future self as a nonsmoker will hopefully crystalize into reality.

Participants practiced cue-controlled relaxation and anchored suggested feelings of empowerment, calm, and confidence by bringing their thumb and a finger together to form a circle. Later, during hypnosis, we returned to this technique connecting the touch of fingers with strength and determination to achieve their goal. We incorporate mindfulness and acceptance-based strategies as we encourage individuals to be aware of an urge, acknowledge it, and accept it without moral judgment. Participants then implement their plan to cope with the urge, distract themselves from it, or engage in another activity to shift attention from the urge until it passes. We argue that smoking urges come and go, similar to negative feelings or frustrations that may arise throughout the day. Susan appreciated the strategy of awareness and acceptance. She acknowledged that she previously felt that she "shouldn't have urges," and if she did it meant that she was doomed to failure. She also welcomed our encouragement to practice self-compassion and to accept and tolerate minor setbacks should they arise.

The hallmark ingredient of our program is hypnosis. We frame hypnosis as "self-hypnosis" because it is the participant doing the work, thinking along with the suggestions, choosing whether to be mentally engaged, and implementing the suggested changes to their life (see Lynn et al., 2017). We note that hypnosis does not force anyone to experience or think about anything that they do not want to experience or think about, that hypnosis requires *active* participation, and a willingness and desire to go along with suggested images and ideas. We discussed several myths and misconceptions about hypnosis (Green, Page, et al., 2006; Lynn et al., 2020) and invited a conversation among group members to address concerns or apprehensions. We discussed how hypnosis can boost focus by providing a means to mentally rehearse coping skills to grapple with smoking urges, withdrawal symptoms, negative affect, counterproductive or self-defeating thoughts, and plans to avoid high risk situations. Our hypnosis scripts reiterate many of the cognitive-behavioral principles and techniques included within the educational component of our program.

Before our first hypnosis session, we presented a video (approximately 8 minutes) of an interview conducted by JPG with a coping model discussing the model's initial uncertainty about hypnosis, later experience of hypnosis, and how she successfully used hypnosis to stop smoking. She discussed how she uses hypnosis to this day to relieve stress and promote her well-being. The model endorses our comprehensive approach and encourages participants to commit to the program. Participants are invited to comment or ask questions about the coping model interview, hypnosis, or anything else before beginning the hypnosis session. The first hypnosis script (approximately 15 minutes) was presented "live" to group members.

At the end of the hypnosis exercise, we encouraged group members to take a little time to reorient themselves to the room and to stretch before standing up. Participants completed a three-item postsession questionnaire about the ease with which they could think along with the suggestions, how absorbed they felt during hypnosis, and how hypnotized they felt during the session. We then discussed experiences and reactions within the group. As was the case when we administered the imagination scale, we stressed that it is not unusual for some individuals to initially report not responding to hypnosis or not feeling *as if* they were hypnotized. Such initial impressions regarding a novel situation are not uncommon and often change with time and practice (Green, 2003). We also shared that initial responses to imagination or hypnotizability scales are not great predictors of achieving smoking cessation. We discuss how some studies have found a connection between initial hypnotizability levels and smoking cessation outcome but others have not (see Green & Lynn, 2019). Given that our multiple-session approach incorporates hypnosis within a suite of strategies for stopping smoking, and because we view hypnosis as an ability that can be learned and honed with practice, we emphasized that initial hypnotizability level is of little concern. Sustained motivation, determination to stop smoking, and commitment to working the program are likely better predictors of a successful outcome. Susan reported feeling "extremely relaxed" during hypnosis, adding "it was very nice." She scored 8 out of 10 on each of the three postsession questions. She disclosed that she probably didn't hear everything said during hypnosis because her mind drifted at various times before coming back to the hypnotist's voice. We noted that this was common and one of many reasons we encourage participants to practice daily with a recording of the session over the next week.

We suggested that the benefit of hypnosis to increase awareness and appreciation of all the strategies embedded within our program would increase with practice. In addition to a copy of the first hypnosis session, we provided participants with a copy of the entire educational presentation through an internet link to either stream or download. We asked that participants review the 1-hour educational component of the program once more before the next meeting, ideally with a supportive family member or friend. Participants were instructed to record how often they listened to their hypnosis as well as continue self-monitoring smoking over the next week. We encouraged participants to begin reducing their smoking frequency over the next week, in anticipation that they will stop smoking completely following the next session.

As part of our ongoing program, we offered participants the opportunity to use nicotine replacement therapy in the form of nicotine patches. We reviewed the benefits of adding nicotine replacement therapy and encouraged its use but did not require it. For those who elected to use nicotine replacement therapy, we determined the proper dose and step-down plan based on their smoking history. We informed the group that we would distribute patches at the next session, on the official *quit date*.

Second Treatment Session

The second session began with a group discussion of the practice sessions using hypnosis, progress made by those who began cutting down consumption, and problems or challenges encountered. With the aid of PowerPoint slides, we reviewed key points inherent to the program (e.g., triggers, effective behavioral substitutions, stress management, hypnosis practice). We then invited participants to go through a *quitting ceremony*. We placed several sheets of paper with different images of cigarettes, ashtrays, lighters, cigarette boxes on a table. Participants took turns coming to the front of the room, selecting one of the papers, and announcing their primary reason (or reasons) for stopping smoking. We provided a list of self-empowering statements on a slide (e.g., *I'm done with cigarettes forever!; I am a nonsmoker!; I'm proud of myself!*) and invited participants to forcefully state one of them while emphatically tearing or crumbling up the paper and throwing it into a trash can. We explained that this exercise symbolized a break from their old smoking status and an embracement of their newfound identity as a nonsmoker. Many of the group members became emotional as they reflected on how important it was for them to stop smoking.

We introduced the second hypnosis script (lasting approximately 32 minutes) as being "longer and stronger" than the first. It focuses on keeping the goal of smoking cessation salient while reviewing major components of our program. Following hypnosis, we invited reactions, discussed experiences, and then instructed participants to listen daily to a copy of the second session for one week. The week after, they could choose to listen to either hypnosis script or both daily. As before, we provided recording forms for listening as well as tracking any smoking they might engage in. For those using nicotine replacement therapy, we reviewed proper use instructions. We provided a 2-week supply of patches with the plan to resupply participants at subsequent meetings as needed. We congratulated participants on completing the treatment phase and encouraged them to continue working the program materials. We informed participants that someone from our team would call them, if they wished, within 5 to 10 days to check in and see how things are going.

Support Sessions

In addition to the brief phone call, we formally met as a group 2 weeks and 4 weeks after the second treatment session. At each meeting, we discussed progress and remained supportive and upbeat, praising any movement toward achieving complete abstinence. Group members were supportive of each other, offering creative solutions to problems or obstacles. We resupplied nicotine replacement therapy as needed during these sessions.

Long-Term Follow-Up Assessments

We contacted participants to schedule an individual appointment 3 months posttreatment. At this meeting, participants completed a progress report, were weighed, and took another carbon monoxide breath test. As an incentive to return, we offered a $25 gift card for completing the 3-month assessment. We later mailed brief assessment forms at 6, 12, and 24 months. We asked participants to return their forms in a self-addressed, stamped envelope.

Concluding Comments About the Case of Susan

Susan reduced her smoking from 10 cigarettes per day (before treatment) to 5 to 8 per day by the time of the first treatment session. She further reduced consumption to 3 to 4 by our second treatment session. She chose not to use nicotine replacement therapy and reported that withdrawal symptoms were disquieting for a couple days but overall tolerable. At the 2-week support session, Susan reported that she had completely stopped smoking since the targeted quit date. She reported listening to her hypnosis recordings as prescribed for the first 2 weeks but then dropped off to about once every second or third day after a week of complete abstinence. She remained abstinent through the 4-week support session. There, she expressed pride in going 1 month without smoking and was highly confident that she could maintain her progress. Susan was attentive and helpful to other group members. For example, in an exchange with another participant who was struggling and whose spouse seemed to undermine her plan to stop smoking, Susan encouraged her to smoke only in one designated area of her home (e.g., the back porch) and to review her reasons to quit smoking before she lit up. She offered to be available by phone should the other participant wish to call for encouragement from someone who "knew what she was going through."

At 3 months follow-up, Susan's carbon monoxide test confirmed her claim of not smoking. Importantly, she was able to achieve smoking cessation without a significant increase in weight (she gained just two pounds between our first session and the 3-month follow-up). She stated that she was careful to monitor her eating and was mindful of snacking. She reported walking regularly in the evenings and using the treadmill that her children bought her. At 6, 12, and 24 months follow-up, Susan reported sustaining her gains and remaining smoke-free. She went on a short vacation with her children to commemorate her first anniversary of being a nonsmoker. She expressed gratitude for our time and assistance and credited the program with helping her "stop smoking for good."

HYPNOSIS PROTOCOL

Below are excerpts from our hypnosis scripts. The first comes from our initial session, showcases part of our induction, and provides examples of deepening suggestions.

"Please close your eyes and begin to think about how nice it'd be to become absorbed in your experience of self-hypnosis and in suggestions that will help you to become a nonsmoker. If you take a few slow,

deep breaths, very slow, deep breaths, and feel the air moving gently in and out, in and out, and if you allow yourself to become more and more absorbed, absorbed in each experience, just as you experience it, as your shoulders rise and fall with each breath, so naturally, then you'll experience a relaxing and comfortable level of hypnosis, where you feel safe and secure and there is nothing to bother, nothing to disturb. If you just settle into your self-hypnosis, a state of absorption in moment-to-moment experiences and suggestions, and if you simply accept whatever goes through your mind and whatever you experience in your body, then you'd discover that you can experience a state of attunement with your intentions and values, acceptance of your experience, with each breath, more and more accepting yet aware on a deep level of your being, of what you want to accomplish, what you're striving for, what you can achieve as you become a nonsmoker. What if you'd allow yourself to the extent possible to stretch yourself in your self-hypnosis? And, what if you would, what if you could get absorbed in going just as deep as you'd like to go with each breath, just as deep and comfortable and absorbed as you allow yourself to be, simply noticing and aware and accepting, then you'd be best able to experience a deep and comfortable level of hypnosis, a level just right for you.

And if you became fully absorbed in your breathing, and in what you'd like to accomplish, then you'd find yourself becoming more and more calm and at ease with each breath, with each breath . . . perhaps feeling any tension from your day draining from your body or breaking up like clouds in the wind. And maybe you'd discover how deep you'd like to go, maybe even deeper, deeper still into your experience of hypnosis, deeper in hypnosis. Scan your body and notice any tension or discomfort, and when you do so, then let any remnants of tension simply flow out with your breath, flow out through your fingertips, and flow out through your toes to enhance your experience of self-hypnosis and go just as deep as you'd like to go" (Green & Lynn, 2019, p. 106).[1]

---

[1]From *Cognitive-Behavioral Therapy, Mindfulness, and Hypnosis for Smoking Cessation: A Scientifically Informed Intervention* (p. 106), by J. P. Green and S. J. Lynn, 2019, Wiley Blackwell (https://doi.org/10.1002/9781119139676). Copyright 2019 by John Wiley & Sons Ltd./Wiley Blackwell. Reprinted here with permission. All rights reserved. No part of this material may be reproduced, stored in a retrieval system, or transmitted, in any form or by any means, electronic, mechanical, photocopying, recording or otherwise, except as permitted by law. Advice on how to obtain permission to reuse material from this title is available at http://www.wiley.com/go/permissions). Portions of this excerpt from Green and Lynn (2019) were reprinted from "A Multifaceted Hypnosis Smoking Cessation Program: Enhancing Motivation and Goal Attainment," by J. P. Green and S. J. Lynn, 2017, *International Journal of Clinical and Experimental Hypnosis*, 65(3), pp. 323–324. (https://doi.org/10.1080/00207144.2017.1314740). Copyright 2017 by Taylor & Francis. Reprinted here with permission.

The next excerpt (also from Session 1) focuses on anchoring the intention to be a nonsmoker.

"Now, what if you went deeper and deeper in hypnosis, and really think about what it is that you wish to accomplish, then perhaps you might move closer to achieving your goal. Let's bring your thumb and forefinger together, and make what I call an anchor . . . anchor your intention, your willingness to let your experiences come and go, to be tolerant and accepting of yourself and others, patient and understanding, more and more in tune with your intentions, your intention to be a nonsmoker, to become absorbed in what you need to do to become a nonsmoker and learn ways to surf discomfort and not avoid doing what you need to do, or just as important, not to do. If you become aware of possibilities within your deepest self, opportunities to live a life in keeping with your best self, your values, then you may discover that you can let any urge pass from your awareness, without your acting on it, becoming nothing more than a mere annoyance that you'll soon forget" (Green & Lynn, 2019, p. 107, *reprinted with permission*).

The final excerpt arises from our second script. Here, we attempt to make salient the goal of smoking cessation and review work recognizing triggers and behavioral substitution.

"Now, get in touch with your intention to preserve your health to be a nonsmoker, your intention to free yourself from this old and tiring habit. Think of all the many reasons you have to stop smoking forever. What if you connect very firmly with each reason to stop and become increasingly aware of all the benefits . . . all you have to gain . . . health . . . money saved . . . loved ones . . . all the benefits. Would you think about all that you have to live for and look forward to? Would it crystallize your motivation to stop smoking? And if you're firm in your intention to stop, then wouldn't it help you to master any passing urge and realize it'll pass and not tug at you? Connect with your future as a nonsmoker with improved health, confidence, and well-being . . . connect with who you want to be and to become, starting today. Now take some time to connect with all your reasons to be a nonsmoker for life!

What if you were to take a moment now to experience just the right level of hypnosis that is comfortable for you? Wouldn't that be nice? Just right for you, just meant for you, just as deep as you'd like to go, comfortable, at ease, safe and secure. How nice it'd be to get even more absorbed in your experiences and the suggestions that will work to give you the edge that you need. Take a few moments to do this now if you like or just sit quietly with nothing to bother, nothing to disturb. I'll be quiet . . . (20 s).

Okay, good. If you make some simple changes in your everyday life, it could increase your awareness and your intention to stop smoking. Perhaps you learned that you lit up and smoked because of cues in your environment. For example, maybe you often smoke first thing in the morning, after dinner, whenever there is an ashtray in front of you, or while working on the computer. Everyone has different cues or triggers in their lives. If you become more aware of those things, or events, that in the past, you associated with smoking, then you could make some simple changes in the short term to change these associations. Couldn't you? For example, you could remove the ashtrays from your living room or kitchen. If you tend to smoke on the back porch, you could place an object on the porch that normally wouldn't be there. For example, you could place a ceramic cat, a broom, or a colorful sign that you made to remind you of your goal of being a nonsmoker. There are endless possibilities.

Try this. When you see the object or become aware of the triggering situation, notice it and then embrace your intention to stop smoking, know it, live it, breathe it, firm it in your resolve. Do the same thing if you smoke at your desk. If you rearrange things on your desk, post a sign stating your goal, put a pillow case over your computer, or do anything different that could signal to you that things are new, things have changed, wouldn't you be changing and controlling your life? Wouldn't you gain the winning edge as you take control of your life and your health? If you smoke in your car, you could change the radio station so that each time you start up your car and drive it, you're consciously aware of your intention to become a nonsmoker. If you make these changes during the first couple of weeks when it's most challenging to achieve your goal, then you'll keep your focus, keep your goal 'fresh,' alive, empowering, and close to your heart.

Now as you continue to experience just the right level of hypnosis that is so comfortable for you, I wonder if you'd be willing to get even more absorbed in your experiences and the suggestions, if that is possible, and go deeper and deeper if you like, calm and at ease. Okay, good. If you think of all the things that you can choose to do, besides picking up a cigarette and smoking, then you position yourself to substitute healthy actions for unhealthy behaviors. Perhaps you'll think of new ones as I speak, or as you think about achieving your intention to be a nonsmoker at different times during the day. If you keep it in mind that urges typically only last for a little while, it'll help you to tolerate them as you let them pass and then do the next right thing. If you take good care of yourself and be the person you want to be, wouldn't you feel empowered? Wouldn't that feel good? Wouldn't it feel good to take this valued action, in keeping with your intentions? Each step closer to being a nonsmoker for life?" (Green & Lynn, 2019, pp. 132–133).[2]

CONCLUSION

We have argued that hypnosis can be a highly promising cost-effective intervention for smoking, although it has not, to date, met the most rigorous standards of scientific evidence. Support for hypnosis appears particularly limited when it is used as a stand-alone treatment. In contrast, hypnosis may compliment cognitive-behavioral and supportive counseling interventions targeting smoking cessation in several ways, including boosting motivation and promoting positive treatment expectancies. We illustrated how hypnosis can be used to reinforce behavioral change strategies and rehearse habit control techniques learned prior to the hypnosis session. Hypnosis remains a popular treatment for smoking. If hypnosis is to gain a seat at the table of empirically established treatments for smoking, we need high quality, large scale, randomized controlled trials showing that hypnosis-based interventions match or exceed the success rates provided by already established approaches for smoking. Much work needs to be done. Let's get to it!

REFERENCES

Abbot, N. C., Stead, L. F., White, A. R., & Barnes, J., & Ernst, E. (2000). Hypnotherapy for smoking cessation. *Cochrane Database of Systematic Reviews, 2000*(2), CD001008. https://doi.org/10.1002/14651858.CD001008.pub2

Agency for Health Care Policy and Research (2008). *Treating tobacco use and dependence: 2008 Update.* Agency for Health Care Policy and Research. https://www.ahrq.gov/prevention/guidelines/tobacco/index.html

---

[2]From *Cognitive-Behavioral Therapy, Mindfulness, and Hypnosis for Smoking Cessation: A Scientifically Informed Intervention* (p. 132–133), by J. P. Green and S. J. Lynn, 2019, Wiley Blackwell (https://doi.org/10.1002/9781119139676). Copyright 2019 by John Wiley & Sons Ltd. / Wiley Blackwell. Reprinted here with permission. All rights reserved. No part of this material may be reproduced, stored in a retrieval system, or transmitted, in any form or by any means, electronic, mechanical, photocopying, recording or otherwise, except as permitted by law. Advice on how to obtain permission to reuse material from this title is available at http://www.wiley.com/go/permissions). Portions of this excerpt from Green and Lynn (2019) were reprinted from "A Multifaceted Hypnosis Smoking Cessation Program: Enhancing Motivation and Goal Attainment," by J. P. Green and S. J. Lynn, 2017, *International Journal of Clinical and Experimental Hypnosis, 65*(3), pp. 322–323. (https://doi.org/10.1080/00207144.2017.1314740). Copyright 2017 by Taylor & Francis. Reprinted here with permission.

Baker, T. B., Piper, M. E., Stein, J. H., Smith, S. S., Bolt, D. M., Fraser, D. L., & Fiore, M. C. (2016). Effects of nicotine patch vs varenicline vs combination nicotine replacement therapy on smoking cessation at 26 weeks: A randomized trial. *Journal of the American Medical Association, 315*(4), 371–379. https://doi.org/10.1001/jama.2015.19284

Bakhshaie, J., Ditre, J. W., Langdon, K. J., Asmundson, G. J. G., Paulus, D. J., & Zvolensky, M. J. (2016). Pain intensity and smoking behavior among treatment seeking smokers. *Psychiatry Research, 237*, 67–71. https://doi.org/10.1016/j.psychres.2016.01.073

Barnes, J., McRobbie, H., Dong, C. Y., Walker, N., & Hartmann-Boyce, J. (2019). Hypnotherapy for smoking cessation. *Cochrane Database of Systematic Reviews, 6*, CD001008. Advance online publication.

Bhattacharyya, R., Sanyal, D., Bhattacharyya, S., Chakraborty, K., Neogi, R., & Banerjee, B. B. (2020). Depression, sexual dysfunction, and medical comorbidities in young adults having nicotine dependence. *Indian Journal of Community Medicine, 45*(3), 295–298. https://doi.org/10.4103/ijcm.IJCM_153_19

Brose, L. S., West, R., McDermott, M. S., Fidler, J. A., Croghan, E., & McEwen, A. (2011). What makes for an effective stop-smoking service? *Thorax, 66*(10), 924–926. https://doi.org/10.1136/thoraxjnl-2011-200251

Bundhun, P. K., Janoo, G., Bhurtu, A., Teeluck, A. R., Soogund, M. Z. S., Pursun, M., & Huang, F. (2019). Tobacco smoking and semen quality in infertile males: A systematic review and meta-analysis. *BMC Public Health, 19*(1), 36. https://doi.org/10.1186/s12889-018-6319-3

Carmody, T. P. (2011). No clear evidence that hypnotherapy for smoking cessation is more effective in the long term than no treatment or other interventions. *Evidence-Based Nursing, 14*(2), 48–49. https://doi.org/10.1136/ebn1138

Carmody, T. P., Duncan, C., Simon, J. A., Solkowitz, S., Huggins, J., Lee, S., & Delucchi, K. (2008). Hypnosis for smoking cessation: A randomized trial. *Nicotine & Tobacco Research, 10*(5), 811–818. https://doi.org/10.1080/14622200802023833

Choi, J., Shin, D. W., Lee, S., Jeon, M. J., Kim, S. M., Cho, B., & Lee, S. M. (2015). Dose-response relationship between cigarette smoking and female sexual dysfunction. *Obstetrics & Gynecology Science, 58*(4), 302–308. https://doi.org/10.5468/ogs.2015.58.4.302

Cinciripini, P. M., Cinciripini, L. G., Wallfisch, A., Haque, W., & Van Vunakis, H. (1996). Behavior therapy and the transdermal nicotine patch: Effects on cessation outcome, affect, and coping. *Journal of Consulting and Clinical Psychology, 64*(2), 314–323. https://doi.org/10.1037/0022-006X.64.2.314

Clair, C., Rigotti, N. A., Porneala, B., Fox, C. S., D'Agostino, R. B., Pencina, M. J., & Meigs, J. B. (2013). Association of smoking cessation and weight change with cardiovascular disease among adults with and without diabetes. *Journal of the American Medical Association, 309*(10), 1014–1021. https://doi.org/10.1001/jama.2013.1644

De Brucker, S., Drakopoulos, P., Dhooghe, E., De Geeter, J., Uvin, V., Santos-Ribeiro, S., Michielsen, D., Tournaye, H., & De Brucker, M. (2020). The effect of cigarette smoking on the semen parameters of infertile men. *Gynecological Endocrinology, 36*(12), 1127–1130. https://doi.org/10.1080/09513590.2020.1775195

Elkins, G., Marcus, J., Bates, J., Hasan Rajab, M., & Cook, T. (2006). Intensive hypnotherapy for smoking cessation: A prospective study. *International Journal of Clinical and Experimental Hypnosis, 54*(3), 303–315. https://doi.org/10.1080/00207140600689512

European Commission Special Eurobarometer. (2017). *Special Eurobarometer 458: Attitudes of Europeans towards tobacco and electronic cigarettes* (v1.00) [Data set]. Directorate-General for Communication. http://data.europa.eu/88u/dataset/S2146_87_1_458_ENG

Glasgow, R. E., & Lichtenstein, E. (1987). Long-term effects of behavioral smoking cessation interventions. *Behavior Therapy, 18*(4), 297–324. https://doi.org/10.1016/S0005-7894(87)80002-3

Gold, P. B., Rubey, R. N., & Harvey, R. T. (2002). Naturalistic, self-assignment comparative trial of bupropion SR, a nicotine patch, or both for smoking cessation treatment in primary care. *The American Journal on Addictions, 11*(4), 315–331. https://doi.org/10.1080/1055049029008811

Gonzales, D., Rennard, S. I., Nides, M., Oncken, C., Azoulay, S., Billing, C. B., Watsky, E. J., Gong, J., Williams, K. E., Reeves, K. R., & the Varenicline Phase 3 Study Group. (2006). Varenicline, an α4β2 nicotinic acetylcholine receptor partial agonist, vs sustained-release bupropion and placebo for smoking cessation: A randomized controlled trial. *Journal of the American Medical Association, 296*(1), 47–55. https://doi.org/10.1001/jama.296.1.47

Gorassini, D. R., & Spanos, N. P. (1986). A social-cognitive skills approach to the successful modification of hypnotic susceptibility. *Journal of Personality and Social Psychology, 50*(5), 1004–1012. https://doi.org/10.1037/0022-3514.50.5.1004

Green, J. P. (1996). Cognitive-behavioral hypnotherapy for smoking cessation: A case study in a group setting. In S. J. Lynn, I. Kirsch, & J. W. Rhue (Eds.), *Casebook of clinical hypnosis* (pp. 223–248). American Psychological Association. https://doi.org/10.1037/11090-011

Green, J. P. (1999). Hypnosis and the treatment of smoking cessation and weight loss. In I. Kirsch, A. Capafons, E. Cardeña-Buelna, & S. Amigó (Eds.), *Clinical hypnosis and self-regulation: Cognitive-behavioral perspectives* (pp. 249–276). American Psychological Association. https://doi.org/10.1037/10282-010

Green, J. P. (2003). Beliefs about hypnosis: Popular beliefs, misconceptions, and the importance of experience. *International Journal of Clinical and Experimental Hypnosis, 51*(4), 369–381. https://doi.org/10.1076/iceh.51.4.369.16408

Green, J. P. (2010). Hypnosis and smoking cessation: Research and application. In S. J. Lynn, J. W. Rhue, & I. Kirsch (Eds.), *Handbook of clinical hypnosis* (2nd ed., pp. 593–614). American Psychological Association. https://doi.org/10.2307/j.ctv1chs5qj.28

Green, J. P., Laurence, J.-R., & Lynn, S. J. (2014). Hypnosis and psychotherapy: From Mesmer to mindfulness. *Psychology of Consciousness: Theory, Research, and Practice, 1*(2), 199–212. https://doi.org/10.1037/cns0000015

Green, J. P., & Lynn, S. J. (2000). Hypnosis and suggestion-based approaches to smoking cessation: An examination of the evidence. *International Journal of Clinical and Experimental Hypnosis, 48*(2), 195–224. https://doi.org/10.1080/00207140008410048

Green, J. P., & Lynn, S. J. (2017). A multifaceted hypnosis smoking cessation program: Enhancing motivation and goal attainment. *International Journal of Clinical and Experimental Hypnosis, 65*(3), 308–335. https://doi.org/10.1080/00207144.2017.1314740

Green, J. P., & Lynn, S. J. (2019). *Cognitive-behavioral therapy, mindfulness, and hypnosis for smoking cessation: A scientifically informed intervention.* Wiley Blackwell. https://doi.org/10.1002/9781119139676

Green, J. P., Lynn, S. J., & Montgomery, G. H. (2006). A meta-analysis of gender, smoking cessation, and hypnosis: A brief communication. *International Journal of Clinical and Experimental Hypnosis, 54*(2), 224–233. https://doi.org/10.1080/00207140500528497

Green, J. P., Lynn, S. J., & Montgomery, G. H. (2008). Gender-related differences in hypnosis-based treatments for smoking: A follow-up meta-analysis. *American Journal of Clinical Hypnosis, 50*(3), 259–271. https://doi.org/10.1080/00029157.2008.10401628

Green, J. P., Page, R. A., Rasekhy, R., Johnson, L. K., & Bernhardt, S. E. (2006). Cultural views and attitudes about hypnosis: A survey of college students across four countries. *International Journal of Clinical and Experimental Hypnosis, 54*(3), 263–280. https://doi.org/10.1080/00207140600689439

Hartmann-Boyce, J., & Livingstone-Banks, J. Ordóñez-Mena, J. M., Fanshawe, T. R., Lindson, N., Freeman, S. C., Sutton A. J., Theodoulou, A., & Aveyard, P. (2021). Behavioural interventions for smoking cessation: An overview and network meta-analysis. *Cochrane Database of Systematic Reviews, 2021*(1). Article No. CD013229. https://doi.org/10.1002/14651858.cd013229.pub2

Hasan, F. M., Zagarins, S. E., Pischke, K. M., Saiyed, S., Bettencourt, A. M., Beal, L., Macys, D., Aurora, S., & McCleary, N. (2014). Hypnotherapy is more effective than nicotine replacement therapy for smoking cessation: Results of a randomized controlled trial. *Complementary Therapies in Medicine, 22*(1), 1–8. https://doi.org/10.1016/j.ctim.2013.12.012

Hughes, J. R. (1995). Combining behavioral therapy and pharmacotherapy for smoking cessation: An update (NIDA Research Monograph no. 150). In L. S. Onken, J. D. Blaine, & J. J. Boren (Eds.), *Integrating behavior therapies with medication in the treatment of drug dependence* (pp. 92–109) U.S. Department of Health and Human Services. https://archives.drugabuse.gov/sites/default/files/monograph150.pdf

Hyland, A., Piazza, K., Hovey, K. M., Tindle, H. A., Manson, J. E., Messina, C., Rivard, C., Smith, D., & Wactawski-Wende, J. (2016). Associations between lifetime tobacco exposure with infertility and age at natural menopause: The Women's Health Initiative Observational Study. *Tobacco Control, 25*(6), 706–714. https://doi.org/10.1136/tobaccocontrol-2015-052510

Jha, P., Ramasundarahettige, C., Landsman, V., Rostron, B., Thun, M., Anderson, R. N., McAfee, T., & Peto, R. (2013). 21st-century hazards of smoking and benefits of cessation in the United States. *The New England Journal of Medicine, 368*(4), 341–350. https://doi.org/10.1056/NEJMsa1211128

Ju, R., Ruan, X., Xu, X., Yang, Y., Cheng, J., Zhang, L., Wang, B., Qin, S., Dou, Z., & Mueck, A. O. (2021). Importance of active and passive smoking as one of the risk factors for female sexual dysfunction in Chinese women. *Gynecological Endocrinology, 37*(6), 541–545. https://doi.org/10.1080/09513590.2021.1913115

Kirsch, I., Montgomery, G., & Sapirstein, G. (1995). Hypnosis as an adjunct to cognitive-behavioral psychotherapy: A meta-analysis. *Journal of Consulting and Clinical Psychology, 63*(2), 214–220. https://doi.org/10.1037/0022-006X.63.2.214

Kokkinidis, D. G., Giannopoulos, S., Haider, M., Jordan, T., Sarkar, A., Singh, G. D., Secemsky, E. A., Giri, J., Beckman, J. A., & Armstrong, E. J. (2020). Active smoking is associated with higher rates of incomplete wound healing after endovascular treatment of critical limb ischemia. *Vascular Medicine, 25*(5), 427–435. https://doi.org/10.1177/1358863X20916526

Kovac, J. R., Labbate, C., Ramasamy, R., Tang, D., & Lipshultz, L. I. (2015). Effects of cigarette smoking on erectile dysfunction. *Andrologia, 47*(10), 1087–1092. https://doi.org/10.1111/and.12393

Kwiatkowski, T. C., Hanley, E. N., Jr., & Ramp, W. K. (1996). Cigarette smoking and its orthopedic consequences. *American Journal of Orthopedics, 25*(9), 590–597. PMID: 8886197. https://pubmed.ncbi.nlm.nih.gov/8886197/

Lavigne, G. L., Lobbezoo, F., Rompré, P. H., Nielsen, T. A., & Montplaisir, J. (1997). Cigarette smoking as a risk factor or an exacerbating factor for restless legs syndrome and sleep bruxism. *Sleep, 20*(4), 290–293. https://doi.org/10.1093/sleep/20.4.290

Law, M., & Tang, J. L. (1995). An analysis of the effectiveness of interventions intended to help people stop smoking. *Archives of Internal Medicine, 155*(18), 1933–1941. https://doi.org/10.1001/archinte.1995.00430180025004

Lynn, S. J., Green, J. P., Accardi, M., & Cleere, C. (2010). Hypnosis and smoking cessation: The state of the science. *American Journal of Clinical Hypnosis, 52*(3), 177–181. https://doi.org/10.1080/00029157.2010.10401717

Lynn, S. J., Green, J. P., Polizzi, C. P., Ellenberg, S., Gautam, A., & Aksen, D. (2019). Hypnosis, hypnotic phenomena, and hypnotic responsiveness: Clinical and research foundations—A 40-year perspective. *International Journal of Clinical and Experimental Hypnosis, 67*(4), 475–511. https://doi.org/10.1080/00207144.2019.1649541

Lynn, S. J., Kirsch, I., Terhune, D., & Green, J. P. (2020). Myths and misconceptions about hypnosis and suggestion: Separating fact and fiction. *Applied Cognitive Psychology 34*(6), 1253–1264. https://doi.org/10.1002/acp.3730

Lynn, S. J., Maxwell, R., & Green, J. P. (2017). The hypnotic induction in the broad scheme of hypnosis: A sociocognitive perspective. *American Journal of Clinical Hypnosis, 59*(4), 363–384. https://doi.org/10.1080/00029157.2016.1233093

Lynn, S. J., Neufeld, V., Rhue, J. W., & Matorin, A. (1993). Hypnosis and smoking cessation: A cognitive behavioral treatment. In J. W. Rhue, S. J. Lynn, & I. Kirsch (Eds.), *Handbook of clinical hypnosis* (pp. 555–585). American Psychological Association. https://doi.org/10.1037/10274-025

McDaniel, J. C., & Browning, K. K. (2014). Smoking, chronic wound healing, and implications for evidence-based practice. *Journal of Wound, Ostomy, and Continence Nursing, 41*(5), 415–423. https://doi.org/10.1097/WON.0000000000000057

Nash, M. R., Perez, N., Tasso, A., & Levy, J. J. (2009). Clinical research on the utility of hypnosis in the prevention, diagnosis, and treatment of medical and psychiatric disorders. *International Journal of Clinical and Experimental Hypnosis, 57*(4), 443–450. https://doi.org/10.1080/00207140903099153

Postol, C. R., Kusin, D. J., Yu, C. C., Du, J. Y., Kim, C. Y., Schell, A. J., Ahn, U. M., & Ahn, N. U. (2020). The relationship between cigarette smoking and the prevalence, frequency, and severity of back pain. *Journal of Surgical Orthopaedic Advances, 29*(3), 165–168. PMID: 33044158 https://pubmed.ncbi.nlm.nih.gov/33044158/#

Schmelzer, A. C., Salt, E., Wiggins, A., Crofford, L. J., Bush, H., & Mannino, D. M. (2016). Role of stress and smoking as modifiable risk factors for nonpersistent and persistent back pain in women. *The Clinical Journal of Pain, 32*(3), 232–237. https://doi.org/10.1097/AJP.0000000000000245

Sood, A., Ebbert, J. O., Sood, R., & Stevens, S. R. (2006). Complementary treatments for tobacco cessation: A survey. *Nicotine & Tobacco Research, 8*(6), 767–771. https://doi.org/10.1080/14622200601004109

Stead, L. F., Perera, R., Bullen, C., Mant, D., Hartmann-Boyce, J., Cahill, K., & Lancaster, T. (2012). Nicotine replacement therapy for smoking cessation. *Cochrane Database of Systematic Reviews*, 2012(11), Article No. CD000146. https://doi.org/10.1002/14651858.cd000146.pub4

Tahiri, M., Mottillo, S., Joseph, L., Pilote, L., & Eisenberg, M. J. (2012). Alternative smoking cessation aids: A meta-analysis of randomized controlled trials. *The American Journal of Medicine, 125*(6), 576–584. https://doi.org/10.1016/j.amjmed.2011.09.028

Tian, J., Venn, A., Otahal, P., & Gall, S. (2015). The association between quitting smoking and weight gain: A systematic review and meta-analysis of prospective cohort studies. *Obesity Reviews, 16*(10), 883–901. https://doi.org/10.1111/obr.12304

Tønnesen, P. (2009). Smoking cessation: How compelling is the evidence? A review. *Health Policy, 91*(Suppl. 1), S15–S25. https://doi.org/10.1016/S0168-8510(09)70004-1

U.S. Department of Health and Human Services. (2010). *How tobacco smoke causes disease: The biology and behavioral basis for smoking attributable disease: A report of the Surgeon General.* U.S. Department of Health and Human Services, Centers for Disease Control and Prevention, National Center for Chronic Disease Prevention and Health Promotion, Office on Smoking and Health. https://www.ncbi.nlm.nih.gov/books/NBK53017/

U.S. Department of Health and Human Services. (2014). *The health consequences of smoking—50 years of progress: A report of the Surgeon General, executive summary.* U.S. Department of Health and Human Services, Centers for Disease Control and Prevention, National Center for Chronic Disease Prevention and Health Promotion, Office on Smoking and Health. https://www.hhs.gov/sites/default/files/consequences-smoking-exec-summary.pdf

Viswesvaran, C., & Schmidt, F. L. (1992). A meta-analytic comparison of the effectiveness of smoking cessation methods. *Journal of Applied Psychology, 77*(4), 554–561. https://doi.org/10.1037/0021-9010.77.4.554

Wilkes, S. (2008). The use of bupropion SR in cigarette smoking cessation. *International Journal of Chronic Obstructive Pulmonary Disease, 3*(1), 45–53. https://doi.org/10.2147/COPD.S1121

Wilson, S. C., & Barber, T. X. (1983). *Inventory of childhood memories and imaginings.* Cushing Hospital.

Wittchen, H. U., Hoch, E., Klotsche, J., & Muehlig, S. (2011). Smoking cessation in primary care—A randomized controlled trial of bupropione, nicotine replacements, CBT and a minimal intervention. *International Journal of Methods in Psychiatric Research, 20*(1), 28–39. https://doi.org/10.1002/mpr.328

World Health Organization. (2017). *WHO report on the global tobacco epidemic, 2017: Monitoring tobacco use and prevention policies.* https://apps.who.int/iris/handle/10665/255874

8 HYPNOSIS WITH CHILDREN AND ADOLESCENTS

LISA LOMBARD AND LEONARD S. MILLING

INTRODUCTION

Hypnosis has long been recognized as a treatment for the psychological and medical challenges that impact children's quality of life and optimal development (Gardner, 1974; Kohen & Olness, 2011; Olness & Gardner, 1978). It is child-centered and rests on connecting with the youngster's imagination and curiosity (Kuttner, 2020). It requires an understanding of child development (Kohen & Olness, 2011; Sugarman & Wester, 2014), as well as recognizing that the child is part of a family system and wider community (Kuttner, 2020; Lyons, 2015). Hypnosis is frequently employed as an intervention for a wide variety of mental health and medical conditions experienced by children and adolescents.

Mental Health Applications

As a stand-alone treatment or when combined with other psychological interventions such as cognitive-behavioral therapy, hypnosis is often used to treat behavioral dysregulation problems (Guyer, 2014) such as developmentally

https://doi.org/10.1037/0000347-008
Evidence-Based Practice in Clinical Hypnosis, L. S. Milling (Editor)

inappropriate temper tantrums and sensation-seeking/avoidant behaviors (Kaiser, 2014), self-harming or age-inappropriate habits such as hair pulling (Zalsman et al., 2001; see also Iglesias, 2003), thumb sucking and nail biting (Wester, 2014), habit coughs (Anbar & Hall, 2004), stuttering and tics (Kohen, 1995; Lazarus & Klein, 2010), and nocturnal enuresis (Gottsegen, 2003; Kohen et al., 1984). It is regularly utilized as a treatment for some very common mental health problems experienced by children and adolescents, such as anxiety (Kaiser, 2017; Kohen & Kaiser, 2014) and depression (Kohen, 2014; Kohen & Murray, 2006). It can be integrated into a comprehensive treatment plan to help children with posttraumatic stress disorder (Wood & Bioy, 2020) and other traumatic syndromes (Cardeña et al., 2009; Linden, 2007). It has also been used to support children with learning differences (Krippner, 1966), attention problems (Barabasz & Barabasz, 2000), and poor executive functioning (Wark, 2011).

Opportunities to address the mental health issues experienced by youngsters using hypnosis are substantial, as eight of the 12 most frequently reported child health concerns are mental, behavioral, or developmental conditions (U.S. Health Resources and Services Administration Maternal and Child Health Bureau, 2020b). Prior to the COVID-19 pandemic, the prevalence of child and adolescent mental disorders (across all mental disorders) was 13.4% (Polanczyk et al., 2015) internationally and 13.2% within the United States (U.S. Health Resources and Services Administration Maternal and Child Health Bureau, 2020a). Of U.S. children age 3 to 17 with a current diagnosed mental or behavioral health condition, anxiety was most common (8.5%), followed by behavior disorder (6.8%) and depression (3.8%; U.S. Health Resources and Services Administration Maternal and Child Health Bureau, 2020a).

Medical Applications

Hypnosis is often used to reduce symptoms and improve quality of life across a range of children's medical issues and pain conditions, including asthma (Anbar, 2017), diabetes (Kihslinger & Sapp, 2006), cancer and related treatment (Hilgard & LeBaron, 1984), burn care (Bernstein, 1965), hemophilia (Swirsky-Sacchetti & Margolis, 1986), and warts (Ewin, 1992). Hypnosis is frequently utilized to reduce the pain associated with invasive medical procedures (Accardi & Milling, 2009) and chronic pain conditions such as headaches (Jong et al., 2019; Kohen, 2017; Kohen & Zajac, 2007). It sometimes has been employed to treat sleep issues (Kuttner, 2009). Finally, hypnosis has been used to support terminally ill children (Gardner, 1976) and as part of comfort care (Kuttner & Friedrichsdorf, 2014).

Hypnosis may be a valuable treatment tool in medical settings, as suggested by its use with very common childhood health concerns like allergies and asthma, which are two of the top three child health conditions, as reported in 2017–2018 (U.S. Health Resources and Services Administration Maternal and Child Health Bureau, 2020a). It also can contribute significantly to the care of children with impactful medical concerns, like cancer, which is the leading cause of death by disease past infancy among children in the United States (Siegel et al., 2021).

Using Hypnosis With Children

Hypnosis with children, although related to adult hypnosis, proceeds differently because the clinician must tailor the experience to the youngster's developmental level. Hypnosis with young children is usually introduced informally or conversationally, using vocabulary that is commensurate with the child's language development and communication skills (Pendergrast, 2017). Since abstract reasoning is immature and developing, suggestions should be clear, concrete, and specific. In a respectful manner, direct suggestions are often given to young children, while indirect suggestions can be interwoven into the older child's hypnotic experience. As children's language develops, and they are exposed to more life situations, the clinician may playfully include puns and humor.

Hypnotic inductions that include stories, especially if they are highly imaginative, engaging, and consistent with the child's interests, hobbies, and fantasy world, can be quite successful. With young children, physical space, and permission to move, spin, and dance may be necessary. Their repetitive movements can be integrated into stories and role playing. They can be engaged by props, figurines, and art supplies, so that therapeutic themes can be explored, confidence strengthened, and self-regulation skills practiced (Linden, 2003).

With young children the hypnotic experience is brief, and although imaginatively engaging, they fluidly go in and out of hypnosis. Younger children rarely close their eyes, have fluctuating attention, and are unlikely to be still for very long. This is evidenced as they look off into the distance while retrieving memories, speak slowly or excitedly about their pretend ideas, and engage the clinician in a shared fantasy world. Relaxation is rarely a primary goal for most children and until about age 10, they usually keep their eyes open (Kohen & Olness, 2011). As youngsters mature, the hypnotic encounter lengthens, and they remain more focused and still.

Novel and fantasy-laden suggestions (like describing imaginary magnets placed on the fingers to draw them together and cue the child to use their imagination for a special purpose, or suggesting a magic carpet ride to a special, safe place that the child then describes) can be enjoyable invitations into hypnosis for many school-age children. Additionally, tweens and teens may enjoy these imaginative experiences when they are enhanced with relaxation activities, such as regulated breathing or progressive muscle relaxation. However, when working hypnotically with adolescents, the clinician must make room for how they navigate the developmental task of establishing their identity and autonomy. Some adolescents, who may be reluctant to "give up" control, keep their eyes open and express considerable skepticism. This can be addressed by respectfully acknowledging their concerns and offering genuine interest in their opinions.

Regardless of the patient's age, the clinician closely observes the child, paces their remarks with the child's breath and behaviors, mirrors verbal and nonverbal communication, and utilizes the interests and objects the child brings to the hypnotic encounter. These practices help build rapport and tailor the experience to the individual, so that hypnotic phenomena like suggestions and imagery are personalized, meaningful, and promote wellness, comfort, and positive change.

REVIEW OF OUTCOME RESEARCH

Historically, the literature on hypnosis with children and adolescents has primarily consisted of case histories (e.g., Roberts, 1998; Wood & Bioy, 2020) and books (e.g., Gardner & Olness, 1981; Hilgard & LeBaron, 1984; Kohen & Olness, 2011) describing the use of this treatment modality. The number of empirical investigations has been small. For example, approximately 20 years ago, one of us conducted a systematic review of all studies with children and adolescents in which hypnosis was compared with a no-treatment, wait list, attention, standard care, or placebo control condition, or an alternative intervention (Milling & Costantino, 2000). Only 16 studies were identified, of which just 10 investigations utilized random assignment to condition in treating a clinical problem (e.g., anxiety, procedural pain, nausea and vomiting associated with chemotherapy).

The number of randomized controlled and randomized comparative studies of the use of hypnosis with children and adolescents has grown over the last 20 years. In the treatment outcome literature, randomized controlled trials are considered the gold standard in part because random assignment increases the chances that individuals assigned to the treatment and control conditions will be equivalent at the outset of a study. This section of the chapter provides a review of randomized controlled studies with children and adolescents in which hypnosis compared favorably with either a control condition or an alternative treatment.

Anxiety

There are a growing number of controlled studies of the use of hypnosis in treating various forms of anxiety (see Valentine et al., 2019). However, only one randomized controlled study has evaluated the efficacy of hypnosis for helping youngsters experiencing anxiety. Stanton (1994) randomly assigned 12- to 15-year-olds who scored in the upper third on a questionnaire measure of test anxiety to hypnosis or attention control conditions. The hypnosis intervention consisted of two 50-minute sessions that included suggestions for imagery associated with relaxation, mastery, and self-efficacy. Youngsters in the hypnosis condition reduced self-reported test anxiety significantly more than those in the control condition at the end of treatment and at a 6-month follow-up. Unfortunately, the impact of hypnosis on actual test performance was not assessed.

Enuresis

Nocturnal enuresis involves urinating in the bed at night beyond the age when children normally gain control of this reflex. Several randomized controlled trials have demonstrated the efficacy of hypnosis in treating nocturnal enuresis (Edwards & van der Spuy, 1985), including its superiority to medication (Banerjee et al., 1993).

Edwards and van der Spuy (1985) randomly assigned children between the ages of 8 and 13 to one of four conditions. The hypnosis condition consisted of six weekly sessions and involved an induction plus suggestions for dry nights. A suggestion-only condition provided suggestions for dry nights without an induction, whereas the induction-only condition offered an induction without suggestions. A wait list control group constituted a fourth condition. Youngsters in the hypnosis and suggestion-only conditions demonstrated significantly more dry nights than those in the control condition at the end of treatment. All three treatment conditions resulted in significantly more dry nights than the control condition at the 6-month follow-up.

Banerjee et al. (1993) randomized youngsters ranging in age from 5 to 16 with nocturnal enuresis to hypnosis or medication conditions. The hypnosis treatment involved three sessions in which children heard suggestions to get up and use the toilet at night when their bladder was full. These patients were taught self-hypnosis and encouraged to practice it before going to sleep. The medication condition consisted of increasing doses of imipramine each week until dry nights were achieved. Both interventions were discontinued after 3 months. Results showed hypnosis produced significantly more dry nights 6 months after treatment was stopped than did imipramine.

Side Effects of Chemotherapy

Chemotherapy is one of the most common treatments for childhood cancers, but it has unpleasant side effects like nausea and vomiting. Hilgard and LeBaron (1984) developed an *imagination-focused* approach to hypnosis for the difficulties commonly experienced by youngsters undergoing cancer treatment. In imagination-focused hypnosis, patients are helped to become highly involved in a story-like fantasy based on their favorite activities (e.g., movies, foods, pets, friends) so they will experience less discomfort when undergoing unpleasant medical interventions like chemotherapy or needle-related procedures. With regard to chemotherapy, several randomized controlled trials have shown that imagination-focused hypnosis is effective for reducing nausea and vomiting (Zeltzer et al., 1991), as well as the use of antiemetic medication (Jacknow et al., 1994).

Zeltzer et al. (1991) randomly assigned youngsters aged 5 to 17 undergoing chemotherapy to hypnosis, distraction, or attention control conditions. During chemotherapy, patients in the hypnosis condition received imagination-focused hypnosis, whereas those in the distraction condition were helped to focus their attention on external objects in the examination room or deep breathing. Children in both treatment conditions experienced a significantly shorter duration of nausea compared with those in the control condition. Only youngsters receiving hypnosis demonstrated a shorter duration of vomiting than controls.

Jacknow et al. (1994) randomized pediatric cancer patients between the ages of 6 and 18 to self-hypnosis or attention control conditions. The self-hypnosis intervention consisted of two to three sessions of training emphasizing a combination of imagination-focused hypnosis, plus suggestions for relaxation, experiencing a special place or activity, as well as direct suggestions to shut off the vomit control center in the brain. During the first and second courses of chemotherapy, there was no difference between the two conditions in episodes of nausea and vomiting, but youngsters in the self-hypnosis condition used significantly less antiemetic medication than those in the control condition. Moreover, 1 to 2 months postdiagnosis, the self-hypnosis group reported significantly less anticipatory nausea than the control group.

Postsurgical Pain

After surgery, patients often complain of pain, nausea (from the anesthesia), and fatigue. Several studies have shown that both hypnotic (Lambert, 1996) and nonhypnotic suggestions (Huth et al., 2004) for imagery can be effective in relieving the pain experienced by youngsters who have undergone surgery.

Huth et al. (2004) randomly assigned 7- to 12-year-olds undergoing tonsillectomy and/or adenoidectomy to imagery (i.e., nonhypnotic suggestion) or attention control conditions. Prior to surgery, youngsters in the imagery condition received training in deep breathing, muscle relaxation, as well as nonhypnotic suggestions for imagery of a park or their favorite place. These patients were also seen by a therapist in the hospital after surgery. Compared with the control condition, the imagery condition reported significantly less sensory (i.e., intensity) and affective (i.e., unpleasantness) pain immediately after surgery.

Lambert (1996) randomized children between the ages of 7 and 12 undergoing elective surgery to hypnosis or attention control conditions. The hypnosis condition consisted of one 30-minute training session a week before surgery that included suggestions to experience an enjoyable image, as well as relaxation and reduced pain. After surgery, youngsters in the hypnosis condition experienced significantly less pain and had shorter hospital stays than those in the control condition.

Needle Pain

Perhaps the mostly extensively studied application of hypnosis with children and adolescents is needle pain. Common needle-related procedures include lumbar punctures (in which a narrow-gauge needle is inserted into the spinal column), bone marrow aspirations (in which a large-gauge syringe is inserted into the hipbone), and venipunctures (in which a vein is punctured with a needle).

Numerous randomized controlled trials have demonstrated the efficacy of hypnosis for relieving the pain and anxiety experienced by children and adolescents undergoing lumbar punctures (Liossi & Hatira, 2003; Liossi et al., 2006), bone marrow aspirations (Kuttner et al., 1988; Liossi & Hatira, 1999), and venipunctures (Liossi et al., 2009; Smith et al., 1996).

Of note, one study found that direct suggestions for pain reduction and indirect suggestions for pleasant or distracting imagery (e.g., suggestions for imagery of the setting sun) were equally effective in reducing the pain and distress produced by lumbar punctures (Liossi & Hatira, 2003).

Moreover, several studies have shown that hypnosis is as effective, if not more effective, than distraction (Kuttner et al., 1988; Smith et al., 1996; Zeltzer & LeBaron, 1982) and cognitive behavioral therapy (Liossi & Hatira, 1999) in reducing the discomfort experienced by youngsters undergoing needle-related procedures. For example, Zeltzer and LeBaron (1982) reported that imagination-focused hypnosis relieved pain and anxiety more than external distraction and deep breathing. Likewise, Liossi and Hatira (1999) found that direct suggestions for pain reduction were more effective in relieving anxiety and distress than a cognitive-behavioral treatment package consisting of relaxation, breathing, and coping self-statements.

Other Forms of Acute Pain

Dental pain is similar to needle-pain because it often (but not always) involves the injection of an anesthetic with a syringe. Huet et al. (2011) randomly assigned 7- to 12- year-olds undergoing dental anesthesia to hypnosis or standard care control conditions. The hypnosis intervention was delivered while children were in the dental chair receiving the anesthetic and involved suggestions to experience stories and activities in which the child was interested. Youngsters receiving hypnosis experienced less pain and anxiety during the dental procedure than those in the control condition.

A voiding cystourethrogram (VCUG) is a radiological evaluation of a child's bladder and urinary tract. It involves the insertion of contrast materials into the bladder and imaging during urination. Butler et al. (2005) randomized youngsters between the ages of 4 and 15 undergoing a VCUG to hypnosis or standard care control conditions. The hypnosis intervention consisted of 1 hour of training in which youngsters received suggestions to imagine floating in a lake, bath, or tub, as well as visiting an amusement park, friend's house, or playground. A therapist was present during the VCUG to help youngsters use the imagery. Observer ratings of distress were significantly lower in the hypnosis condition than the control condition.

Chronic Pain

Irritable bowel syndrome is a chronic condition that involves abdominal pain, cramping, bloating, gas, diarrhea or constipation, and abnormal bowel movements. Vlieger et al. (2007) randomly assigned 8- to 18-year-olds diagnosed with irritable bowel syndrome or functional abdominal pain for at least 1 year to hypnosis or attention control conditions. The hypnosis intervention, referred to as *gut-directed hypnotherapy*, consisted of six 50-minute sessions over 3 months and included suggestions for relaxation, control of abdominal pain, normalization of gut functions, improved sleep, and ego-strengthening. Patients were given a recording of a standardized hypnosis session and encouraged to listen to it each day. Youngsters in the hypnosis condition reported significantly lower pain intensity and frequency than those in the control condition 1 year after the conclusion of therapy. These differences were maintained at a 5-year follow-up (Vlieger et al., 2012).

Summary of Reviewed Studies

Generally, the treatment outcome literature indicates hypnosis can be a useful clinical tool in working with children and adolescents. The research base supporting the effectiveness of hypnosis as an intervention for anxiety, enuresis, chemotherapy, postsurgical pain, dental pain, voiding cystourethrograms, and irritable bowel syndrome is promising, but modest in size. In contrast, a substantial number of randomized controlled trials have established the efficacy of hypnosis for relieving needle pain. Considered as a group, the vast majority of methodologically sound studies with youngsters have addressed medical conditions. More randomized controlled studies are greatly needed verifying the efficacy of hypnosis as a treatment for childhood mental health issues.

CASE EXAMPLES

Although it is not unusual for children to occasionally experience anxiety, when it becomes excessive and interferes with daily functioning, intervention is indicated. Childhood anxiety has implications for parents, siblings, and others, and about six in 10 children receive treatment (Centers for Disease Control and Prevention, 2021). Families often struggle to reconfigure their child's environment to avoid anxiety-producing experiences. This strategy, albeit well-intentioned, does not help the child learn coping skills and may escalate the problem by reinforcing the message that there is something dangerous that needs to be avoided. Regardless of the origins of the anxiety, it can be characterized as a set of interconnected physical, psychological, and behavioral experiences that are uncomfortable and fuel avoidance. Because avoidance is not an effective coping strategy and can be quite limiting, children's self-confidence weakens, cognitive distortions strengthen, and associated physical expressions of anxiety intensify. This problematic cycle should be the focus of clinical intervention, not the content of the child's worries. Using hypnosis, the clinician and child build or rediscover skills that foster ego strength, coping, and mastery.

The use of hypnosis to help children cope with anxiety is presented below in four case examples ranging in age from 4 to 19 years old. (Each case example includes a hypnosis protocol.) The specific content of the anxiety, although interesting, is often not the explicit target of the hypnotic interventions. The clinician selects hypnotic invitations and intensifications that are most suitable for *this child at this moment*, to reach treatment goals like symptom reduction, relaxation and tension release, cognitive-behavioral growth, better insight, and positive behavioral lifestyle changes.

Case Example 1

Kevin (pseudonym) is a 4-year-old boy with a dairy allergy and associated food avoidance behaviors, visceral hypersensitivity after eating, unexplained vomiting into his mouth, and recent weight loss. He reached developmental milestones within normal limits. Apart from the weight loss and vomiting, he is generally healthy. As an infant he had torticollis, which resolved on its own. Several medical workups have taken place, and he is under the care of pediatric specialists. Psychotropic medication and a visit to a chiropractor have not helped. There is a positive family history of obsessive-compulsive disorder. Kevin lives with his parents in an urban community. He attends preschool regularly, and there are no concerns about social or academic performance. He is fascinated by trucks and much of his play centers on transportation-related topics.

Parents sought hypnotherapy to help Kevin cope with the visceral sensations he has after eating and to reduce his general distress about meals. Their primary concern is Kevin's dysregulated, negative behavior during meals and his growing preoccupation with avoiding foods. He coughs, hits, and verbally lashes out at parents during meals. Because of his weight loss, parents carefully measure food portions to ensure he consumes enough calories throughout the day. They also rearrange their work schedules so someone can be with him for extended periods, to coax him to eat, reassure him that he is not going to vomit, manage his behavior, and clean up after he vomits. Mother is highly attentive to his needs, and because she sometimes anticipates problems before they occur, her responses can magnify his fears and sense of losing control. Father is slightly rigid and verbally expresses his frustration with his son. If Kevin gets emotionally overwhelmed and physically aggressive toward mother during a meal, she leaves the room and father continues to feed him, stopping when the measured portion is consumed. Then, father cancels the family's evening activities, in anticipation of Kevin vomiting and because he finds it difficult to enjoy time together after these disturbances. Although parents have introduced the iPad as distraction during meals, it is inconsistently helpful and not a long-term solution. Kevin recognizes that meals are a problem, but willingly cooks in the kitchen with mother and does not find food odors aversive. He stated, "I never vomit when helping mommy cook, I like to mix (the food)." Parents report he has a poor appetite and dislikes many foods. His favorite foods are pepperoni and hot dogs, which he eats in bite-size pieces and tolerates well.

The clinician met with mother to gather a developmental history and then separately with Kevin to build rapport and learn more about his interests. He explained that he was meeting with a "talking and feelings doctor," so he could have "better meals." This he explained, meant feeling better while eating and not fighting with his parents. Belly breathing was discussed, demonstrated, and practiced (with mother watching and taking notes), to facilitate relaxation before the meal and to introduce a positive experience that would be incompatible with the ritualized negative mealtime routine his family had created. Over time, it was hoped his hypervigilance would decrease as his body became more comfortable. He was taught belly breathing, pretended a balloon was in his tummy, and quickly became engrossed in inflating the pretend balloon to see his tummy grow larger (inhale) and smaller (exhale). He repeated this pattern several times, became still in his seat, and demonstrated a smooth natural rhythm of inhaling and exhaling. Next, he practiced regulated breathing with a small stuffed animal on his belly so that he could later teach this method to his father. Finally, we practiced blowing a pretend feather, an additional practice for him to share with dad.

We developed a graduated incentive plan to encourage specific behaviors during meals and to ignore (as much as possible) nontargeted behaviors. He earned firetruck stickers, first by coming to the table (regardless of whether he ate). Every few days, additional steps were added (like a sticker for doing belly breathing before the meal), so that eventually he earned stickers for bringing food to his mouth without a fuss and putting food in his mouth while noticing enjoyable textures, flavors, temperature, and good aroma. He retrieved a prize from a treasure box at home for earning three stickers in a 5-day period. This graduated reward plan encouraged parents to notice small, incremental successes rather than battle over an entire meal.

Hypnosis Protocol
Kevin was invited to use his imagination in special ways in this conversationally based hypnosis. The therapist simply described how Kevin was moving colorful wooden beads at different speeds and in different directions through a large maze.

"So, you see all of those beads and they're all different colors, aren't they? (Utilizing what he is doing and offering a truism to begin the process

of joining with Kevin.) *They go to different parts, and they go around in circles and straight and up and down.* (He spontaneously names some of the colors, showing he is already participating in the back-and-forth dialogue with the therapist.) *You're right.* (Confirming his perspective and capacity.) *There's blue and yellow and red and green . . . and around and around they go, and up and down and all around.* (Repetition of words, pacing in time with his movements as the beads slide down, describing what he makes the beads do.)

When you just watch them go around and around, maybe you listen to the sound of them too, as they fall down, as they slide down [the metal path]. (Adding indirect suggestion to bring in more sensory details by listening.) *And they go around and around and down, down, down, down, down.* (Therapist repeats words and sounds, drawing out the word with her voice to nonverbally invite him to slow down, listen, go deeper into the playful experience.) *Oh, I see they are going slower and lower, they sound softer . . . gentle.* (Observing and utilizing the change in speed that he produced.) *And when they all get to the end . . . when you hear every bead get to the end . . . that's going to be your special signal to put your bottom on the rug and just . . . sit . . . down next to all the beads.* (Suggestion for changing his behavior and posture, to be like the beads slowing down and stopping, in preparation for listening and turning his focus inward.) *When they all get down there, that'll be your signal to have your bottom sit still on the rug . . .* (He sits down.) *You knew the signal!* (Praise and exaggerated positive verbal reinforcement to acknowledge his capabilities.)

We can touch them, and you can look at the colors and you can listen. (A yes response set to encourage collaboration; a multi-sensory experience.) *You might find it fun to imagine that those colors are like cans of paint.* (Therapist invites him to be curious.) *Cans of paint . . . and there could be a red paint and a yellow paint or a blue paint or green paint. Which paint do you want to dip your paintbrush into?"* ("Yellow," he answers.) *"Okay, great choice. You picked the yellow paint and maybe you dip your pretend paint brush into that paint can and then take the paint.* (He does this gesture and therapist remains quiet for a moment.) *It might be fun to brush it on . . . to . . .* (Therapist pauses, hopes the delay further engages his attention, curiosity, and anticipation of what happens next.) *. . . your toes!* (He does the motion of painting.) *Yes, what fun, paint the yellow paint onto your toes . . . take the yellow paint brush in your imagination and paint your toes yellow. Good job! Feel the yellow going on.* (Mixing sensory input of visual color with tactile sensation, perhaps unexpected, again hoping to heighten his absorption in the imaginative experience.)

Feel it begin to go up, up your legs . . . I wonder what that's like? It might not even be on your toes anymore, right? And, it might feel ticklish, it might feel tingly . . . I don't know." (Therapist offers some permissive suggestions for changing sensation.) ("Tingle," he specifies.) *"So let that tingle feeling go up . . . and to . . . those knees now.* (Therapist implies dissociation by talking about the tingle feeling from an observational perspective.) *Help it move into your knees: up, up, up, up, up . . . into your knees! Yes, wow, you're really good at this.* (Therapist's voice rises with each word, to emphasize mastery and control over a sensation in his own body—not typical experiences for him.) *Let the tingle feeling grow bigger and stronger in your knees.* (He gestures with his hands, as if he is now painting his fingernails.) *Sure, paint your nails. Okay . . . doing it. What color is the tingle?"* ("Yellow," he replies and then places his hands back on his knees and resumes motion of painting his legs. Note the importance of closely observing the child.) *"Let the tingle grow bigger and stronger, if you'd like, and move up your leg: up, up, up till it gets up the whole leg.*

And it might be interesting to do your belly button and feel the tingle. (The therapist has taken quite a bit of time to establish this activity as fun, interesting, and safe, before focusing on the belly, where his symptoms take place.) *Yes, Kevin, and take that color or another color."* (He is invited to choose his own paint color for the tummy, to exercise some age-appropriate control. "Red," he reports.) *"Okay, you got red* (Therapist remains neutral about whether this is positive or negative, because there is not enough information yet.) *Is there still yellow going into the tingle?* (Nods yes.) *Wonderful, Kevin.*

And with the next breath in that you take, notice the air at the tip of your nose, as it goes inside your nose and then you can, when you're ready, let the breath out through your mouth. (Therapist has shifted the conversation to focus on his breathing, to add regulated breathing and comfort to this focus on his belly.) *It might be neat to pretend that when the breath goes in and goes out, your colors go in and out too. The red and yellow you feel.* (Permissive suggestion.) *Would you like the tingle and the colors to go up into your shoulders? Even up into your head and brain?* (He nods yes.) *Sure then, move it up, go ahead bring it in . . . and then out.* (Therapist pauses during his inhale and speaks again when he exhales, pacing to deepen the experience and to nonverbally guide him to coordinate breathing and moving his tingling feeling in his body.)

I can see you are really very good at moving that tingling feeling. (Ego strengthening.) *That's so good. And as you do this, your body, legs, tummy, arms are . . . there . . . and may feel more and more comfortable. From the tippy top down to the toes.* (Therapist offers a suggestion for a positive physical transformation, using age-appropriate language and matching the sequence that's been followed.) *And maybe you imagine the red and yellow washing all around your hair.* (Therapist introduces a familiar and practical way to apply the colors to his head.) *What would it look like if you had red and yellow hair?!"* (Using humor to keep his interest and to add positive elements to this activity. The therapist and Kevin giggle at this silly image. "It would look tingly," he says.) *"And how does your whole body feel when everything turns red and yellow? Is that a lovely, good feeling?* (Therapist suggests that this transformation is positive. He nods yes.) *And so, take a moment and enjoy the tingly feeling.*

That's good. Feel the tingles all around and inside of you. (The therapist has generalized the tingly feeling and associated color wash to be both inside and outside. The feeling inside is tingly, not painful or distressing. He holds out a hand, as if to ask for the hand to be included, too.) *Oh yes, the fingertips. Look at the fingertips. What do they look like?"* ("Red," he answers.) *"They do look red and let them go together and rub one another and let the tingle get bigger and stronger and then take your hands please, and put them on the outside of your belly, on your tummy . . . and let all the tingly good feelings soak inside your tummy so it feels especially good right now. And isn't it cool* (deliberately using the word cool to add a potentially comforting sensation to the experience) *how you can make your tummy feel better by putting your hands on it and letting the tingling feeling go inside?* (This suggestion summarizes the goals of this hypnotic experience: ego strengthening, mastery, and learning a new skill to change unpleasant sensations.) *And every time you listen to this recording at home, you'll get better and better at doing this, and it gets easier and faster to let your belly and your tummy feel good and tingly!* (Therapist offers a posthypnotic suggestion to encourage him to practice self-hypnosis.) *And that will be a nice thing to do for yourself. All right! Good job, Kevin!"*

This session was followed by one in which he drew multiple pictures of red swirls representing stomach sensations and then changed them by scribbling over them in gray. He spontaneously shouted, "And send off the red to stay away from me!" The therapist agreed enthusiastically and complimented HIS excellent idea. As Kevin drew, the therapist again narrated and described how his drawings matched his plan to change his tummy sensations, and how understandably proud he seemed to feel. A posthypnotic suggestion was offered, reminding him that when he looked at his drawings, he could feel growing confidence and pride that his tummy and body are healthy and work very well. This pleased Kevin.

As the session ended, he spontaneously reported that at a recent meal, his father went from being angry to calm. Due to time limitations, the therapist quickly commented, *"Wow, daddy changed too!"* As Kevin left the therapy room, he gave the therapist an unexpected hug (rather than the usual high five), nonverbally communicating that he felt understood and perhaps comforted by hearing this. Two weeks later, mother reported that Kevin's demeanor and eating habits were improving. He had successfully managed stomach discomfort in the car, when he verbally labelled a tummy sensation, did not vomit, asked for the window to be opened so he could get fresh air, and described using his color changing strategy!

Case Example 2

Susanna (pseudonym) is an 8-year-old girl in second grade who came to therapy because of her fear of extreme weather and difficulty falling asleep. Together, we quickly determined that better sleep was the first goal of therapy. She appreciated hearing that she was going to learn more about how to "invite yourself to fall asleep." She is a middle child in a sibship of three girls. The busy family lives in a suburban area outside of a large city in the Midwest. Both parents work and father travels considerably for his job. Susanna reached developmental milestones within normal limits. Her health is very good. She has many friends and is quite sociable, but mother described her as "shy" and "moody . . . doesn't know how to bounce back" when something does not go her way. Susanna is very involved in ballet and gymnastics. Although she does well in school, mom reports that she struggles to finish her homework in the evening because she is easily distracted. She prefers to sleep with mom and dad (because "they have a very large bed that fills the room"); her baby sister also sleeps with parents. When Susanna is in her own room at night, she awakens very early in the morning to hear father leave for work because she worries he will be late. After he leaves, she climbs into bed with mother and baby. Her father had given her a book about how to fall asleep by remembering things that happened during the day. We decided to adapt the idea for Susanna and record a story, for her to listen to at home as she imagines going to her "remembering place" to review the pleasant events of the day and fall asleep. She decided the main character would be a fish named Samantha. The modified story about Samantha, tailored to include details from Susanna's life, becomes the hypnotic experience.

Hypnosis Protocol
"I'm going to tell you the story about Samantha and it's pretty similar to one you've heard before, but there might be some differences too. She has

a very busy day, doesn't she, with her friends and going to school. What grade should she be in?" (The patient answers, "Second grade.") "Okay. And then sometimes she plays outside, and she loves to do gymnastics and she does it all the time, whenever she has free time, she just does flips wherever she can. Sometimes she even flips in her own living room. Some days Samantha is so busy she doesn't have much time to sit and rest, so then after dinner she's very ready to slow down and get calm and comfortable for the night. Samantha loves to get calm and comfortable because that is when she can have her quiet time, quiet time with her mom or with her dad or her babysitter.*

It's interesting, she enjoys spending time being busy and *she loves to have quiet time and to listen to special stories about falling asleep at bedtime. Then she gets cuddles and hugs in her cozy bed. Samantha is so tired and sleepy after a busy day that she loves to get comfortable and cozy and to settle into sleep. Sometimes Samantha is so very, very tired but she needs a bit of help getting comfortable and cozy so that she can fall asleep easily. She likes it when a grown up helps her slow down and get comfortable and do all the things she knows how to do, to drift into sleep. So, every night when Samantha is in her pajamas and has her blankets and pillows and finds just the right place in her bed, someone special helps.*

And then she pretends she's taking a walk or perhaps, because Samantha is a salmon, she pretends she is swimming and floating to a special remembering place where she can remember everything that happened that day. When Samantha goes to the special remembering place, she can see herself playing with her friends at school. She can see herself doing gymnastics. She can see herself drawing and coloring and reading stories and books. She sees herself doing favorite activities at her favorite spots. She sees it all, and of course she sees herself the clearest. She sees herself with her teacher at school and she sees herself with her mom and her big sister and her little baby sister and her dad. And Samantha remembers the day. She also likes to remember all the good feelings she has had.

Sometimes Samantha likes to close her eyes and remember her classroom and her table spot and her locker, and all the good feelings there. Sometimes she likes to close her eyes and remember sounds, like singing or gentle breathing. Sometimes she likes to remember how things feel, like how soft her earmuffs are or how firm the mattress is when she does a flip on it. Or she remembers how cool her sheets are when she first gets into bed until she warms them up. And sometimes she likes to remember how good it smells when her mom cooks dinner or when she smells beautiful roses outside in the summer. Samantha can be busy, by being still and remembering so many good feelings.

She loves the way she lets her busy mind drift happily through all the nice things she was remembering. . . . As Samantha floats, she moves a bit more slowly and after a little while moves even more slowly than before. Samantha starts to feel her body beginning to get a little tired and then she moves even more slowly. She feels comfortable floating and drifting at her own slow speed. Sometimes she goes up a little and then down again even deeper and then up again and down again. Samantha can feel how her breathing starts to slowly match the way she is moving . . . up and down . . . slower and slower . . . until everything is easy. She feels like she's a bird gliding in the sky or a lovely fish swimming smoothly in the water. She feels so happy . . . just enjoying how good it feels to be moving slowly and to easily adjust the pace, so it all . . . feels . . . just . . . right.

After a little while Samantha decides to take a bit of a rest. She looks around for a place that will feel just right and sure enough she finds the place she knows is just the right place for her, because she sees her favorite things there—her favorite books, favorite pillow, favorite stuffed animal, her favorite sweater, her favorite pictures from the wall, her favorite toys, her favorite pieces of clothing, all there for Samantha in just the right size and shape. It looks as if they've been waiting there for her all along. She can feel her breathing becoming calm and slow, calm and slow. Samantha loves the feeling of being so comfortable that she wants to go to sleep. Samantha knows that when she goes to sleep, she can hold onto all her lovely feelings all through the night. She is safe and soon it will be another day."

Case Example 3

John (pseudonym), an 11-year-old boy in fifth grade, attends private school in a large Midwestern city. He lives with his parents, who own a new business, and an older and younger sibling. Parents brought him to therapy when he shared that he is sometimes bothered by sounds and clicking noises. His visit to the pediatrician was unremarkable and no further intervention was recommended, but John and his parents notice he is developing the habit of opening his mouth to "pop" his ears. John is capable, hard-working, has close friends, does well in school, and participates in karate, swimming, basketball, baseball, cross-country, and choir. He likes to keep a journal. He is healthy and reached developmental milestones within normal limits. He is described as "even-tempered" but has difficulty relaxing, according to his mother. Privately, he acknowledged many worries and asked many "what if" questions. He shared that his anxiety sometimes interferes with his ability to go to new places, although he recognized that he usually enjoys them once there. He especially liked going to a local amusement park and riding the roller coaster. John presented with an open, friendly, and curious demeanor. He reported using regulated breathing and mindfulness apps to manage his anxiety and added that by counting to 10 he could "train his brain" to not think about his worries. This had been effective for about a month, but he began to over-focus on counting to 10 and now worries he is doing something incorrectly. He hopes to learn alternative coping skills, despite remarking that he might not "do it right." John is also interested in learning hypnosis so he can be more relaxed and perform better during athletic and musical events. The session excerpt that follows describes his introduction to hypnotic relaxation and contains preparatory ideas for how he might ignore sounds (and thoughts) that are not important. The imaginative experience pertains to feeling positive and carefree, not to traditional relaxation. As he sits in a reclining chair the therapist begins to speak.

Hypnosis Protocol

"So, if you are comfortable, and it's OK, you can get even more comfortable. Lean back even further and put your feet up on that footstool, so you can be as comfortable as you'd like to be. Whatever you need to do. (Not explicitly using the word relax, because he is rather self-critical about this, but suggesting he might get more comfortable.) *You might already notice that you can feel the seat behind you with the coolness of the chair underneath your neck and head and back.* (Noticing these sensations are easy and not likely to judge himself as doing it wrong.) *And that your feet are dangling down a little bit. And as you notice that and pay closer and closer attention to the words that I'm saying, maybe all the other sounds in the background begin to fade away, and you don't even notice them happening, as you listen more and more to the words that I say and the ones that are right for you.* (Invitation to select what he pays attention to.) *And then you can keep them in that special place in your memory where you remember things clearly. Very, very good job, John.*

And just let your body sink into the chair, more and more. It might be fun to use that good imagination of yours, so I invite you to imagine with that good imagination what you described earlier. . . . Being in a special place, maybe some place that you've been to before or maybe somewhere where you really wish you could go. Some place where the stress fades. And when you have that special place in your imagination go ahead and either nod your head or let me know you found it. (He nods.) *Okay! And as we talk and you see yourself in that special place, it might be interesting to hear what you can hear there, while you're here.* (Word play.) *And to see as you look around in that special place, what does it look like?"* (He responds, "Big, a big fun roller coaster.") *"Great! A big, fun one.*

You might imagine you're on a roller coaster right now . . . the roller coaster goes up, up, up or is it going down, down, down?" (He clarifies, "Going straight.") *"Okay, thanks. And you're all buckled in* (Therapist adds this to remind him that he knows how to stay safe.) *and you're at the amusement park and you're on the roller coaster and it's going straight and of course sometimes roller coasters are very quiet and sometimes they're kind of noisy, right? Which one is more like the roller coaster you're on?"* (He says, "Noisy.") *"Noisy, so go ahead and listen to the sound of the roller coaster from the car, but I don't know if you're at the front or in the middle or the back."* (He says, "Second row.") *"You're in the second row and it's going along and it's kind of noisy and maybe you begin to feel the breeze, the wind in your face. The speed might change because roller coasters do go fast and slow and medium. All different speeds, all are right for different times and different parts of the roller coaster. Perhaps you notice the different speeds because it feels different on your face and skin, as some of the air or breeze touches you. And every time you feel the breeze it's another signal for you to enjoy this special place even more.* (Therapist offers suggestion to enjoy and make this a positive experience.)

Because as you enjoy the special place and feel the breeze and hear the sounds, you might also notice other . . . fun things happening. Sometimes people laugh when that happens, don't they? Sometimes people shout out on a roller coaster. (Therapist encourages a sense of autonomy, by noting that "some" people, not "all" people, feel this way and wondering how he feels.) *I don't know exactly what you do on a roller coaster, but it can really feel like unexpected things are about to happen, fun unexpected things.* (Therapist predicts the unexpected AND that they can be fun) *That's right, just let your memory of a roller coaster ride get clearer and clearer, noticing more of what is fun and whatever else you want to notice. And of course, as you close those eyes things do become clearer in your imagination.* (Therapist mentions this to confirm that his eyes have closed, although there was no direct suggestion for this to happen.) *You're doing this very well, just right for you.* (Adding positive reinforcement and ego strengthening.)

Feel the breeze, the wind, hear the sounds, it looks like so much fun and you're confident this ride is a fun one. Maybe talking to someone near you or maybe not talking. Maybe smelling some treats like popcorn or cotton candy. Maybe there's music going on at the amusement park and laughing in the background. And you're feeling like, oh I don't know. . . .

(A smile begins to form on his face.) *Yes, you're smiling and smiling and smiling. That's a great smile, as you enjoy this little vacation in your imagination. A special place, a treat for yourself, like giving yourself a gift or a present in the present moment. And you get faster and better at imagining the roller coaster in just the right way for you, the more you listen to this recording and picture everything in your imagination.* (Post-hypnotic suggestion for practicing self-hypnosis and building confidence.)

In fact, you may be pleasantly surprised just how easy it is to hear the sounds, feel the breeze, notice the smile, and have these fun feelings again! How fun to be there and to bring that fun feeling here . . . now, or sometime later. So, I'll be silent for a moment so that you can continue to enjoy this good feeling and bring forward with you all the cool things you saw in your imagination and enjoyed so much. Bring them all with you, just like you keep other important things with you, safe and with you, so they'll be with you in the coming days and weeks as you listen to the recording and remember this fun roller coaster and the enjoyable experience of being somewhere special like this."

Case Example 4

Amy (pseudonym) is a 19-year-old young woman who just completed her first semester of college away from home. She is the oldest of three children. She came to therapy because of "compulsive knuckle biting." Her hands looked red, and the skin was cracked and broken in several places. She was fashionably dressed and well groomed. She was referred by her dermatologist for brief treatment while back home for a 3-week winter break. Several years earlier, she participated in intensive psychotherapy with another therapist because of anxiety and depression. She continues taking Prozac under the care of a psychiatrist. She does not self-harm, nor does she have thoughts or wishes to die. Her mood and affect were stable and positive. At college, she consumed four to eight alcoholic drinks on weekends; she does not use drugs. She reports having good friends, despite some social drama in her group. She described herself as very healthy and fit, but mentioned two car accidents and concussions, as well as migraines. She is frustrated that she seems to have weakened her immune system by nail and knuckle biting. In high school she was not interested in academics but is motivated to succeed in college. She reported being messy and disorganized, but prides herself on her sense of style and interest in design. Her new hobby is cooking, and she has been doing this quite a bit recently. Her nail and knuckle-biting habit deeply distress her and her family. It is also expensive because she spends so much money on nail polish and skin-care treatments. She participated in two hypnotherapy sessions. This portion of the first session introduces her to hypnosis and guides her as she develops alternative behaviors to replace her nail-biting habit, while promoting a healthy self-image as an emerging adult.

Hypnosis Protocol

"Let yourself get as comfortable as you can in your chair. Whatever position works for you is fine and there's no one single right or wrong way. (Mindful of working with a young adult.) *You can listen to me as much as you'd like to, or you can begin to let my words drift off and just experience what it's like to sit, seeing your feet rest on the footstool and your hands in your lap, listening to the sound of my voice and letting all the other sounds just drift off into the background. You might notice that your breathing has shifted a little bit. You might notice that it's slowing.* (Therapist observes and mentions what is happening.) *That's right.*

And as you notice that, you might also be noticing that your eyelids begin to feel a little different, as if they're heavier and heavier. (Her eyes had started to blink and she nods her head.) *And your feet are resting, your hands there in your lap, and your eyelids . . . are . . . feeling heavier. And if you would like to be a little more comfortable, they may gently drift . . . closed, and you might notice that they do that all . . . by . . . themselves as you continue to let your breathing become easier and slower.* (Therapist slows pace of speech and softens voice.)

You may wish to release tension and tightness . . . that's right. Your hands are in your lap and your breathing continues to be just right for you, so that with the next breath in you can feel even more comfortable than before. (Some attention given to her hands, but not directly to her nail-biting. Truisms followed by a suggestion to intensify the relaxation.) *Those muscles across your forehead, so soft and smooth. Perhaps your tongue drops low in your mouth.*

As you breathe it may be as if there's a stone going deep inside the well of your body, finding that still calm place. So that just a few moments of this sort of rest and relaxation can allow you to take in the benefits of many minutes of a relaxed healing experience. (Associating relaxation with healing because her skin needs to heal.) *That's right, you're doing this very nicely.* (Positive reinforcement and ego strengthening.) *Your feet are resting on the footstool. The hands are in your lap and a part of your mind that is so resourceful and creative may already be making note of the steps that you used to find a little bit of stillness and calm, to enjoy the beautiful elements of your own imagination.* (Utilizing her interest in design and beauty to support her confidence.)

Being aware of the beauty of your body and your thoughts in a way that really builds your self-confidence as you adopt behaviors that are healthy . . . for you, that help you create just the look that you want in your wardrobe, your make-up, your hands and nails, knuckles. It allows you to enjoy the beauty that you can see in ways that are really quite perfect for you: healthy and right for you. As your feet are resting on the footstool, your hands are in your lap, and that designing part of your mind is creating the recipe for success to keep your hands, skin, nails looking nicely made up. (Using cooking terms to amplify and reinforce her interests.)

In a moment I'll be quiet, allowing you time to just enjoy this relaxation and sense of confidence that you've created. A few moments of relaxation to allow you to find the recipe for healthy, confident behavior that will last long after you leave here. What ingredients will you notice, like a good chef noting the steps and ingredients, if there's an urge—like you used to have—to bite your knuckles? (Past tense, the urge is in the past.) *I wonder how you will mix it up, to turn the page and choose to do something else or to skip that page and not even notice the urge? I don't know exactly what will be right for you, but you'll know what's right as you continue to make such good progress and create this new pattern of behavior for yourself.* (Reinforcing her capacity and adult status, while utilizing her creative interests and design talents, to suggest she'll create and design new, healthier patterns of behavior.)

Now, with this change in the ingredients you have available, you are ready to simply be 'on automatic' and mix it up so those hands no longer wish, no longer desire to continue that outgrown and unwanted habit that used to damage your knuckles. It used to draw attention and embarrass you in front of your family, but now as you continue to discontinue the habit you feel such a growing and beautiful sense of well-being and a sense of approval for yourself. (Therapist promotes themes of growing up, uses language of cooking and creating, references the habit as in the past, and plays with language.)

There are so many benefits to staying healthy. Your hands don't introduce germs and colds or sickness into your general immune system as often. You will be stronger and healthier . . . healthier and stronger. And of course, there's also the exciting positive outcome of saving some money, not spending as much money on your nails, nail polish. And that money can be redirected toward other things that you find beautiful and affirming and useful for you. You know how to take care of yourself on the outside . . . and on the inside.

You use that wonderful helpful part of your mind for remembering what you need to remember and forgetting what used to bother you so much. *That's right, you may be pleasantly surprised how quickly your skin heals and the color returns to its ordinary healthy color, and how smooth the knuckles become and how little attention you even need to pay to them and your hands, as you care for yourself on the inside and the outside. So beautiful! And perhaps you'll enjoy a few moments now to imagine something utterly pleasing. Perhaps a place you've been to in the past or somewhere you'd like to visit in the future, where you experience success and joy and remind yourself of the many ways you take care of yourself. I'll be quiet for a few moments so that you can fully enjoy this."*

At the second session, Amy reported "big success," as she had dramatically reduced nail and knuckle biting. She proudly showed off her hands, which looked significantly healthier. She was applying lotion to them and using her imagination to envision them "healed and looking good." She was enthusiastic about these changes and proud that she was taking better care of her health by not putting her hands in her mouth.

CONCLUSION

In clinical practice, hypnosis is used to treat a very wide range of mental health and medical conditions experienced by children and adolescents. The number of randomized controlled trials supporting the efficacy of hypnosis with this population has grown in recent years, although the vast majority of studies have addressed medical issues. The evidence base supporting the effectiveness of this treatment modality for relieving needle pain is especially impressive. More randomized controlled studies are needed evaluating mental health applications of hypnosis with young people. The four case examples presented in this chapter illustrate how hypnosis can be employed to help youngsters suffering from anxiety. These case examples highlight the potential of hypnosis for alleviating mental health problems experienced by many children and adolescents.

REFERENCES

Accardi, M. C., & Milling, L. S. (2009). The effectiveness of hypnosis for reducing procedure-related pain in children and adolescents: A comprehensive methodological review. *Journal of Behavioral Medicine, 32*(4), 328–339. https://doi.org/10.1007/s10865-009-9207-6

Anbar, R. D. (2017). Asthma. In G. R. Elkins (Ed.), *Handbook of medical and psychological hypnosis: Foundations, applications, and professional issues* (pp. 161–168). Springer Publishing.

Anbar, R. D., & Hall, H. R. (2004). Childhood habit cough treated with self-hypnosis. *The Journal of Pediatrics, 144*(2), 213–217. https://doi.org/10.1016/j.jpeds.2003. 10.041

Banerjee, S., Srivastav, A., & Palan, B. M. (1993). Hypnosis and self-hypnosis in the management of nocturnal enuresis: A comparative study with imipramine therapy. *American Journal of Clinical Hypnosis, 36*(2), 113–119. https://doi.org/10.1080/ 00029157.1993.10403053

Barabasz, A., & Barabasz, M. (2000). Treating AD/HD with hypnosis and neurotherapy. *Child Study Journal, 30*(1), 25–42.

Bernstein, N. R. (1965). Observations on the use of hypnosis with burned children on a pediatric ward. *International Journal of Clinical and Experimental Hypnosis, 13*(1), 1–10. https://doi.org/10.1080/00207146508412920

Butler, L. D., Symons, B. K., Henderson, S. L., Shortliffe, L. D., & Spiegel, D. (2005). Hypnosis reduces distress and duration of an invasive medical procedure for children. *Pediatrics, 115*(1), e77–e85. https://doi.org/10.1542/peds.2004-0818

Cardeña, E., Maldonado, J. R., Hart, O. V. D., & Spiegel, D. (2009). Hypnosis. In E. B. Foa, T. M. Keane, M. J. Friedman, & J. A. Cohen (Eds.), *Effective treatments for PTSD: Practice guidelines from the International Society for Traumatic Stress Studies* (pp. 427–457). Guilford Press.

Centers for Disease Control and Prevention. (2021). *Data and statistics on children's mental health.* https://www.cdc.gov/childrensmentalhealth/data.html

Edwards, S. D., & van der Spuy, H. I. (1985). Hypnotherapy as a treatment for enuresis. *The Journal of Child Psychology and Psychiatry, 26*(1), 161–170. https://doi.org/ 10.1111/j.1469-7610.1985.tb01635.x

Ewin, D. M. (1992). Hypnotherapy for warts (verruca vulgaris): 41 consecutive cases with 33 cures. *American Journal of Clinical Hypnosis, 35*(1), 1–10. https://doi.org/ 10.1080/00029157.1992.10402977

Gardner, G. G. (1974). Hypnosis with children. *International Journal of Clinical and Experimental Hypnosis, 22*(1), 20–38. https://doi.org/10.1080/00207147408412981

Gardner, G. G. (1976). Childhood, death, and human dignity: Hypnotherapy for David. *International Journal of Clinical and Experimental Hypnosis, 24*(2), 122–139. https://doi.org/10.1080/00207147608405603

Gardner, G. G., & Olness, K. (1981). *Hypnosis and hypnotherapy with children.* Grune & Stratton.

Gottsegen, D. N. (2003). Curing bedwetting on the spot: A review of one-session cures. *Clinical Pediatrics, 42*(3), 273–275. https://doi.org/10.1177/000992280304200312

Guyer, C. G. (2014). Hypnotic treatment of behavior disorders. In L. I. Sugarman & W. C. Wester (Eds.), *Therapeutic hypnosis with children and adolescents* (2nd ed., pp. 265–296). Crown House Publishing.

Hilgard, J. R., & LeBaron, S. (1984). *Hypnotherapy of pain in children and adolescents with cancer.* William Kaufmann.

Huet, A., Lucas-Polomeni, M.-M., Robert, J.-C., Sixou, J.-L., & Wodey, E. (2011). Hypnosis and dental anesthesia in children: A prospective controlled study. *International Journal of Clinical and Experimental Hypnosis, 59*(4), 424–440. https:// doi.org/10.1080/00207144.2011.594740

Huth, M. M., Broome, M. E., & Good, M. (2004). Imagery reduces children's post-operative pain. *Pain, 110*(1–2), 439–448. https://doi.org/10.1016/j.pain.2004. 04.028

Iglesias, A. (2003). Hypnosis as a vehicle for choice and self-agency in the treatment of children with trichotillomania. *American Journal of Clinical Hypnosis*, *46*(2), 129–137. https://doi.org/10.1080/00029157.2003.10403583

Jacknow, D. S., Tschann, J. M., Link, M. P., & Boyce, W. T. (1994). Hypnosis in the prevention of chemotherapy-related nausea and vomiting in children: A prospective study. *Journal of Developmental and Behavioral Pediatrics*, *15*(4), 258–264. https://doi.org/10.1097/00004703-199408000-00007

Jong, M. C., Boers, I., van Wietmarschen, H. A., Tromp, E., Busari, J. O., Wennekes, R., Snoeck, I., Bekhof, J., & Vlieger, A. M. (2019). Hypnotherapy or transcendental meditation versus progressive muscle relaxation exercises in the treatment of children with primary headaches: A multi-centre, pragmatic, randomised clinical study. *European Journal of Pediatrics*, *178*(2), 147–154. https://doi.org/10.1007/s00431-018-3270-3

Kaiser, P. (2014). Childhood anxiety and psychophysiological reactivity: Hypnosis to build discrimination and self-regulation skills. *American Journal of Clinical Hypnosis*, *56*(4), 343–367. https://doi.org/10.1080/00029157.2014.884487

Kaiser, P. (2017). Anxiety in children and teens. In G. R. Elkins (Ed.), *Handbook of medical and psychological hypnosis: Foundations, applications, and professional issues* (pp. 477–484). Springer Publishing.

Kihslinger, D., & Sapp, M. (2006). Hypnosis and diabetes: Applications for children, adolescents, and adults. *Australian Journal of Clinical Hypnotherapy and Hypnosis*, *27*(1), 19–27.

Kohen, D. P. (1995). Ericksonian communication and hypnotic strategies in the management of tics and Tourette syndrome in children and adolescents with Tourette syndrome. In S. R. Lankton & J. K. Zeig (Eds.), *Difficult contexts for therapy—Ericksonian monographs* (Vol. 10, pp. 117–142). Brunner/Mazel.

Kohen, D. P. (2014). Depression. In L. I. Sugarman & W. C. Wester (Eds.), *Therapeutic hypnosis with children and adolescents* (2nd ed., pp. 187–208). Crown House Publishing.

Kohen, D. P. (2017). Headache—Children. In G. R. Elkins (Ed.), *Handbook of medical and psychological hypnosis: Foundations, applications, and professional issues* (pp. 259–271). Springer Publishing.

Kohen, D. P., & Kaiser, P. (2014). Clinical hypnosis with children and adolescents—What? Why? How?: Origins, applications, and efficacy. *Children*, *1*(2), 74–98. https://doi.org/10.3390/children1020074

Kohen, D. P., & Murray, K. (2006). Depression in children and youth: Applications of hypnosis to help young people help themselves. In M. D. Yapko (Ed.), *Applying hypnosis in treating depression: Innovations in clinical practice* (pp. 189–216). Routledge Press.

Kohen, D. P., & Olness, K. (2011). *Hypnosis and hypnotherapy with children* (4th ed.). Routledge.

Kohen, D. P., Olness, K. N., Colwell, S. O., & Heimel, A. (1984). The use of relaxation-mental imagery (self-hypnosis) in the management of 505 pediatric behavioral encounters. *Journal of Developmental and Behavioral Pediatrics*, *5*(1), 21–25. https://doi.org/10.1097/00004703-198402000-00005

Kohen, D. P., & Zajac, R. (2007). Self-hypnosis training for headaches in children and adolescents. *The Journal of Pediatrics*, *150*(6), 635–639. https://doi.org/10.1016/j.jpeds.2007.02.014

Krippner, S. (1966). The use of hypnosis with elementary and secondary school children in a summer reading clinic. *American Journal of Clinical Hypnosis, 8*(4), 261–266. https://doi.org/10.1080/00029157.1966.10402503

Kuttner, L. (2009). Treating pain, anxiety and sleep disorders with children and adolescents. In D. C. Brown (Ed.), *Advances in the use of hypnosis in medicine, dentistry, pain prevention and management* (pp. 177–194). Crown House Publishers.

Kuttner, L. (2020). Pediatric hypnosis: Treatment that adds and rarely subtracts. *International Journal of Clinical and Experimental Hypnosis, 68*(1), 16–28. https://doi.org/10.1080/00207144.2020.1685329

Kuttner, L., Bowman, M., & Teasdale, M. (1988). Psychological treatment of distress, pain, and anxiety for young children with cancer. *Journal of Developmental and Behavioral Pediatrics, 9*(6), 374–381. https://doi.org/10.1097/00004703-198812000-00010

Kuttner, L., & Friedrichsdorf, S. J. (2014). Hypnosis and palliative care for children and their families. In L. I. Sugarman & W. C. Wester (Eds.), *Therapeutic hypnosis with children and adolescents* (2nd ed., pp. 491–509). Crown House Publishing.

Lambert, S. A. (1996). The effects of hypnosis/guided imagery on the postoperative course of children. *Journal of Developmental & Behavioral Pediatrics, 17*(5), 307–310. https://doi.org/10.1097/00004703-199610000-00003

Lazarus, J. E., & Klein, S. K. (2010). Nonpharmacological treatment of tics in Tourette syndrome adding videotape training to self-hypnosis. *Journal of Developmental and Behavioral Pediatrics, 31*(6), 498–504. https://doi.org/10.1097/DBP.0b013e3181e56c5d

Linden, J. H. (2003). Playful metaphors. *American Journal of Clinical Hypnosis, 45*(3), 245–250. https://doi.org/10.1080/00029157.2003.10403530

Linden, J. H. (2007). Hypnosis in childhood trauma. In L. I. Sugarman & W. C. Wester (Eds.), *Therapeutic hypnosis with children and adolescents* (2nd ed., pp. 143–166). Crown House Publishing.

Liossi, C., & Hatira, P. (1999). Clinical hypnosis versus cognitive behavioral training for pain management with pediatric cancer patients undergoing bone marrow aspirations. *International Journal of Clinical and Experimental Hypnosis, 47*(2), 104–116. https://doi.org/10.1080/00207149908410025

Liossi, C., & Hatira, P. (2003). Clinical hypnosis in the alleviation of procedure-related pain in pediatric oncology patients. *International Journal of Clinical and Experimental Hypnosis, 51*(1), 4–28. https://doi.org/10.1076/iceh.51.1.4.14064

Liossi, C., White, P., & Hatira, P. (2006). Randomized clinical trial of local anesthetic versus a combination of local anesthetic with self-hypnosis in the management of pediatric procedure-related pain. *Health Psychology, 25*(3), 307–315. https://doi.org/10.1037/0278-6133.25.3.307

Liossi, C., White, P., & Hatira, P. (2009). A randomized clinical trial of a brief hypnosis intervention to control venepuncture-related pain of paediatric cancer patients. *Pain, 142*(3), 255–263. https://doi.org/10.1016/j.pain.2009.01.017

Lyons, L. (2015). *Using hypnosis with children: Creating and delivering effective interventions*. W. W. Norton.

Milling, L. S., & Costantino, C. A. (2000). Clinical hypnosis with children: First steps toward empirical support. *International Journal of Clinical and Experimental Hypnosis, 48*(2), 113–137. https://doi.org/10.1080/00207140008410044

Olness, K., & Gardner, G. G. (1978). Some guidelines for uses of hypnotherapy in pediatrics. *Pediatrics, 62*(2), 228–233. https://doi.org/10.1542/peds.62.2.228

Pendergrast, R. A. (2017). Incorporating hypnosis into pediatric clinical encounters. *Children, 4*(3), 18. https://doi.org/10.3390/children4030018

Polanczyk, G. V., Salum, G. A., Sugaya, L. S., Caye, A., & Rohde, L. A. (2015). Annual research review: A meta-analysis of the worldwide prevalence of mental disorders in children and adolescents. *The Journal of Child Psychology and Psychiatry, 56*(3), 345–365. https://doi.org/10.1111/jcpp.12381

Roberts, D. (1998). The use of hypnosis and brief strategic therapy with a case of separation anxiety and school refusal. *Contemporary Hypnosis, 15*(4), 219–222. https://doi.org/10.1002/ch.138

Siegel, R. L., Miller, K. D., Fuchs, H. E., & Jemal, A. (2021). Cancer Statistics, 2021. *CA: A Cancer Journal for Clinicians, 71*(1), 7–33. https://doi.org/10.3322/caac.21654

Smith, J. T., Barabasz, A., & Barabasz, M. (1996). Comparison of hypnosis and distraction in severely ill children undergoing painful medical procedures. *Journal of Counseling Psychology, 43*(2), 187–195. https://doi.org/10.1037/0022-0167.43.2.187

Stanton, H. (1994). Self-hypnosis: One path to reduced test anxiety. *Contemporary Hypnosis, 11*(1), 14–18.

Sugarman, L. I., & Wester, W. C. (2014). *Therapeutic hypnosis with children and adolescents* (2nd ed.). Crown House Publishing.

Swirsky-Sacchetti, T., & Margolis, C. G. (1986). The effects of a comprehensive self-hypnosis training program on the use of factor VIII in severe hemophilia. *International Journal of Clinical and Experimental Hypnosis, 34*(2), 71–83. https://doi.org/10.1080/00207148608406973

U.S. Health Resources and Services Administration, Maternal and Child Health Bureau. (2020a). *Mental and Behavioral Health NSCH Data Brief.* https://mchb.hrsa.gov/sites/default/files/mchb/data-research/nsch-data-brief-2019-mental-bh.pdf

U.S. Health Resources and Services Administration, Maternal and Child Health Bureau. (2020b). *National Survey of Children's Health NSCH Data Brief.* https://mchb.hrsa.gov/sites/default/files/mchb/about-us/nsch-data-brief.pdf

Valentine, K. E., Milling, L. S., Clark, L. J., & Moriarty, C. L. (2019). The efficacy of hypnosis as a treatment for anxiety: A meta-analysis. *International Journal of Clinical and Experimental Hypnosis, 67*(3), 336–363. https://doi.org/10.1080/00207144.2019.1613863

Vlieger, A. M., Menko-Frankenhuis, C., Wolfkamp, S. C. S., Tromp, E., & Benninga, M. A. (2007). Hypnotherapy for children with functional abdominal pain or irritable bowel syndrome: A randomized controlled trial. *Gastroenterology, 133*(5), 1430–1436. https://doi.org/10.1053/j.gastro.2007.08.072

Vlieger, A. M., Rutten, J. M. T. M., Govers, A. M. A. P., Frankenhuis, C., & Benninga, M. A. (2012). Long-term follow-up of gut-directed hypnotherapy vs. standard care in children with functional abdominal pain or irritable bowel syndrome. *American Journal of Gastroenterology, 107*(4), 627–631. https://doi.org/10.1038/ajg.2011.487

Wark, D. M. (2011). Traditional and alert hypnosis for education: A literature review. *American Journal of Clinical Hypnosis, 54*(2), 96–106. https://doi.org/10.1080/00029157.2011.605481

Wester, W. C. (2014). Hypnotic treatment of habit disorders. In L. I. Sugarman & W. C. Wester (Eds.), *Therapeutic hypnosis with children and adolescents* (2nd ed., pp. 167–186). Crown House Publishing.

Wood, C., & Bioy, A. (2020). Early hypnotic intervention after traumatic events in children. *American Journal of Clinical Hypnosis, 62*(4), 380–391. https://doi.org/10.1080/00029157.2019.1659128

Zalsman, G., Hermesh, H., & Sever, J. (2001). Hypnotherapy in adolescents with trichotillomania: Three cases. *American Journal of Clinical Hypnosis, 44*(1), 63–68. https://doi.org/10.1080/00029157.2001.10403457

Zeltzer, L., & LeBaron, S. (1982). Hypnosis and nonhypnotic techniques for reduction of pain and anxiety during painful procedures in children and adolescents with cancer. *The Journal of Pediatrics, 101*(6), 1032–1035. https://doi.org/10.1016/S0022-3476(82)80040-1

Zeltzer, L. K., Dolgin, M. J., LeBaron, S., & LeBaron, C. (1991). A randomized, controlled study of behavioral intervention for chemotherapy distress in children with cancer. *Pediatrics, 88*(1), 34–42. https://pubmed.ncbi.nlm.nih.gov/2057271/

9 EVIDENCE-BASED PRACTICE IN CLINICAL HYPNOSIS

Current Status and Future Directions

LEONARD S. MILLING

Evidence-based practice in health care is rooted in the assumption that clinical practice should be informed by scientific evidence. In psychology, *evidence-based practice* is defined as "the integration of the best available research with clinical expertise in the context of patient characteristics, culture, and preferences" (American Psychological Association, 2006, p. 273). In turn, *best research evidence* refers to "scientific results related to intervention strategies, assessment, clinical problems, and patient populations in laboratory and field settings as well as to clinically relevant results of basic research in psychology and related fields" (American Psychological Association, 2006, p. 274). Indeed, *clinical expertise* is said to be essential for integrating the best research evidence with clinical information in order to achieve the best outcome for the patient. This chapter builds upon the treatment outcome research reviewed in the main section of the book to appraise the current status of the efficacy of hypnosis as a treatment or intervention. The chapter concludes with suggestions designed to strengthen the evidence base supporting the use of hypnosis as a clinical tool.

https://doi.org/10.1037/0000347-009
Evidence-Based Practice in Clinical Hypnosis, L. S. Milling (Editor)

CURRENT STATUS OF EVIDENCE-BASED PRACTICE
IN HYPNOSIS

This section of the chapter presents a summary of the evidence of the efficacy of hypnosis as a treatment or intervention for the problems and symptoms addressed earlier in this book.

Anxiety

Anxiety symptoms and the anxiety disorders are among the most pervasive of mental health problems. For example, the anxiety disorders as a group rank as the most common of the mental disorders in the United States (American Psychiatric Association, 2013), with a lifetime prevalence of 29% (Kessler et al., 2005). In Chapter 2 of this book, Reid's narrative review of 14 controlled studies reveals hypnosis is effective for alleviating a range of anxiety conditions, including the anxiety associated with dental procedures, surgery and medical interventions, test taking and performance situations, as well as general anxiety.

Meta-analysis offers a method for statistically combining the results of different studies on a particular topic. In the case of treatment outcome research, a meta-analysis can quantify the overall impact of a treatment (e.g., hypnosis) on an outcome variable (e.g., anxiety). Meta-analysis yields a statistic referred to as an *effect size*. Cohen (1988) classifies effect sizes of 0.20 as a small effect, 0.50 as a medium effect, and 0.80 as a large effect. It should be remembered that meta-analysis shows the effect of a *class* of interventions on an outcome variable. Hypnosis is a general term that encompasses many specific interventions and suggestions. Thus, a reported effect size quantifies the impact of hypnosis averaged across all of the specific interventions and suggestions included in the studies contained in a meta-analysis.

Not long ago, Valentine et al. (2019) reported the findings of a meta-analysis of all controlled studies of the efficacy of hypnosis for relieving the symptoms of anxiety. The overall mean weighted effect size for 17 trials of hypnosis at the end of active treatment was 0.79. An effect size of 0.79 falls toward the top of the medium range (Cohen, 1988) and suggests the average patient receiving hypnosis reduced anxiety more than about 79% of untreated individuals. The overall mean weighted effect size for seven trials of hypnosis at the longest follow-up was 0.99. This would be classified as a large effect and indicates the average patient treated with hypnosis showed more improvement than about 84% of control participants at follow-up.

The methodological quality of the 17 trials in Valentine et al. (2019) could be described as good. Randomized controlled trials are said to be the gold standard in appraising the efficacy of an intervention. Including both a treatment group and a control group that have the same experience other than the intervention under consideration makes it more likely that differences in outcome can be ascribed to the treatment. Randomly assigning participants to the treatment and control groups makes it less likely there will be differences between the two groups at the beginning of a study on variables (e.g., attitudes toward hypnosis) that could affect the findings. All but two of the 17 controlled trials in Valentine et al. were randomized controlled trials.

More generally, it has recently become the norm to formally assess the methodological quality of the trials included in a meta-analysis using a standardized measure (Moher et al., 2009). We would have more confidence in a meta-analysis that was derived predominantly from methodologically sound studies. The 17 trials in Valentine et al. (2019) were evaluated using the Cochrane Risk of Bias Tool (Higgins & Green, 2011). Each trial was rated as having a high risk, low risk, or unclear risk on five Risk of Bias domains. *Sequence generation* examines whether the method of assigning participants to condition resulted in random assignment. A related dimension is *allocation concealment* or whether the researcher enrolling participants into a study was in a position to interfere with the random assignment process (e.g., unsealed random assignment envelopes). *Incomplete outcome data at post* and *incomplete outcome data at follow-up* evaluate the extent of participant attrition due to withdrawing, no-showing, or not providing data. Finally, *selective outcome reporting* is concerned with whether all of all key outcome variables mentioned in the Method section of a study are analyzed and reported in the Results section.

Eleven of the 17 trials (65%) included in Valentine et al. (2019) did not receive high risk ratings on any of the five Risk of Bias dimensions that were assessed. Therefore, based on a group of studies of good methodological quality, the findings of Valentine et al. show that hypnosis has a medium to large effect when used as a treatment for anxiety symptoms. Together, the Valentine et al. meta-analysis and Reid's narrative review in Chapter 2 argue that clinicians should regard hypnosis as an evidence-based treatment option when working with patients and clients who experience anxiety.

Depression

The depressive disorders (e.g., major depressive disorder, persistent depressive disorder) are arguably the second most prevalent group of mental disorders, according to the fifth edition of the *Diagnostic and Statistical Manual of Mental Disorders* (*DSM-5*; American Psychiatric Association, 2013). The common features of the depressive disorders include sad or irritable mood, along with anhedonia, hopelessness, difficulty concentrating, low energy, as well as changes in appetite and sleep (American Psychiatric Association, 2013). One recent survey showed that between 2013 and 2016, approximately 8.1% of U.S. adults age 20 or older had experienced clinically significant levels of depression symptoms (Brody et al., 2018).

In Chapter 3, Yapko and Criswell assert that hypnosis can be helpful in treating depression by increasing positive affect and hopefulness, encouraging effective thinking and social interaction, taking positive action, as well as focusing on the positive. These experts reviewed 14 controlled studies in which hypnosis specifically targeted depression symptoms, as well as one benchmarked feasibility study and several relevant meta-analyses. Yapko and Criswell conclude that treating depression with hypnosis is effective and that adding hypnosis to other psychological interventions augments the efficacy of those interventions.

How effective is hypnosis in treating depression? In a recent meta-analysis, Milling et al. (2019) reported a mean weighted effect size of 0.71 for 13 trials at the end of treatment, indicating the average participant receiving hypnosis reduced depression symptoms more than about 76% of control participants. At the longest follow-up, four trials produced a mean weighted effect size of 0.52, suggesting the average participant in the hypnosis condition showed more improvement than about 51% of those in the control condition. Effect sizes of 0.71 and 0.52 fall in the medium range according to Cohen's (1988) guideline.

Nine of the 13 controlled trials included in Milling et al. (2019) utilized random assignment to condition. Moreover, eight of the 13 trials (62%) received no high risk ratings on any of the five Risk of Bias dimensions (Higgins & Green, 2011) that were evaluated. The findings of the Milling et al. meta-analysis, derived from studies of good methodological quality, suggest hypnosis has a medium effect when used as a treatment for depression symptoms. However, any conclusions should be qualified by the relatively small number of trials ($n = 13$) in this meta-analysis. All in all, the research literature appears to provide moderate support for the efficacy of hypnosis as a treatment for depression symptoms.

Clinical Pain

Physical pain is the most common of medical complaints. It is also the most extensively studied application of clinical hypnosis. Pain can be classified as acute or chronic. *Acute* pain tends to develop suddenly, is time-limited, and linked to an identifiable injury, illness, or event (Institute of Medicine, 2011). *Procedural* pain is a subtype of acute pain that is associated with an invasive medical procedure (e.g., lumbar punctures). *Chronic* pain is said to be pain lasting 3 to 6 months beyond the time associated with normal healing (Merskey & Bogduk, 1994).

In Chapter 4, Milling's narrative review of 36 randomized controlled trials concludes hypnosis is effective for relieving many forms of acute and procedural pain. This includes the pain connected with burn wound care, labor and delivery, cancer, dental procedures, radiological procedures, biopsies, surgery, and needle-related pain. In the 36 trials, when hypnosis was not more effective than a control condition, it appeared to be a function of low statistical power, the use of audio recordings as the primary intervention, or when there was a long time gap between the provision of hypnosis and the experience of pain.

Similarly, McKernan and Connor's narrative review in Chapter 5 finds that hypnosis is helpful for reducing pain and improving functioning in a variety of chronic pain conditions, including *nociceptive* pain (i.e., pain associated with tissue damage), *neuropathic* pain (i.e., pain associated with damage to the somatosensory nervous system), and *nociplastic* pain (i.e., widespread pain with no identifiable pathology). More specifically, this review concludes hypnosis may be more effective with *neuropathic* pain (e.g., chronic brachial neuralgia, spinal cord injuries, complex regional pain syndrome) than *nociceptive* pain (e.g., temporomandibular disorders, hemophilia, arthritis, Crohn's disease, low back pain) and *nociplastic* pain (e.g., irritable bowel syndrome, fibromyalgia, chronic widespread pain), although all three chronic pain conditions do seem to benefit.

Evidence-based practice is not synonymous with *empirically supported therapies*. However, there are links between the two frameworks. More than 25 years ago, the American Psychological Association Division 12 (Clinical Psychology) Task Force on Promotion and Dissemination of Psychological Procedures (American Psychological Association, 1995) developed research criteria for identifying a psychological treatment as *empirically supported* for particular problems and populations. These research criteria were later refined by Chambless and Hollon (1998). Recognizing a particular treatment as empirically supported can be an important source of the *best research evidence,* which is a component of the process of evidence-based practice.

A few years later, Montgomery et al. (2000) published the first comprehensive meta-analysis of the efficacy of hypnotic analgesia. This seminal meta-analysis reported an overall mean weighted effect size of 0.67 for 27 trials of hypnosis. This included mean weighted effect sizes of 0.64 for 17 experimental pain trials and 0.74 for 10 clinical pain trials. These effect sizes fall in the medium range of magnitude (Cohen, 1988). Relative to the Chambless and Hollon (1998) framework for empirically supported therapies (ESTs), Montgomery et al. concluded that hypnotically suggested analgesia met the EST criteria for a *well-established treatment.*

In the years since Montgomery et al. (2000) was published, the number of controlled studies of hypnosis and clinical pain has more than quadrupled! In a new comprehensive meta-analysis, Milling et al. (2021) reported mean weighted effect sizes of 0.60 for 40 trials of hypnosis at the end of active treatment and 0.61 for nine trials at the longest follow-up. These effect sizes fall in the medium range according to Cohen's (1988) guideline and suggest the average participant treated with hypnosis reduced pain more than about 73% of control participants. Moreover, when the analysis was limited to studies with the most robust methodology (i.e., studies with no high risk ratings on any of the five Risk of Bias dimensions), 19 trials yielded a mean weighted effect size of 0.77 at the end of treatment. Hypnosis had a similar benefit for different types of pain. More specifically, at the end of treatment, mean weighted effect sizes were 0.55 for 17 trials of procedural pain, 0.63 for 11 trials of acute, nonprocedural pain, and 0.64 for 12 trials of chronic pain.

Just as the number of controlled studies of hypnosis with clinical pain has grown through the years, the method by which empirically supported therapies are identified has evolved. Tolin et al. (2015) advanced a revised set of criteria for empirically supported therapies that utilizes the results of existing meta-analyses and systematic reviews. According to the revised criteria, empirical support for a particular therapy is classified as *weak, strong,* or *very strong.* Based on the studies with the most robust methodology in the Milling et al. (2021) meta-analysis, the effect of hypnosis on clinical pain would appear to be consistent with a classification of *strong* or *very strong* according to the Tolin et al. criteria. In any event, meta-analytic evidence in combination with narrative reviews provided in Chapters 4 and 5 of this book suggests clinicians should have a high level of confidence when using hypnosis to treat clinical pain.

Other Behavioral Medicine Applications

Besides pain, hypnosis has many other useful applications in behavioral medicine. In Chapter 6, Elkins and Snyder identify five applications with promising empirical support. Based on several randomized controlled trials, these scholars conclude there is strong research support for the use of hypnosis with irritable bowel syndrome, as well as menopause and hot flashes. Furthermore, there appears to be preliminary evidence of the effectiveness of hypnosis as a treatment for hypertension (i.e., high blood pressure) and sleep problems. Finally, Elkins and Snyder assert there is moderate research support for employing hypnosis as an intervention with cancer-related symptoms, including the nausea and vomiting associated with chemotherapy, stress management, as well as improving immune functioning.

Meta-analytic reviews of the efficacy of these five behavioral medicine applications are scarce. The few that do exist include either a very small number of trials (thereby raising questions about the representativeness of the results) or effect sizes calculated from pre to post changes in outcome variables in the hypnosis condition (which can inflate effect sizes). Nevertheless, based on Elkins and Snyder's narrative review in Chapter 6, hypnosis appears to hold much promise for addressing these five behavioral medicine problems. More randomized controlled studies of behavioral medicine applications of hypnosis seem warranted.

Smoking Cessation

Tobacco use continues to be a serious health problem in the United States. For example, the 2018 National Survey on Drug Use and Health found that approximately 47 million U.S. adults smoked cigarettes, including 27 million who were daily smokers and 11 million who smoked a pack or more per day (Substance Abuse and Mental Health Services Administration, 2019). In Chapter 7, Green and Lynn maintain hypnosis can help patients to stop smoking by boosting motivation, enhancing self-efficacy, promoting self-acceptance, providing a vehicle for mentally practicing alternatives to smoking, and visualizing behaviors designed to cope with urges to smoke, as well as the discomfort of withdrawal symptoms.

In their review of controlled studies, Green and Lynn paint a mixed picture of the efficacy of hypnosis for smoking cessation. On the one hand, these experts question the benefits of hypnosis when used as the primary or sole intervention. On the other hand, the empirical literature appears to indicate hypnosis can be effective when coupled with other established interventions for this problem, such as cognitive-behavioral therapy, counseling, and nicotine replacement therapy. Therefore, clinicians should have confidence using hypnosis to help patients stop smoking when it is employed in combination with other well-accepted interventions for smoking cessation.

Hypnosis With Children and Adolescents

It is well-known that children and adolescents love the world of the imagination. The strong imaginative capacity of youth may help to explain why they tend to be more responsive to hypnosis than adults. For example, on equivalent standardized measures of hypnotic suggestibility, children are more likely than adults to pass each of the test suggestions (London, 1962). Developmentally, hypnotic suggestibility has been shown to increase up to age 8, peak between the ages of 8 and 12, decline somewhat through age

16, and thereafter remain stable into adulthood (London, 1965; Morgan & Hilgard, 1978/1979).

In Chapter 8, Lombard and Milling contend that hypnosis must be tailored to a youngster's developmental level. Hypnosis with younger children tends to be more conversational and less reliant upon a formal induction than is the case with adults. Investigations of the effectiveness of hypnosis with children and adolescents mirror the treatment outcome literature with adults. The majority of studies demonstrating the efficacy of hypnosis with youngsters involve clinical pain, particularly procedure-related pain. More generally, the focus of this body of research has been on medical applications, including the side effects of chemotherapy and enuresis. More randomized controlled studies are greatly needed investigating mental health applications of hypnosis with children and adolescents.

Other Promising Applications of Hypnosis

A small, but growing literature suggests hypnosis may be an efficacious treatment for the symptoms of trauma. Psychological distress is common following exposure to stressful or traumatic events. In the U.S., the lifetime prevalence of posttraumatic stress disorder (PTSD) is estimated to be about 8.7% (American Psychiatric Association, 2013) and trauma symptoms (e.g., re-experiencing the trauma, avoidance, alterations in cognitions and mood, hyperarousal) can occur outside of a formal diagnosis of PTSD. In a recent meta-analysis of five randomized controlled studies of the effectiveness of hypnosis for alleviating trauma symptoms, Rotaru and Rusu (2016) obtained mean weighted effect sizes of 1.17 for four trials at the end of treatment and 1.58 for three trials at a 4-week follow-up. These effect sizes fall in the large range according to Cohen (1988). Although these encouraging findings must be qualified by the small number of trials in this meta-analysis, they also draw attention to the need for more studies of the use of hypnosis in treating trauma.

The enhancement of sports performance is another application of hypnosis for which there is growing empirical support. Rather than relying upon randomized controlled trials, this research literature is typified by carefully executed *single case design* studies. For example, in a single case design study, the performance of one golfer might be tracked prior to receiving hypnosis (i.e., baseline phase) and after the intervention (i.e., postintervention phase), with multiple assessment points during both phases to establish a stable trend for the target behavior of interest (e.g., putting accuracy).

Hypnosis has been shown to be effective for improving performance in a variety of sports, with strongest support for its use in basketball, golf, soccer, and badminton (reviewed in Milling & Randazzo, 2016). Of note,

Pates and colleagues have consistently demonstrated that a hypnosis intervention designed to increase *flow state* (sometimes called "being in the zone") was useful for enhancing performance in golf (Pates, 2013; Pates & Maynard, 2000; Pates, Oliver, & Maynard, 2001) and basketball (Pates et al., 2002; Pates, Maynard, & Westbury, 2001). Similarly, Barker and his colleagues have repeatedly shown that a hypnosis intervention intended to increase efficacy expectations was useful for bettering soccer skills (Barker et al., 2010; Barker & Jones, 2008). In any event, based on this expanding research literature, hypnosis appears to be a useful tool for enhancing sports performance.

Moderators of Treatment Outcome

A *moderator* is a variable that affects the strength or direction of relations between an independent variable and a dependent variable (Baron & Kenny, 1986). In the case of treatment outcome research, a moderator variable could explain the conditions when an intervention is most likely to affect the outcome variable. For example, if research shows cognitive-behavioral therapy reduces anxiety symptoms more in females than in males, then gender would be said to moderate the effect of cognitive-behavioral therapy on anxiety. Identifying moderator variables (e.g., characteristics of interventions and clients) in treatment outcome research is important because it tells us *when* a treatment is more likely to be beneficial.

The treatment outcome research reviewed in this book indicates with some consistency there are at least two moderators of the effectiveness of hypnosis. One of these moderators involves a characteristic of clients or patients. There are large individual differences in the tendency to respond to hypnosis and hypnotic suggestions (Gwynn & Spanos, 1996). As noted by Lynn and Green in Chapter 1, these individual differences are variously referred to as hypnotic suggestibility, hypnotizability, hypnotic susceptibility, etc.

Hypnotic suggestibility can be assessed with standardized measures consisting of a hypnotic induction and a series of test suggestions. Research with these scales indicates the majority of people respond to some, but not all of the test suggestions, placing them in the *medium* range of suggestibility. A smaller number of individuals respond to most or all of the test suggestions, positioning them in the *high* range of suggestibility. An equally small number of people respond to few or none of the test suggestions, classifying them in the *low* suggestibility range.

In the first comprehensive meta-analysis of the effectiveness of hypnotic analgesia, Montgomery et al. (2000) observed the impact of hypnosis on pain varied substantially by level of hypnotic suggestibility. For individuals in the low range of suggestibility, the benefits of hypnosis were inconsequential, with a mean weighted effect size of -0.01. However, for participants in the medium suggestibility range, hypnosis produced a mean weighted effect size of 0.64, which would be classified as a medium effect (Cohen, 1988). Finally, for those in the high suggestibility range, hypnosis yielded a mean weighted effect size of 1.16, which would be considered a large effect. That is, hypnotic suggestibility moderated the effect of hypnosis on pain.

Later in a meta-analysis of the association between hypnotic suggestibility and the efficacy of hypnosis in treating a range of problems encountered in clinical care settings, Montgomery et al. (2011) reported an overall mean weighted correlation (i.e., effect size) of $r = 0.24$, which would be classified as a small effect according to Cohen (1992). Moreover, in a recent meta-analysis of the impact of hypnosis on clinical pain, Milling et al. (2021) observed a mean weighted correlation (i.e., effect size) of $r = .53$ for the association between suggestibility and hypnotic pain reduction, which would be considered a large effect.

The findings of these meta-analyses have important clinical implications. Specifically, patients and clients who fall in the high range of suggestibility are likely to profit the most from treatment with hypnosis. For these individuals, hypnosis may be the treatment of choice. In contrast, patients and clients in the low range of suggestibility are least likely to benefit from intervention with hypnosis.

Nevertheless, it is not recommended that clinicians screen clients and patients using standardized measures of hypnotic suggestibility to identify who might be a good candidate for intervention with hypnosis. It takes time to administer standardized suggestibility measures and the results are unlikely to conclusively predict whether a specific individual will respond to a hypnotic intervention. Instead, it is recommended that clinicians include hypnosis in the treatment plan for clients and patients who are receptive to it. If a patient responds well, continue with hypnosis. If a patient does not respond well, consider nonhypnotic interventions for the problem or symptoms.

A second possible moderator involves a characteristic of hypnosis interventions. Three separate lines of research converge to argue that for some problems and symptoms, hypnosis is more likely to be effective when combined with other psychological treatments than when used as a stand-alone intervention. First, in Chapter 7, Green and Lynn provide a narrative review of the treatment outcome literature on smoking cessation in which they conclude hypnosis is more likely to help patients stop smoking when paired with other established interventions for this problem (e.g., cognitive-behavioral therapy, counseling, nicotine replacement therapy) than when employed as a monotherapy.

Second, Kirsch et al. (1995) conducted the first meta-analysis of the impact of adding hypnosis to cognitive-behavioral therapy (CBT) for a range of problems and symptoms. These scholars reported a mean weighted effect size of 0.66 in 18 studies comparing CBT with the same treatment augmented by hypnosis. This would be classified as a medium effect (Cohen, 1988) and indicates the average client receiving CBT with hypnosis showed more improvement than about 75% of clients receiving CBT without hypnosis. Recently, Ramondo et al. (2021) published an update to the original meta-analysis, this time involving 49 studies. This latest meta-analysis produced significant mean weighted effect sizes of 0.29 for 48 trials at the end of active treatment and 0.65 for 25 trials at follow-up, which fall in the low to medium range of magnitude. Together, the findings of Kirsch et al. and Ramondo et al. contend that CBT supplemented by hypnosis may be significantly more effective than CBT alone.

The Kirsch et al. (1995) and Ramondo et al. (2021) meta-analyses included only studies in which CBT was compared with the same treatment augmented by hypnosis. In actuality, there are a variety of ways that hypnosis and other psychological therapies can be combined. Valentine et al. (2019) addressed this issue in a meta-analysis of the efficacy of hypnosis as a treatment for anxiety. Valentine and her colleagues reported a mean weighted effect size of 0.70 for 13 trials in which hypnosis was employed as a stand-alone treatment. However, the four trials in which hypnosis was combined with some other psychological therapy yielded a mean weighted effect size of 1.25. The difference between these effect sizes was statistically significant.

Thus, for some problems like anxiety and smoking cessation, hypnosis may be more effective when combined with other psychological interventions than when used as a stand-alone treatment. There are at least two ways that hypnosis and other psychological interventions can be combined. First, hypnosis and other treatments like CBT could be employed as side-by-side interventions. Alternatively, CBT could be provided in a *hypnotic context* (Kirsch et al., 1995) by first delivering a hypnotic induction and then relabeling the CBT procedures as hypnotic in nature. For example, stress inoculation training (SIT) is a well-known form of CBT that is sometimes used to treat pain (Turk et al., 1983). SIT includes techniques like progressive muscle relaxation, guided imagery, and coping self-statements. To help create a hypnotic context, progressive muscle relaxation could be labeled *hypnotic relaxation*. Guided imagery could be described as *hypnotic imagery*. Coping self-statements could be called *coping self-suggestions*.

Additional research is needed to identify the problems that are more likely to be responsive to a combination of hypnosis and other treatments like CBT. In practice, clinicians may wish to consider whether integrating hypnosis with other psychological techniques could be of benefit to their clients and patients.

FUTURE DIRECTIONS FOR RESEARCH ON THE EFFICACY OF HYPNOSIS

This section of the chapter offers suggestions intended to strengthen the evidence base supporting the use of hypnosis as a clinical tool. Some of the suggestions are meant to promote the use of sound research methodology in hypnosis outcome studies. These recommendations are not an exhaustive treatise on research methodology, but instead focus on some of the most common methodological issues noted in the hypnosis literature. Other suggestions are designed to facilitate the use of meta-analysis to evaluate the efficacy of clinical hypnosis.

1. **Randomized controlled trials.** In treatment outcome research, randomized controlled trials are considered the gold standard for evaluating the impact of an intervention. In designing hypnosis outcome studies, if possible, compare hypnosis with a control group and utilize random assignment to condition. As explained earlier in this chapter, including a control group makes it more likely that differences in outcome can be attributed to the hypnosis intervention. Random assignment makes it more likely that at the outset of a study, participants in the hypnosis and control conditions will be comparable on variables that could affect outcome (e.g., attitudes towards hypnosis).

2. **Method of random assignment.** A related issue is the method by which participants are assigned to condition. For assignment to be random, participants must have an equal chance of being allocated to either the hypnosis or control condition. A random numbers table, flipping a coin, throwing dice, or shuffling assignment envelopes are accepted ways of randomly assigning participants to condition. Assigning patients to condition by odd/even date of birth or date of admission are not random. Journal articles should clearly describe the method of assigning participants to condition and state whether it was random. All too often, articles in the hypnosis literature state, "participants were assigned to condition" without clarifying whether the process was random. In a meta-analysis, utilizing random assignment minimizes the possibility a study will be classified as high risk on the risk of bias dimension of *sequence generation* (Higgins & Green, 2011). Where feasible, a researcher should design the method of random assignment so that they cannot interfere with

the random allocation process. If a researcher has knowledge of the next condition assignment, they could potentially influence whether a particular patient or client actually receives that assignment. Having a third party conduct the allocation process or utilizing sealed assignment envelopes are ways of concealing the random assignment process. In the context of a risk of bias assessment in meta-analysis, this will reduce the chances a study will be rated as high risk on the dimension of *allocation concealment*.

3. **Specification of hypnosis treatment.** At the outset of a study, specify the hypnosis intervention in a treatment manual. This increases the likelihood all members of an investigative team will deliver the treatment in the same way and makes it possible for other investigative teams to replicate the intervention. Journal articles should clearly describe the hypnosis intervention, including the total amount of time involved in treatment, as well as the modes of delivery (e.g., individual sessions, group sessions, audio recordings). If self-hypnosis is used, indicate whether instructions and opportunities for practice in self-directed hypnosis skills are provided (see Eason & Parris, 2019). Clearly describe the types of hypnotic suggestions that were used (e.g., direct suggestions for symptom reduction, relaxation, ego-strengthening, pleasant imagery, etc.) and include examples of important suggestions in a brief appendix to the journal article (see Barker & Jones, 2006, for an example).

4. **Specification of sample.** In a journal article, clearly describe the nature of the problem or symptoms targeted by hypnosis, as well as the sample included in the study. The sample description should include breakdowns by age, gender, and race (e.g., White, Black, Hispanic, Asian or Pacific Islander, Native American or Alaskan native, etc.). Describing the demographic characteristics of the sample will enable readers to determine the population to which the results may generalize. For some problems or symptoms (e.g., anxiety, depression), it may be important to specify whether and how participants were screened for clinically significant levels of dysfunction.

5. **Sample size.** Include an adequate number of participants in a study. Chambless and Hollon (1998) recommended that treatment outcome studies incorporate 25 to 30 participants per condition. In the hypnosis literature, some otherwise excellent outcome studies produced inconclusive findings because they included only 8 to 10 participants per condition, potentially resulting in low statistical power. For example, Chapter 4 reviewed a number of dissertations investigating the use of hypnosis for

alleviating acute pain. Some of these studies failed to produce statistically significant results—and it is impossible to know whether this was because the hypnosis intervention has no effect on pain or because the studies incorporated 10 or fewer participants in each condition. Researchers can conduct a power analysis to estimate the number of participants needed to detect statistical significance in a study if a treatment effect actually exists.

6. **Outcome variables.** Utilize outcome measures that reflect not only symptom reduction, but also functional consequences. In the revised criteria for empirically supported therapies, Tolin et al. (2015) contended that "symptom reduction is important in determining the efficacy of a treatment, but the value of symptom reduction is greatly diminished if functional improvement is not also demonstrated" (pp. 4–5). For example, in their review of the chronic pain literature in Chapter 5, McKernan and Connors note that hypnosis has been shown to not only relieve pain severity, but also benefit such functional outcomes as sleep quality, emotional distress, quality of life, overall social functioning, medication use, and physical disability.

   In journal articles, report the statistical analyses of all relevant primary and secondary outcome measures, including the results that are not statistically significant. Failing to report the findings for all outcome measures that were mentioned in the Method section can raise questions about whether nonsignificant results were withheld from publication and lead to a high risk classification on the risk of bias dimension of *selective outcome reporting*.

7. **Long-term follow-up.** In the original criteria for empirically supported therapies, Chambless and Hollon (1998) emphasized that "information regarding the long-term effects of treatment is highly desirable but difficult to come by . . . it is important to know whether treatment has an enduring effect" (p. 10). This may be especially true in the case of hypnosis. Some meta-analytic studies have pointed to the possibility that the effects of hypnosis may be as great as or even greater at follow-up than at the end of active treatment. Furthermore, if self-hypnosis is taught as a self-directed skill, it would make sense the benefits of hypnosis might extend beyond the conclusion of treatment. For some problems and symptoms (e.g., anxiety, depression, smoking cessation), including a follow-up assessment would seem to provide very valuable information about the efficacy of hypnosis.

8. **Attrition of research participants.** In a journal article, describe the attrition of research participants due to withdrawing, no-showing,

and failing to provide data. Accordingly, researchers should track the number of participants who (a) are enrolled in the study, (b) are assigned to each condition, (c) provide data at the end of treatment (i.e., at posttreatment), and (d) provide data at follow-up. This will enable the calculation of attrition rates at each stage of a study. Where possible, determine the reasons for missing data in each of the treatment conditions and assess whether these reasons might be associated with outcome. In meta-analysis, this will diminish the likelihood a study will be designated as high risk on the dimension of *incomplete outcome data* at post and follow-up.

9. **Present complete descriptive data.** In the Results section of a journal article, present complete descriptive data (e.g., means, standard deviations, and sample size) for each of the key outcome variables by condition at baseline, posttreatment, and follow-up. This information is needed if the study is to be included in a meta-analysis.

10. **Consider a single case design study.** At this point in the chapter, some readers will undoubtedly conclude the preceding suggestions have little relevance for them. Even those who are interested in contributing to the treatment outcome literature may say they do not have the resources needed to carry out a randomized controlled trial. In many settings, it simply is not possible to recruit enough participants to make a randomized controlled trial feasible. However, Borckardt and Nash (2002) contend there is another well-accepted research design that is compatible with real world clinical practice. This design is sometimes referred to as a *single case design* or *time series design*.

As described earlier in this chapter, in a single case design study, the behavior of one patient or client is assessed before (i.e., baseline phase) and after treatment (i.e., postintervention phase), with multiple assessment points during both phases to establish a stable trend for the outcome variable. Indeed, the original Chambless and Hollon (1998) criteria for empirically supported therapies state that as few as three well-executed single case design studies are sufficient to identify an intervention as empirically supported. The literature on hypnosis and enhancing sports performance provides excellent examples of the use of single case design studies. Of note, single case design studies do not need to be complex to be meaningful. Almost anyone can make an important contribution to the hypnosis treatment outcome research literature using simple single case design studies.

CONCLUSION

All in all, the treatment outcome literature provides strong empirical support for the efficacy of hypnosis as a treatment for clinical pain and at least moderate support for its use as an intervention for other behavioral medicine problems, smoking cessation, as well as anxiety and depression symptoms. Furthermore, the research literature appears to offer preliminary to moderate support for the effectiveness of hypnosis in relieving the symptoms of trauma and enhancing sports performance. These applications of clinical hypnosis would seem to be a vehicle for engaging in evidence-based practice. No doubt, there are other problems and symptoms for which hypnosis is an effective intervention. More research on these untested applications is greatly needed.

The research literature indicates people who fall in the high range of hypnotic suggestibility may show the strongest response to treatment with hypnosis, whereas those in the low suggestibility range may demonstrate the weakest response. Patients and clients in the medium suggestibility range are likely to exhibit a meaningful response to clinical hypnosis and even those in the low range may derive some benefit. However, for highly suggestible patients and clients, hypnosis may be a treatment of choice.

For at least some problems and symptoms (e.g., anxiety symptoms, smoking cessation), combining hypnosis with other psychological interventions may be more beneficial than utilizing it as a stand-alone treatment. Perhaps combining hypnosis with other interventions provides a more extensive set of tools that can address a broader array of symptoms than when hypnosis is used as a stand-alone treatment. More research is needed to identify the problems that are most responsive to a combination of hypnosis and other interventions.

Of course, evidence-based practice is not an inventory of efficacious treatments. Evidence-based practice is a decision-making process that involves three elements—the best available research evidence; the expertise of the clinician; and patient characteristics, culture, and preferences (American Psychological Association, 2021). The aim of evidence-based practice is to achieve the best outcome for the patient. To engage in evidence-based decision-making, clinicians are encouraged to cultivate an understanding of the research literature in their area of practice. The reviews of the outcome research presented in the chapters in the main section of this book strive to present some of the best research evidence needed to participate in evidence-based practice in clinical hypnosis. The case histories and hypnosis protocols in these chapters offer examples of how these applications of hypnosis might be carried out. It is my fervent hope this material will serve to enrich both future practice and research in clinical hypnosis.

REFERENCES

American Psychiatric Association. (2013). *Diagnostic and statistical manual of mental disorders* (5th ed.). https://doi.org/10.1176/appi.books.9780890425596

American Psychological Association. (1995). *Template for developing guidelines: Interventions for mental disorders and psychosocial aspects of physical disorders.*

American Psychological Association. (2021). *Professional practice guidelines for evidence-based psychological practice in health care.* https://www.apa.org/about/policy/psychological-practice-health-care.pdf

American Psychological Association, Presidential Task Force on Evidence-Based Practice. (2006). Evidence-based practice in psychology. *American Psychologist, 61*(4), 271–285. https://doi.org/10.1037/0003-066X.61.4.271

Barker, J., Jones, M., & Greenlees, I. (2010). Assessing the immediate and maintained effects of hypnosis on self-efficacy and soccer wall-volley performance. *Journal of Sport & Exercise Psychology, 32*(2), 243–252. https://doi.org/10.1123/jsep.32.2.243

Barker, J. B., & Jones, M. V. (2006). Using hypnosis, technique refinement, and self-modeling to enhance self-efficacy: A case study in cricket. *The Sport Psychologist, 20*(1), 94–110. https://doi.org/10.1123/tsp.20.1.94

Barker, J. B., & Jones, M. V. (2008). The effects of hypnosis on self-efficacy, affect, and soccer performance: A case study. *Journal of Clinical Sport Psychology, 2*(2), 127–147. https://doi.org/10.1123/jcsp.2.2.127

Baron, R. M., & Kenny, D. A. (1986). The moderator–mediator variable distinction in social psychological research: Conceptual, strategic, and statistical considerations. *Journal of Personality and Social Psychology, 51*(6), 1173–1182. https://doi.org/10.1037/0022-3514.51.6.1173

Borckardt, J. J., & Nash, M. R. (2002). How practitioners (and others) can make scientifically viable contributions to clinical-outcome research using the single-case time-series design. *International Journal of Clinical and Experimental Hypnosis, 50*(2), 114–148. https://doi.org/10.1080/00207140208410095

Brody, D. J., Pratt, L. A., & Hughes, J. P. (2018). Prevalence of depression among adults aged 20 and over: United States, 2013–2016. *NCHS Data Brief, No. 303*, 1–8. https://www.cdc.gov/nchs/products/databriefs/db303.htm

Chambless, D. L., & Hollon, S. D. (1998). Defining empirically supported therapies. *Journal of Consulting and Clinical Psychology, 66*(1), 7–18. https://doi.org/10.1037/0022-006X.66.1.7

Cohen, J. (1988). *Statistical power analysis for the behavioral sciences* (2nd ed.). Lawrence Earlbaum Associates.

Cohen, J. (1992). A power primer. *Psychological Bulletin, 112*(1), 155–159. https://doi.org/10.1037/0033-2909.112.1.155

Eason, A. D., & Parris, B. A. (2019). Clinical applications of self-hypnosis: A systematic review and meta-analysis of randomized controlled trials. *Psychology of Consciousness: Theory Research, and Practice, 6*(3), 262–278. https://doi.org/10.1037/cns0000173

Gwynn, M. I., & Spanos, N. P. (1996). Hypnotic responsiveness, nonhypnotic suggestibility, and responsiveness to social influence. In R. G. Kunzendorf, N. P. Spanos, & B. Wallace (Eds.), *Hypnosis and imagination* (pp. 147–175). Baywood Publishing.

Higgins, J. P. T., & Green, S. (Eds.). (2011). *Cochrane handbook for systematic reviews of interventions* (v. 5.1.0). The Cochrane Collaboration. http://handbook.cochrane.org/

Institute of Medicine. (2011). *Relieving pain in America: A blueprint for transforming prevention, care, education, and research.* National Academies Press. https://doi.org/10.17226/13172

Kessler, R. C., Berglund, P., Demler, O., Jin, R., Merikangas, K. R., & Walters, E. E. (2005). Lifetime prevalence and age-of-onset distributions of *DSM-IV* disorders in the National Comorbidity Survey Replication. *Archives of General Psychiatry, 62*(6), 593–602. https://doi.org/10.1001/archpsyc.62.6.593

Kirsch, I., Montgomery, G., & Sapirstein, G. (1995). Hypnosis as an adjunct to cognitive-behavioral psychotherapy: A meta-analysis. *Journal of Consulting and Clinical Psychology, 63*(2), 214–220. https://doi.org/10.1037/0022-006X.63.2.214

London, P. (1962). Hypnosis in children: An experimental approach. *International Journal of Clinical and Experimental Hypnosis, 10*(2), 79–91. https://doi.org/10.1080/00207146208415867

London, P. (1965). Developmental experiments in hypnosis. *Journal of Projective Techniques & Personality Assessment, 29*(2), 189–199. https://doi.org/10.1080/0091651X.1965.10120197

Merskey, H., & Bogduk, N. (1994). *Classification of chronic pain* (2nd ed.). IASP Press.

Milling, L. S., & Randazzo, E. S. (2016). Enhancing sports performance with hypnosis: An ode for Tiger Woods. *Psychology of Consciousness: Theory, Research, and Practice, 3*(1), 45–60. https://doi.org/10.1037/cns0000055

Milling, L. S., Valentine, K. E., LoStimolo, L. M., Nett, A. M., & McCarley, H. S. (2021). Hypnosis and the alleviation of clinical pain: A comprehensive meta-analysis. *International Journal of Clinical and Experimental Hypnosis, 69*(3), 297–322. https://doi.org/10.1080/00207144.2021.1920330

Milling, L. S., Valentine, K. E., McCarley, H. S., & LoStimolo, L. M. (2019). A meta-analysis of hypnotic interventions for depression symptoms. High hopes for hypnosis? *American Journal of Clinical Hypnosis, 61*(3), 227–243. https://doi.org/10.1080/00029157.2018.1489777

Moher, D., Liberati, A., Tetzlaff, J., Altman, D. G., & The PRISMA Group. (2009). Preferred reporting items for systematic reviews and meta-analyses: The PRISMA statement. *PLOS Medicine, 6*(7), e1000097. https://doi.org/10.1371/journal.pmed.1000097

Montgomery, G. H., DuHamel, K. N., & Redd, W. H. (2000). A meta-analysis of hypnotically induced analgesia: How effective is hypnosis? *International Journal of Clinical and Experimental Hypnosis, 48*(2), 138–153. https://doi.org/10.1080/00207140008410045

Montgomery, G. H., Schnur, J. B., & David, D. (2011). The impact of hypnotic suggestibility in clinical care settings. *International Journal of Clinical and Experimental Hypnosis, 59*(3), 294–309. https://doi.org/10.1080/00207144.2011.570656

Morgan, A. H., & Hilgard, J. R. (1978/1979). The Stanford Hypnotic Clinical Scale for children. *American Journal of Clinical Hypnosis, 21*(2–3), 148–169. https://doi.org/10.1080/00029157.1978.10403969

Pates, J. (2013). The effects of hypnosis on an elite senior European Tour golfer: A single-subject design. *International Journal of Clinical and Experimental Hypnosis, 61*(2), 193–204. https://doi.org/10.1080/00207144.2013.753831

Pates, J., Cummings, A., & Maynard, I. (2002). The effects of hypnosis on flow states and three-point shooting performance in basketball players. *The Sport Psychologist, 16*(1), 34–47. https://doi.org/10.1123/tsp.16.1.34

Pates, J., & Maynard, I. (2000). Effects of hypnosis on flow states and golf performance. *Perceptual and Motor Skills, 91* (Suppl. 3), 1057–1075. https://doi.org/10.2466/pms.2000.91.3f.1057

Pates, J., Maynard, I., & Westbury, T. (2001). An investigation into the effects of hypnosis on basketball performance. *Journal of Applied Sport Psychology, 13*(1), 84–102. https://doi.org/10.1080/10413200109339005

Pates, J., Oliver, R., & Maynard, I. (2001). The effects of hypnosis on flow states and golf-putting performance. *Journal of Applied Sport Psychology, 13*(4), 341–354. https://doi.org/10.1080/104132001753226238

Ramondo, N., Gignac, G. E., Pestell, C. F., & Byrne, S. M. (2021). Clinical hypnosis as an adjunct to cognitive behavior therapy: An updated meta-analysis. *International Journal of Clinical and Experimental Hypnosis, 69*(2), 169–202. https://doi.org/10.1080/00207144.2021.1877549

Rotaru, T.-Ș., & Rusu, A. (2016). A meta-analysis for the efficacy of hypnotherapy in alleviating PTSD symptoms. *International Journal of Clinical and Experimental Hypnosis, 64*(1), 116–136. https://doi.org/10.1080/00207144.2015.1099406

Substance Abuse and Mental Health Services Administration. (2019). *Key substance use and mental health indicators in the United States: Results from the 2018 National Survey on Drug Use and Health* (HHS Publication No. PEP19-5068, NSDUH Series H-54). https://www.samhsa.gov/data/

Tolin, D. F., McKay, D., Forman, E. M., Klonsky, E. D., & Thombs, B. D. (2015). Empirically supported treatment: Recommendations for a new model. *Clinical Psychology: Science and Practice, 22*(4), 317–338. https://doi.org/10.1037/h0101729

Turk, D. C., Meichenbaum, D., & Genest, M. (1983). *Pain and behavioral medicine: A cognitive–behavioral perspective.* Guilford Press.

Valentine, K. E., Milling, L. S., Clark, L. J., & Moriarty, C. L. (2019). The efficacy of hypnosis as a treatment for anxiety: A meta-analysis. *International Journal of Clinical and Experimental Hypnosis, 67*(3), 336–363. https://doi.org/10.1080/00207144.2019.1613863

Index

About the Editor

Leonard S. Milling, PhD, is the recently retired Professor of Psychology at the University of Hartford. He is a Fellow of the American Psychological Association (APA) through Division 30 (Society of Psychological Hypnosis). He received the Distinguished Contributions to Scientific Hypnosis award from APA Division 30 in 2020.

He is best known for his peer-reviewed journal articles on the mediator and moderator variables associated with hypnotic pain reduction, as well as on the efficacy of hypnosis as a treatment or intervention.